Progress in Drug Research
Fortschritte der Arzneimittelforschung
Progrès des recherches pharmaceutiques
Vol. 46

Progress in Drug Research
Fortschritte der Arzneimittelforschung
Progrès des recherches pharmaceutiques
Vol. 46

Edited by / Herausgegeben von / Rédigé par
Ernst Jucker, Basel

Authors / Autoren / Auteurs
Norman K. Hollenberg and Steven W. Graves · Robert B. McCall ·
William T. Jackson and Jerome H. Fleisch · M. Margaglione, E. Grandone,
F.P. Mancini and G. Di Minno · N. Seiler, A. Hardy and J.P. Moulinoux ·
James Claghorn and Michael D. Lesem · Eric J. Lien, Arima Das and Linda
L. Lien

1996   Birkhäuser Verlag
                        Basel · Boston · Berlin

Editor:

Dr. E. Jucker
Steinweg 28
CH-4107 Ettingen
Switzerland

© 1996 Birkhäuser Verlag, P.O. Box 133, CH-4010 Basel, Switzerland
Softcover reprint of the hardcover 1st edition 1996
Printed on acid-free paper produced from chlorine-free pulp. TCF ∞

ISBN-13: 978-3-0348-9861-4   e-ISBN-13: 978-3-0348-8996-4
DOI: 10.1007/978-3-0348-8996-4

9 8 7 6 5 4 3 2 1

Contents · Inhalt · Sommaire

Foreword

Volume 46 of "Progress in Drug Research" contains seven reviews and the various indexes which facilitate its use and establish the connection with the previous volumes. The articles in this volume deal with endogenous sodium pump inhibition, with neurotransmitters involved in the central regulation of the cardiovascular system, with leukotrienes and development of novel anti-inflammatory agents, with antithrombotic strategies and drugs affecting the plasma fibrinogen levels, with natural aminoglycosides and polyamines and their effects in the mammalian organism, with the latest developments in antidepressant agents and with immunopharmacological and biochemical bases of Chinese herbal medicine. These reviews provide valuable information on several new developments in the complex domain of drug research.

In the 37 years that PDR has existed, the Editor has enjoyed the valuable help and advice of many colleagues. Readers, the authors of the reviews and, last but not least, the reviewers have all contributed greatly to the success of this series of monographs. Although the comments received so far have generally been favorable, it is nevertheless necessary to analyze and to reassess the current position and the future direction of such publications.

So far, it has been the Editor's intention to help disseminate information on the vast and fast growing domain of drug research, and to provide the reader with a tool with which to keep abreast of the latest developments and trends. The reviews in PDR are useful to the nonspecialist, who can obtain an overview of a particular field of drug research in a relatively short time. The specialist readers of PDR will appreciate the reviews' comprehensive bibliographies, and, in addition, they may even get fresh impulses for their own research. Finally, the readers can use the 46 volumes of PDR as an encyclopedic source of information.

It gives me great pleasure to present this new volume to our readers. At the same time I would like to extend my gratitude to the authors who willingly accepted the task of preparing extensive reviews. My sincere thanks also go to Birkhäuser Verlag, and in particular to Mrs. L. Koechlin and Mssrs. H.-P. Thür, E. Mazenauer and G. Messmer. Without their personal commitment, assistance and advice, editing PDR would be a nearly impossible task.

Basel, April 1996   DR. E. JUCKER

Vorwort

Der vorliegende 46. Band der Reihe «Fortschritte der Arzneimittelforschung» enthält sieben Beiträge sowie die verschiedenen Register, wel-
che das Arbeiten mit diesem Band erleichtern und den Zugriff auf die
vorhergehenden Bände ermöglichen.

Die Artikel des 46. Bandes behandeln wiederum verschiedene aktuelle
Themen des komplexen Gebietes der Arzneimittelforschung. Der erste
Beitrag befasst sich mit den noch zu lösenden Problemen der Hyperto-
nie im Zusammenhang mit den den Digitalis-Glykosiden analogen Sub-
stanzen und Natrium. Alsdann wird die Regulierung des kardiovaskulären
Systems auf der Basis der Neurotransmitter beschrieben, und im näch-
sten Beitrag werden Leukotriene und ihre Rezeptoren im Zusammenhang mit der Entwicklung von neuen Entzündungshemmern behandelt.
Die Probleme der Thrombose im Zusammenhang mit dem Fibrinogen
des Plasma bilden den Gegenstand einer Übersicht, und natürliche Ami-
noglykoside und Polyamine werden aus der Sicht ihres Einflusses im Säu-
getierorganismus beschrieben. Die beiden letzten Beiträge befassen sich
mit den neuesten Entwicklungen auf dem Gebiet der Antidepressiva, bzw.
mit den immunopharmakologischen und biochemischen Grundlagen der
in der chinesischen Medizin verwendeten Heilpflanzen. Alle sieben Über-
sichten vermitteln dem Leser ein aufschlussreiches Bild der neuesten Entwicklungen einiger Gebiete der Arzneimittelforschung.

Seit der Gründung der Reihe sind 37 Jahre vergangen. In dieser langen
Zeit konnte der Herausgeber immer auf den Rat der Fachkollegen, der
Leser und der Autoren zählen. Manche Anregungen empfing ich auch von
den Rezensenten. Obwohl die grosse Mehrzahl der Besprechungen posi-
tiv war, stellt sich doch immer wieder die Frage nach dem Sinn und Zweck
der «Fortschritte». Nach wie vor ist es unser Ziel, neueste Forschungen
in Form von Übersichtsreferaten darzustellen und dem Leser auf diese
Weise zu ermöglichen, sich verhältnismässig rasch und mühelos über be-
stimmte aktuelle Richtungen der Arzneimittelforschung zu informieren.
Er erhält damit die Möglichkeit, sich in diesem komplexen und rasant sich
entwickelnden Fachgebiet auf dem Laufenden zu halten. Dem Spezia-
listen hingegen bieten die «Fortschritte» eine wertvolle Quelle der Origi-
nalliteratur dar, erlauben ihm Vergleichsmöglichkeiten und können u.U.
seine eigenen Untersuchungen befruchten. Für alle Leser stellt die Serie
mit ihren umfangreichen Registern eine nützliche Quelle von enzyklo-
pädischem Wissen dar, so dass das gesamte Werk auch als Nachschlage-
werk dienen kann.

Ich freue mich, diesen neuen Band der «Fortschritte» der Fachwelt über-
geben zu dürfen. Zugleich möchte ich auch meinen Dank den Autoren
für ihre grosse Arbeit aussprechen. Dem Birkhäuser Verlag, insbesondere
Frau L. Koechlin und den Herren H.-P. Thür, E. Mazenauer und Gregor
Messmer gebührt der Dank für die ausgezeichnete Zusammenarbeit, für
das Eingehen auf die Wünsche des Herausgebers und für die sorgfältige
Ausstattung des Bandes.

Basel, April 1996   DR. E. JUCKER

Progress in Drug Research, Vol. 46 (E. Jucker, Ed.)
© 1996 Birkhäuser Verlag, Basel (Switzerland)

Endogenous sodium pump inhibition: Current status and therapeutic opportunities

By Norman K. Hollenberg and Steven W. Graves

Brigham and Women's Hospital and Harvard Medical School, Departments of Medicine and Radiology, 75 Francis Street, Boston, MA 02115, USA

Correspondence to: Norman K. Hollenberg, M.D., Ph.D., Brigham and Women's . Hospital, 75 Francis Street, Boston, MA 02115, USA

1 Introduction: Historical perspectives

Controversy is a favorite term among reviewers. How better can one justify a review of a subject than to indicate that the subject is controversial? Sometimes the term is employed to indicate that consensus has not been achieved on all of the details, a synonym for disagreement. At other times, the term is used more appropriately to indicate passionate advocacy and equally impassioned denial, as evidenced in recent Letters to the Editor [1–3]. There is continuing interest in the possibility that a circulating sodium pump inhibitor, believed to be digitalis-like, contributes to sodium homeostasis and the pathogenesis of sodium-sensitive hypertension, as evidenced by a series of recent review articles [4–13]. In general, the tone of these review articles could be described as cautious but optimistic. The continued controversy is better indicated by the specific wording of one of the recent Letters to the Editor [1]. "After approximately twenty years of a fruitless search for endogenous digitalis-like factors, interest has declined considerably among scientists occupied with theoretical aspects of the sodium pump... Among clinicians, however, judging from the great number of articles in clinical journals... the interest is undiminished... The number of publications on the topic, however, seems inversely related to the facts and realities of the subject." Similar views, perhaps with a more balanced expression, have been expressed by other authorities in this field [14]. Although some of the recent reviews appeared to have been based on acceptance of the possibility that ouabain is the putative endogenous digitalis-like factor [6, 8, 9], most of the reviews have expressed a more guarded position, and several groups have indicated that the postulated sodium, potassium ATPase inhibitor that circulates in plasma is not ouabain [15–17]. Even the balanced reviews acknowledge that the most fundamental issues remain to be resolved.

Our goal in this essay is not to provide yet another detailed review of the available information that has been obtained from what has become a prodigious literature: Indeed, one of the truly excellent reviews appeared recently in this publication [11]. Rather, we wish to use that information in several alternative ways. Our first goal is to analyze the factors that have contributed to the controversy. Our second goal is to develop guidelines as a step to resolving the issues. We acknowledge that the attempt to develop guidelines must, inevitably, contribute to the controversy as not all will agree. On the other hand, the field would be much improved if the center of debate could be moved to the issue of the standards to be applied. Our final goal is to paint with broad strokes a picture of the potential therapeutic implications of this effort beyond renal sodium handling and salt-sensitive hypertension.

This is not the first time, of course, that a voluminous literature and substantial confusion have grown out of sustained controversy. Our decision to open our essay on the digitalis-like factor with the review of medical events in the mid-to-late nineteenth century reflects our belief that lessons learned well before the nineteenth century closed still carry an important message for us as the twentieth century comes to an end.

During the past year, two editorials appeared on the contribution of Robert Koch to biology and medicine. One editorial was by Thomas Weller [18] whose Nobel Prize was awarded for cultivation of the poliomyelitis virus. That achievement, in turn, was based on the successful development of viral tissue culture techniques. To Dr. Weller in that editorial, Koch's major contribution was that "...he revolutionized bacteriology by introducing solid and semi-solid culture media and by improving staining techniques". Few would argue that advances in technique and technology have been an important path to advances in science.

The second editorial provided a different – we think larger – perspective on Koch and his contribution to Nineteenth Century science [19]. Koch's major contribution involved the recognition and formulation of a series of rules of logic required to establish causal relationships in a complex situation. That story evolved over several decades, not unlike our current situation with the digitalis-like factor.

In a chapter with the intriguing title "The Germ Theory Before Germs", Nuland [20] pointed out that one of the problems faced by Ignac Semmelweis involved unfortunate timing: His ingenuity uncovered the importance of hand washing to prevent puerperal sepsis nine years before Pasteur demonstrated that bacteria caused putrefaction. Indeed, it was to be another twenty years until Lister demonstrated in the 1860s that wound infections, since they are caused by bacteria, can be transmitted by doctor's hands [20–22]. In a remarkable shift of "informed opinion", bacteria during the next decade moved from a stage in which they could explain nothing to a stage in which they could explain everything. They are ubiquitous.

The genius of Robert Koch created order from the chaos with his publication of the "Etiology of Traumatic Infective Diseases" in 1879 [21]. Although his paper dealt with wound infections, as had that of Lister, he considered the more general problem of connecting specific bacteria with specific effects. The issue involved whether the bacteria were a consequence of the infection, or its cause, or an innocent bystander. To address these issues, Koch developed a series of principles which were expanded and refined to form what came to be known as "Koch's Postulates" [21]. As obvious as they are today, they were revolutionary in their time – and as pointed out above – too often have been forgotten.

Koch identified four logical requirements. The first was that the organism must be present in every case of the disease. The second was that the organism could be identified in pure culture. The third involved transfer of the organism to another animal, which reproduced the disease. Fourth, the organism could then be recovered from the inoculated animal and again grown in pure culture. Koch's application of these criteria to the anthrax bacillus led Julius Cohnheim, one of the giants of the 19th century medicine to conclude: "It leaves nothing more to be proved. I regarded it as the greatest discovery ever made with bacteria." [20]

These rules of logic are applicable broadly and have thereby influenced much of the evolution of medicine [20–23]. With appropriate modification, they have been crucial in the research on hormones. As pointed out by Haber [23], the element involving transfer of the vector in Koch's postulates became the ablation-replacement experiment in endocrinology: In this experiment, the investigator first documents the physiological implications of absence of the hormone following gland ablation, and then the response to hormone replacement. When that experiment is impossible, pharmacological interruption of the system or immuno-neutralization has provided an analogous pivotal element.

In the case of endogenous hormonal systems, an additional logical element must involve documentation of the endogenous biosynthesis – both the location and enzymatic pathway. When these criteria are met, one is left – like Julius Cohnheim – with no doubt concerning the role of a hormone in the body economy.

Our goal in this essay is to develop this theme and apply it to the problem of the digitalis-like factor – a putative hormone which many consider to mediate normal sodium homeostasis and volume control, and contribute to the pathogenesis of sodium-sensitive hypertension. Despite an enormous and growing literature, the subject remains highly controversial – in large part, we believe, because the principles so carefully delineated by Koch have often not been applied

2   Identification of the digitalis-like factor: Statement of the problem

We would argue that because the rules of logic have not been applied adequately, there has been not only an extraordinary number of individual chemical species suggested as the candidate, there has been a remarkable number of chemical classes: Table 1 enumerates several of the proposed chemical classes, with a few examples of each, and is not intended to be exhaustive. The primary references for each candidate can be found in the series of recent review articles [4–14]. What factors led to this unusual literature?

Table 1
Candidates as a circulating digitalis-like sodium pump inhibitor

I	Lipids	
	(i)	Fatty acids
	(ii)	Lysophophatidyl choline
	(iii)	HETE pathway
II	Steroids	
	(i)	DHEA-S
	(ii)	Progesterone
	(iii)	Ouabain
	(iv)	Digoxin
	(v)	Bufalin, 19-norbufalin
	(vi)	Bile salts
III	Peptides	
	(i)	MSH
	(ii)	Endotoxin

2.1   Pitfalls

One important contributor to this diversity of candidates is the fact that single assays of limited specificity were often employed to monitor DLF purification. Typically, this has been either a chemical assay of sodium, potassium ATPase activity or a radioimmunoassay for digoxin (Table 2). The chemical assay of sodium, potassium ATPase activity is sensitive to an array of specific and nonspecific interfering influences. For example, claims that free fatty acids, lysophophatidyl choline and dehydroepiandrosterone sulfate (DHEAS) should be considered candidates depended largely on their activity in a biochemical assay. Figure 1 compares inhibition of sodium, potassium ATPase induced by these three proposed candidates. The information used to construct the figure was taken from the

Table 2
Pitfalls

(1)	Inadequate assay specificity and range
(2)	Ignoring potency of known candidates
(3)	Problems reflecting the source of the material
(4)	Assumption of stability
(5)	Inadequate purification

relevant publications [24, 25]. Note that although ouabain is relatively inactive compared to most hormones – with a Ki well above 10^{-7}M, the relation between ouabain concentration and enzyme inhibition followed a typical sigmoid, mass action relationship, developing over several orders of concentration, as expected of a hormone. The other candidates are far less potent and show a precipitous onset and narrow range of activity, a concentration effect suggestive of a nonspecific, physical action. In the case of the lipids, it may represent a "detergent" effect.

Radioimmunoassay (RIA) for digoxin or another digitalis glycoside has also been employed as a single assay in attempts to isolate and purify DLF. RIA does not measure bioactivity. Moreover, it examines only a portion of the molecule, and crossreactivity with a host of interfering molecules has led to misleading results when RIA was employed alone [7, 26]. To complicate matters further, antisera directed against digoxin vary widely in their sensitivity to the endogenous crossreactive agent and this appears not to have been considered in many research strategies.

Many investigators consider it crucial not only that multiple assays be employed, but also that at least one relevant bioassay system be employed as part of the strategy in attempts to isolate DLF [5, 7, 11–13]. Unfortunately, bioassay systems are complex and often poorly understood. For example, if one assumes that the candidate acts as the natriuretic agent, and makes bioassay of natriuresis a crucial criterion, the fact that blockade of sodium reabsorption in one portion of the nephron can be offset by increased reabsorption elsewhere might limit the information obtained from this bioassay. In the case of vascular smooth muscle, it has been recognized only recently that the contractile response resulting from sodium pump inhibition differs dramatically from the contractile response resulting from other known agonists [27]. In the case of sodium pump inhibition there is a striking delay in the contractile response, often measured in hours. Virtually every research strategy, involving vascular smooth muscle contraction employed to study DLF then, would have missed the rel-

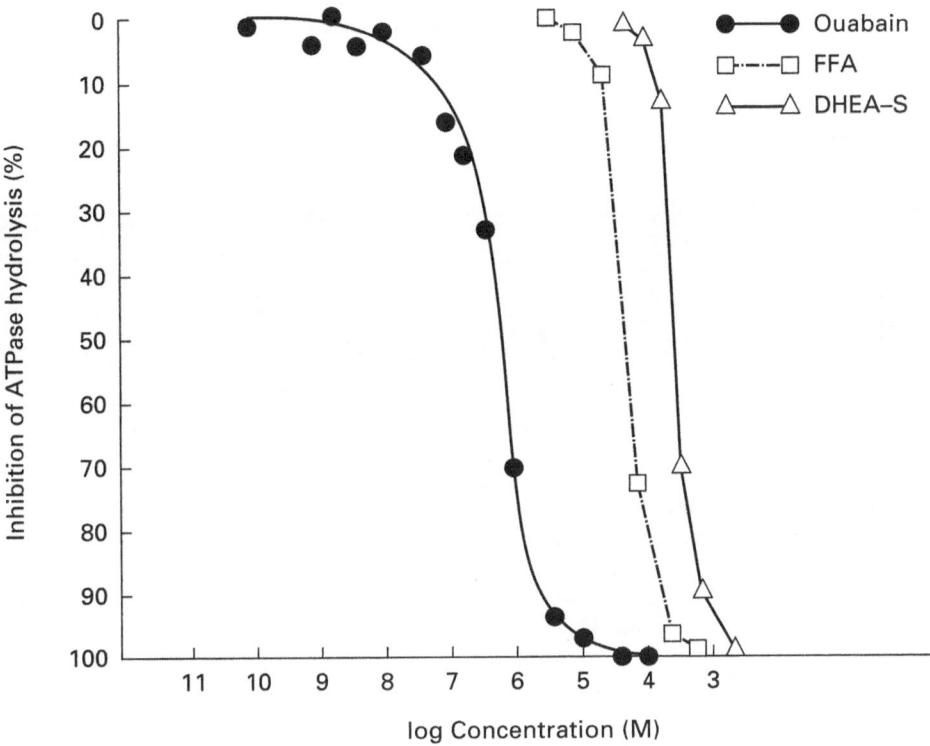

Fig. 1
Relation between sodium pump inhibitor concentration and inhibition. Note the typical mass action kinetics shown by ouabain, and the precipitous inhibition shown by free fatty acids (FFA) and by dehydroepiandrosterone sulphate (DHEA-S) (from reference [19]).

evant contractile response because the experiment was discontinued prematurely.

The decision concerning the source of the material to be purified has also been crucial. Plasma and urine as a source are discussed in the next section. In some cases, the investigators have ignored the physiological role of the putative agent, and did not employ volume expansion as a stimulus before the samples were collected. Indeed, a comparison of samples collected from volume-expanded and volume-contracted individuals can serve as a useful criterion for candidacy (Figure 2). As an alternative to attempts to isolate and purify a candidate from a biological source, a second approach involves assessing defined pure biochemicals as candidates.

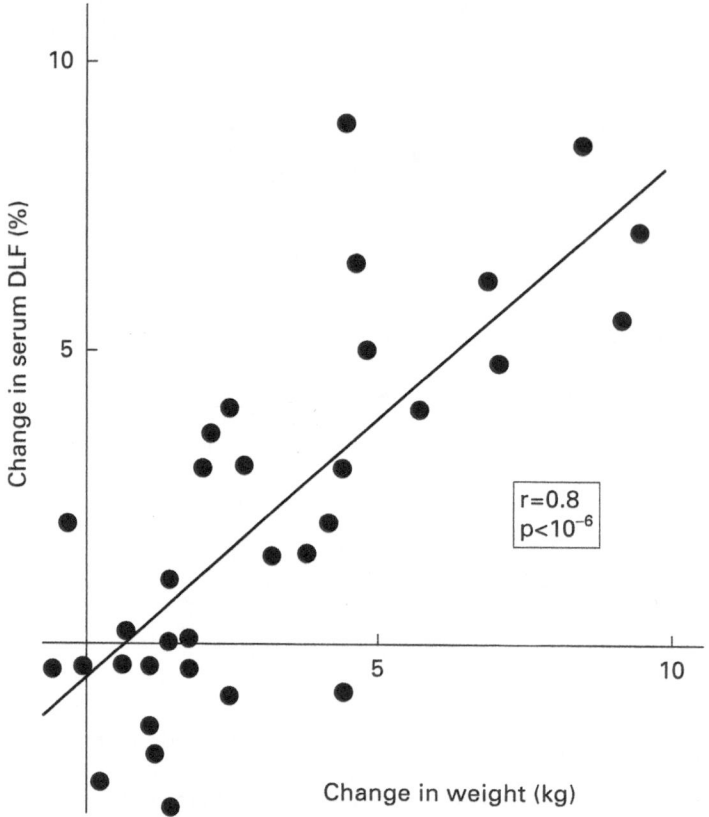

Relationship of change in serum DLF
[Na, K] ATPase inhibition to body weight change

Fig. 2
Relation between change in body weight, as an index of extracellular fluid volume expansion, and serum digitalis like factor (DLF) activity during liberalization of salt and water intake in patients on chronic ambulatory peritoneal dialysis (PD). The increase in digitalis-like activity, reflecting increases in the specific inhibitor molecule only during volume expansion should be a crucial criterion for candidates as the endogenous digitalis-like agent (from reference [40]).

In many cases, especially the endogenous steroids with an already known alternative hormonal function, some weak digitalis-like activity has been found in one or more assay systems. Too often investigators have ignored the fact that high concentrations were required for "DLF" activity in the assay systems, and that these high concentrations are never achieved *in vivo* – see, for example, Figure 1.

2.2   Unstated assumptions

Every research strategy reported has made a fundamental assumption, although it is rarely stated. In each case, the approach has assumed that the putative hormone is sufficiently stable that techniques commonly employed to protect a labile agent or minimize the influence of lability have not been employed. Prolonged intervals between collection and purification steps and in some cases assay as well as exposure to harsh chemicals to precipitate plasma protein before further purification may well have complicated the process [23]. At least one candidate is extremely labile, with a half life measured in hours [29]. We identified a labile sodium pump inhibitor in peritoneal dialysate from dialysis patients, which was unstable in aqueous solution despite attempts to reduce its degradation by storage under argon at –70°C (Figures 3 and 4). This candidate lost approximately 50% of its activity overnight [29].

Assumptions regarding the appropriateness of the specimen used in DLF isolation were mentioned earlier. Plasma as the source has the advantage that the material obtained must be in the circulation, but also a series of disadvantages in efforts to isolate DLF. Only a limited amount of plasma can be collected from each individual and so samples must be pooled and stored [30]. Moreover, protein binding can be a complicating factor: In one study, a candidate was found to show substantial protein binding, and required harsh, potentially modifying conditions to remove the agent from the protein [26]. Urine is an attractive source because it is freely available and abundant, but many hormones reach urine only in limited quantities because of prior metabolism. Moreover, urine may contain factors that interfere in the assay systems [5].

Tissues as an alternative source have been considered in detail in the section on biosynthesis below. Several lines of evidence have suggested that the tissue source could be the hypothalamus [31] or the adrenal [7, 32], and investigators have exploited these observations to attempt to isolate candidates from these tissues. Although this approach might ultimately prove to be productive, the large number of steroids found in the adrenal that appear to have at least weak sodium, potassium ATPase inhibitory activity or crossreactivity in digoxin or ouabain RIA has complicated efforts [32]. In the case of the hypothalamus, the small amount of tissue obtained from each animal and the time required to collect that material might prove to be crucial for a labile factor.

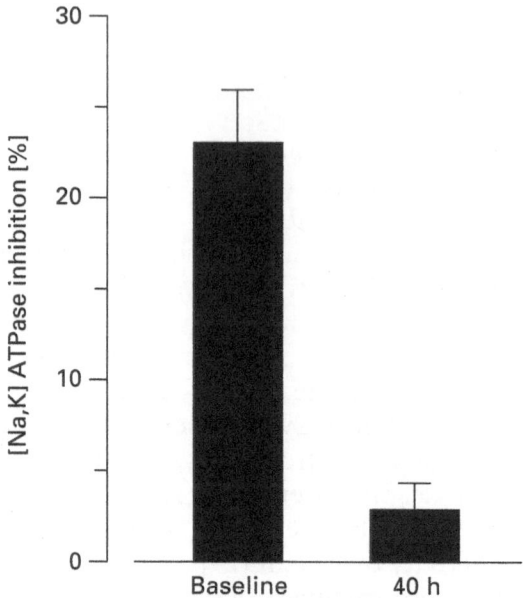

Fig. 3
Stability of the DLF isolated from PD. The sample was divided and half of the sample
was assayed immediately by a chemical assay for sodium potassium ATPase activity. The
second half was stored for about 40 hours at −70°C (from reference [40]).

Claims of isolation of a pure agent often have been based on inadequate
purification. Application of several HPLC steps has led to a description
of "purified to a single HPLC peak" or "purified to homogeneity by
HPLC", with the unstated assumption that this meant that a single chemical species had been isolated. We have found (Figure 5) that application
of supercritical fluid chromatography to a single active fraction that was
the product of three HPLC steps, and that appeared to be pure, revealed
several residual peaks, probably reflecting multiple chemical species [33].

2.3   Is there more than one DLF?

One logical explanation for the multiplicity of candidates put forward is
that there is more than one agent. Redundancy of mechanisms is a general feature of mechanisms governing sodium homeostasis, but there are

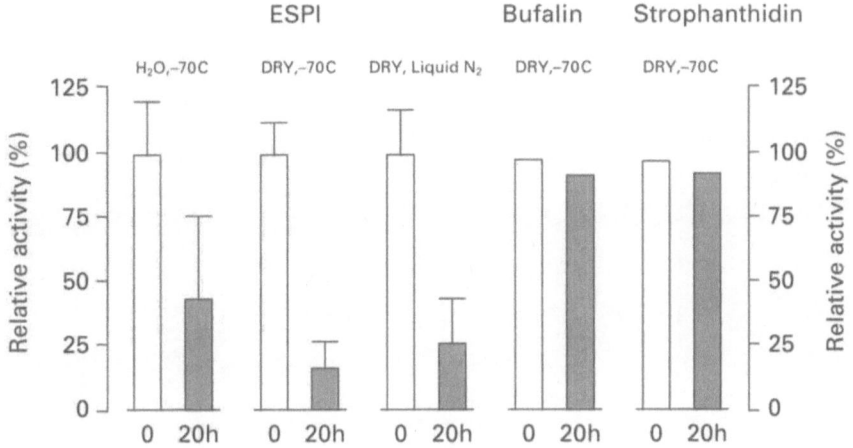

Fig. 4
The labile endogenous sodium pump inhibitor (ESPI) was unstable under argon, and despite conditions that are frequently employed to stabilize labile compounds. Note, by comparison, the stability of other cardiac glycosides, bufalin and strophantidin (from reference [29]).

no examples of two or more hormones that regulate a process via a single receptor site.

As one approach to addressing that fundamental problem, we exploited the observation that commercial antisera directed against digoxin displayed a wide range of affinity for the endogenous DLF despite essentially identical affinity for digoxin. The use of seven antisera provided an "immunochemical fingerprint" for DLF (Figure 6), and revealed striking concordance in serum from pregnant women and patients with advanced renal failure or hepatic disease [34]. The pattern in a fourth source, fetal cord blood, was very similar but not identical, probably reflecting a very high local concentration of DHEAS. The application of antisera directed against digitoxin – a glycoside that differs from digoxin in one additional hydroxyl group – confirmed and extended that observation [35]. Although the criterion of immunochemical specificity cannot, by itself, be considered absolute, the only available evidence on the point favors rather strongly the existence of a single chemical species. An attractive alternative possibility is that a single chemical species – one hormone – is found in the circulation, but that other moieties exist in the

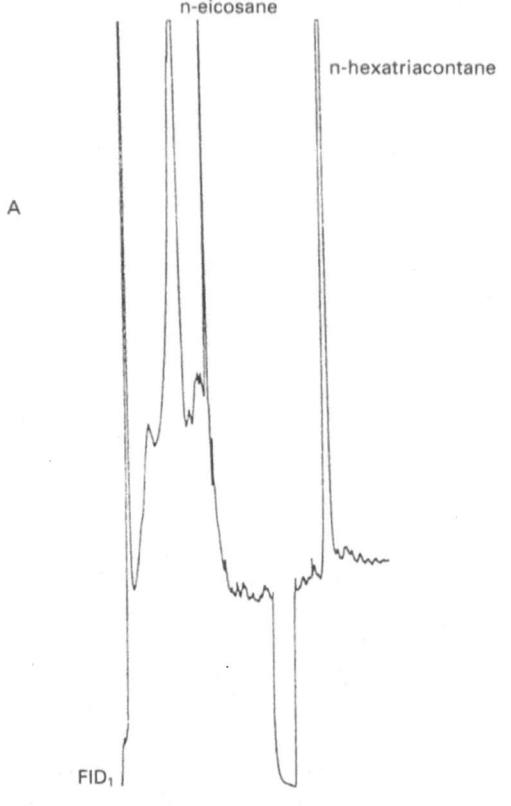

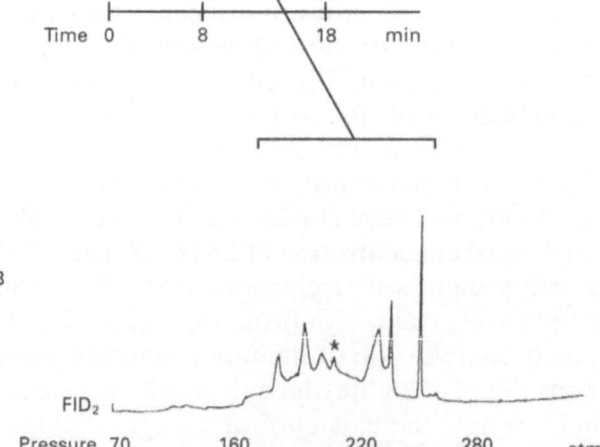

Fig. 5

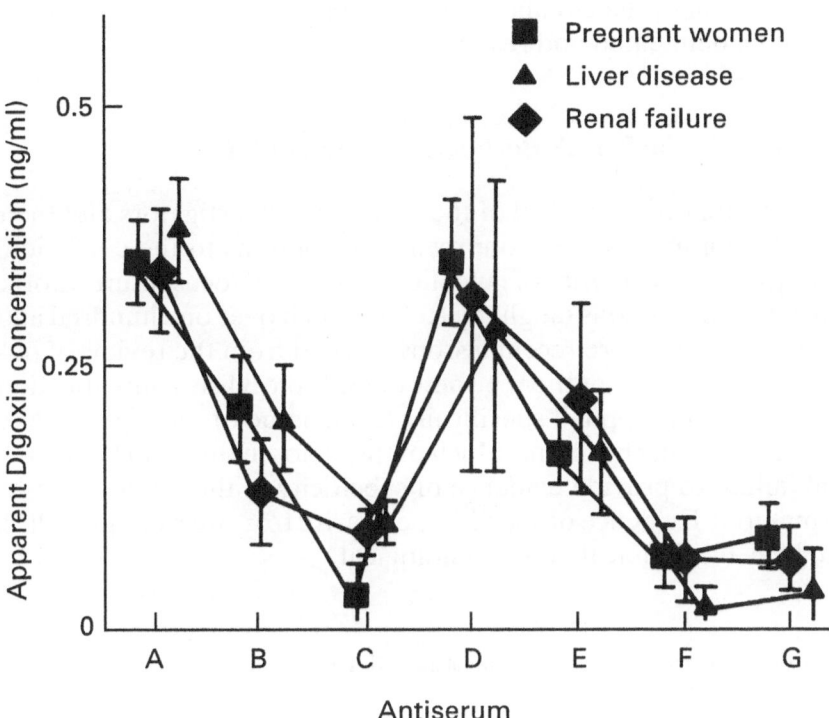

Fig. 6
Seven antisera directed against digoxin, and with equivalent affinity for digoxin, showed a striking variation in their affinity for the endogenous DLF. Note the essential identity of the immunochemical profile in samples obtained from patients with renal failure, patients with liver disease, and pregnant women (from reference [34]).

Fig. 5
Supercritical fluid chromatograms of a PD apparently purified to homogeneity following ultrafiltration, solid phase extraction, and two HPLC steps. On supercritical fluid chromatography (SFC), the apparently homogeneous fraction contained multiple fractions. "FID" represents flame ionization detection, a quantitative measure of the mass of the material in the chromatogram. "ATM" represents atmospheres of CO_2 pressure. Eicosane and N-Hexatricotane were employed as internal standards. All of the activity in the first chromatographic phase (A) was found in the area indicated, between 150 and 160 atmospheres. Note that even after this first SFC chromatographic purification, that there are at least seven residual peaks (B). The star indicates the zone in which the activity was found (from reference [33]).

tissues, and serve an as yet unknown local autocrine or paracrine function, especially in the central nervous system [31, 36]. Certainly, the more tractable problem of the circulating agent must be resolved before local actions can be delineated and resolved.

3   The criteria: Koch's Postulates applied to DLF

It is not our intent to be critical of the individual investigators and their efforts, including in retrospect our own contributions to the confusion, but rather to establish a series of guidelines which will focus future efforts, exploiting both the lessons taught by Robert Koch over one hundred and thirty years ago, and more recent lessons learned from the review of pitfalls. If errors are made, let them be new ones. Table 3 lists a modification of Koch's Postulates applied specifically to the issue of the digitalis-like factor – or indeed, any hormone. Much of the chaos in this field has arisen from the failure to provide evidence of specificity in the attempt to isolate the material. Evidence of specificity can arise from many approaches, physiological, biochemical, or immunological.

Table 3
Criteria required to prove that a candidate is an endogeneous hormone –
The digitalis-like factor

(1)	Action at a physiological concentration
(2)	Relevant physiological and clinical correlates
(3)	Appropriate biochemical activity
(4)	Appropriate bioactivity
(5)	Surgical, pharmacological, or immunological reversal
(6)	Biosynthesis

3.1   Potency and adequate concentration

The first criterion, that the candidate be present in blood or other body fluids in a concentration adequate to induce the biological response of interest is so obvious that one might be tempted to omit it. On the other hand, examination of the literature makes it clear that this criterion has often been ignored. As one example, the very high concentrations of the candidates shown in Figure 1 are not achieved in plasma. This topic merits a more detailed presentation.

Elegant evidence suggests that a material identical to or very similar to ouabain can be found in normal human plasma [6,30]. On the other hand, the concentrations of ouabain reported in the early studies were very low. Initial estimates of ouabain concentration made by Hamlyn and his group were approximately 50 pmol/L in normal individuals, which rose with volume expansion to about 130 pmol/L: Subsequent measurement led to about a 10-fold higher estimate, which was up to 50-fold higher in the occasional patient [30,36]. Even the much higher estimates of concentration, however, would seem to be too little to produce the levels of inhibition of the sodium pump measured in the serum of patients with essential hypertension reported by this group [23]. Indeed, there appears to be far too little to lead to vascular smooth muscle contraction *in vitro* in most tissues [27], although it has been suggested that these concentrations reach the threshold for contraction of small human arteries [12]. Similarly, although progesterone and other progestins have some actions suggestive of an endogenous sodium pump inhibitor [37], the concentration required to act in most assay systems is 100-to-1,000 fold higher than the usual endogenous concentration [33]. In contrast, another steroid, DHEAS, might achieve levels in cord blood required to act in some assay systems (see [34] for references).

3.2   Relevant clinical and physiological correlation

The second criterion involves relevant clinical or physiological correlations. Specifically, is the concentration of the material elevated under appropriate circumstances in affected individuals, and does the concentration vary in appropriate direction and magnitude with the appropriate stimulus? In the case of the digitalis-like factor, the appropriate stimulus must include volume expansion and an increase in total body sodium, although other stimuli might also prove to be effective [4]. In the many hypertension models examined by Haddy and his coworkers, a volume-dependent factor was a common theme [4]. Some investigators have documented an influence of rapid volume expansion with saline [39]. Whether acute and rapid volume changes or more gradual and sustained changes are more effective as a stimulus is not yet known. Development of an appropriate model that includes this criterion should be helpful in attempts to isolate the hormone. Some would argue that it should be a crucial element. Our group has employed as a useful model, and source of material, the patient with chronic renal failure who is maintained by peritoneal dialysis. In such patients a programmed and predictable shift in total body sodium can be achieved easily with changes in salt and water intake [40]. In this situation, we have been able to show close correlations between short-term changes in body weight, as the index of volume expansion, and both changes in arterial blood pressure and changes in the activity of the putative hormone in plasma and in peritoneal dialysate (Figure 2). Such an observation provides substantial confidence to the investigator that the material under investigation is, indeed, a viable candidate.

3.3   Appropriate activity in multiple assays

Appropriate activity in multiple assays is the third criterion. The term "appropriate" includes a requirement that the agent under consideration show affinity for the digitalis-binding site of ATPase, that the action be reversible, that there be substantial potency, and that the pattern of inhibition display features suggesting an appropriate mass action relationship. Specificity for the binding site for digitalis glycosides includes appropriate sensitivity to the ionic milieu [41]. Indeed, incubation conditions prior to initiating hydrolysis can provide additional information on the mechanism of action for DLF – enzyme interactions [42]. Equally important is the requirement that the agents show consistent activity in a range of assay systems. As a minimum, the chemical assay systems should include inhibition of [Na,K]ATPase hydrolysis, the function of the enzyme, and an assessment of binding.

The use of RIA employing antisera directed against digoxin or other known cardiac glycosides is convenient, but has often led to controversial and possibly misleading data. For example, specificity of the antiserum employed to measure ouabain might have contributed to current confusion. A recent report by Ludens et al. [32] described the use of the same antiserum as Hamlyn and coworkers used to estimate plasma concentration in humans [6, 30] to probe for the tissue source of ouabain. Eluate

---

Fig. 7
Dose response curves for the inhibitory effects of ouabain (top), bufalin (middle), and the endogenous sodium pump inhibitor (ESPI) from PD (bottom) obtained from two assays. The open circles represent standard assay conditions. Conventional conditions included a sodium concentration of 100, potassium of 5, and magnesium of 3 mM. Open circles represent modified assay condition in which sodium and potassium have been removed, magnesium concentration has been increased to 10, and phosphorous has been added at a concentration of 10 mM. These conditions favor binding of digitalis glycosides to the active site, which is evident in a much more sensitive assay (data from reference [115]).

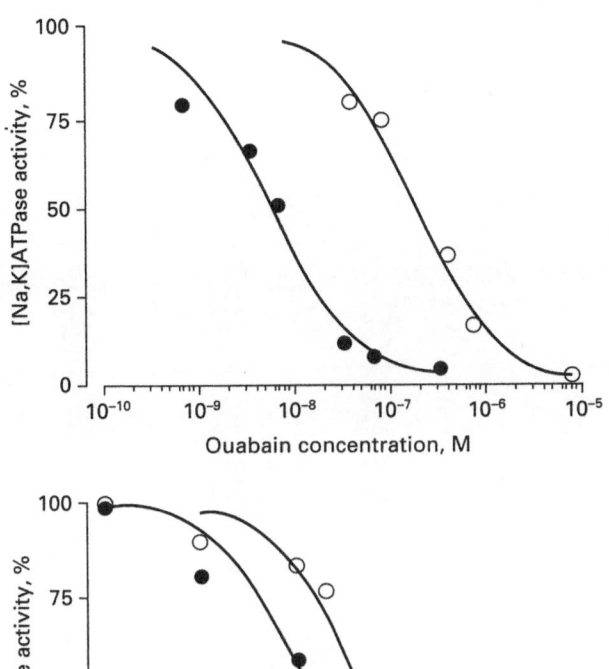

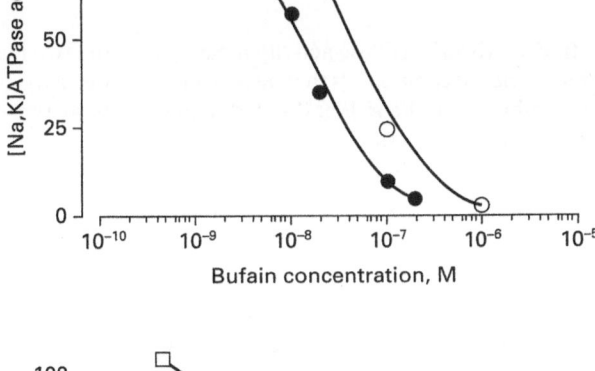

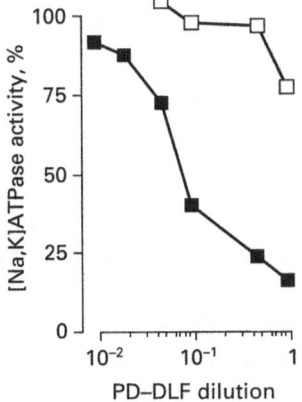

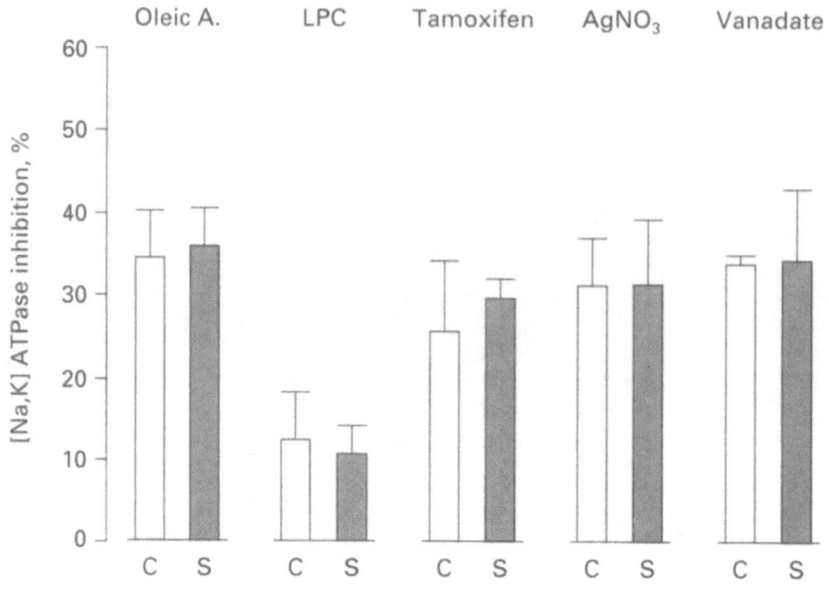

Fig. 8
Comparison of the inhibitor effect on [Na,K]ATPase activity measured by the two methods demonstrated in Figure 7 on a series of compounds that have been described as sodium pump inhibitors. Note that preincubation in the milieu that led to greater assay sensitivity (Figure 7) did not influence their inhibitory effect, indicating the nonspecificity of their action via a step unrelated to the digitalis binding site (data from reference [115]).

from high performance liquid chromatography fractionated rat adrenal homogenates demonstrated many peaks with ouabain-like immunoreactivity: indeed several had elution times close to that of ouabain. Should RIA be employed, we believe that it should be applied in conjunction with at least two other DLF assays – a chemical assay and a bioassay.

3.4 Bioactivity

Appropriate bioassay we believe is an absolute requirement, best performed in conjunction with appropriate biochemical assays of activity. Failure to document an appropriate action on vascular smooth muscle, renal sodium handling, or blood pressure at concentrations that can be achieved *in vivo* would have dismissed many candidates at an early stage, and thereby would have saved much confusion and avoided much waste. In the case of many digitalis glycosides their cardiac toxicity might well have led to death of an assay animal well before an acute pressor response occurred. Although it has been difficult to demonstrate a sustained elevation in blood pressure in response to cardiac glycoside administration alone, recent work has suggested that ouabain may contribute to hypertension when employed in conjunction with other maneuvers. Sekihara et al. [43] demonstrated that the administration of ouabain for six weeks in a dose of 1 mg/week did not influence blood pressure directly but did double the pressor response to a subthreshold dose of DOCA. Yuan et al. [44] employed ouabain at much lower doses, approximately 4 µg/day, for the same six week interval in rats with a surgical reduction in renal mass. This much smaller dose induced hypertension, which varied with the mass of kidney removed. According to this study, the heminephrectomy employed by Sekihara et al. should have led to hypertension with the much larger ouabain dose employed. The complexity of these protocols makes it clear that identification of a sustained blood pressure rise with an endogenous agent goes beyond what most laboratories could sustain. Certainly, acute pressor responses are not a feature of the digitalis glycosides.

Identification of a smooth muscle contraction has not been a feature in many studies. One possible explanation involves the delayed myogenic vascular smooth muscle response to sodium pump inhibition [27]. A delay of several hours before an unambiguous contractile response occurred had not been appreciated until recently [27]. In Figure 9 the gradual VSM contractile response to the DLF found in PD is shown.

3.5   Surgical, pharmacologic, or immunologic reversal

The term "surgical, pharmacologic, or immunologic reversal", employed in Table 3 requires explanation. Earlier, we emphasized the point made by Haber [23] that the ablation:replacement experiment is crucial evidence that a candidate represents an endogenous hormone. In the classical experiment, the biological influence of ablation of the source is documented, and reversal of that influence by replacement with the candidate closes the logic loop [23]. Ablation of portions of the hypothalamus indeed led to biological responses consistent with the thesis that an endogenous sodium pump inhibitor from this region participates in sodium homeostasis [45]. Unfortunately, both in the case of the hypothalamus and in the case of the adrenal, ablation creates an extraordinarily complex situation for blood pressure control and sodium homeostasis. Encouraging preliminary efforts have been made with antisera directed against digoxin as

VSM response to labile ESPI and Digibind

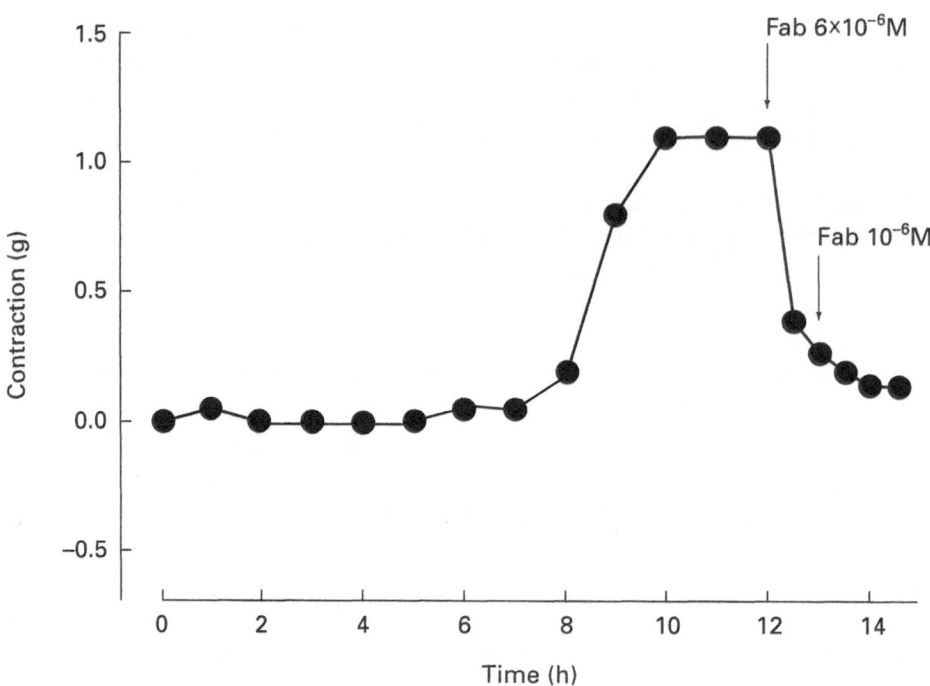

Fig. 9
VSM contractile response to the DLF isolated from PD. This assay was performed on rabbit aorta *in vitro*. Note the delay of several hours before a contractile response occurred, and the rapid evolution of that contractile response once initiated. The response is similar to that induced by ouabain. Note also the reversal of the contractile response induced by the Fab fragment of an antiserum directed against digoxin, Digibind (data from reference [116]).

pharmacological probes [46–50] (Figure 9), although questions of specificity have been raised [51].

3.6   Biosynthesis

Finally, given the large number of candidates identified, the ubiquitous distribution of steroids in many varieties of plants with at least some action on the sodium pump and growing evidence that these are absorbed and even taken up by tissues such as the adrenal, there is an additional criterion that is likely to be required before investigators interested in this field will accept a candidate. We believe that delineation of the biosynthetic pathway is a crucial step in proving that a candidate is an endogenous hormone, and therefore merits detailed review.

The available data concerning where such a factor is made are more suggestive than conclusive, but two potential sites of biosynthesis have emerged as leading possibilities, the adrenal and the hypothalamus, although other tissues including the kidney [52] and the heart [53] have been considered.

The common first step in establishing a biosynthetic pathway has been the attempt to localize its site of production. For the sodium pump inhibitor this has meant the procurement of tissue from animals (sometimes on a high-salt diet), homogenization, and screening the supernatants for the factor using an anti-digoxin (and more recently anti-ouabain) antiserum [32, 54–56]. Occasionally, there have been attempts to measure biochemical activity in conjunction with a chromatographic separation technique [55, 57–59] and rarely have both an immunological and bioassay been employed together [60]. Many studies have suggested relatively high levels of digoxin-like immunoreactivity (DLI) and ouabain-like immunoreactivity (OLI) in the adrenal and in the brain, particularly the hypothalamus [4–12], but other studies have localized activity to only the hypothalamus [61] or only the adrenal [62]. Despite these controversies, most investigators have focused on either one of the other tissue as a potential source.

3.6.1   The hypothalamus

Early experiments demonstrated the requirement for an intact hypothalamus for the development of certain volume-sensitive forms of hypertension [63]. In addition there appeared to be a natriuretic factor regulated by that center [64]. Further studies suggested the presence of sodium pump inhibitory activity in hypothalamic extracts [31, 57, 58], and the ablation of the anteroventral third ventricle (AV3V) region, which adjoins the pituitary/hypothalamic region of the brain, prevented both the elaboration of this hypothalamic pump inhibitor and the rise in blood pressure in DOCA:salt hypertension [45, 65].

The chemical nature of this factor has divided into two experiences. There are a few laboratories which have obtained data consistent with the factor produced in the pituitary/hypothalamic region being peptidic [66–70]. Others have found evidence of a hypothalamic factor having a physical and chemical nature closer to that of a steroid digitalis glycoside [31, 58]. The accumulating and impressive biochemical evidence has demonstrated that this compound has a range of activities that is almost identical to that of ouabain, with two exceptions [73–75]. The most prominent difference is the hypothalamic factor's facile ability to inhibit rat renal [Na,K]ATPase [74] which is known to be very ouabain resistent [75]. Recently, Haupert and coworkers isolated and characterized convincingly an isomer of ouabain obtained from bovine hypothalamus [73]. A fuller comparison of this new, purified isomer with ouabain is eagerly awaited. Immunohistochemical staining, using ouabain-specific antiserum, suggested that ouabain-like immunoactivity is limited to specific morphological elements within the brain [76, 77]. However, the evidence for this factor originating in the hypothalamus is tentative. The absence of well established hypothalamic cell lines continues to hamper a more direct approach to the question of secretion and biosynthesis.

Additional controversy has been created by the observation that common rat chow contains a substance with chromatographic properties and bioactivity indistinguishable from the isomer of ouabain [73]. Studies designed to assess the contribution of this dietary factor found that feeding rats on chow selected for low factor levels resulted in Milan hypertensive animals having more of the hypothalamic [Na,K]ATPase activity than the normotensive Milan animal controls. Hamlyn et al. [6] recognized this problem and attempted to resolve it by identifying the ouabain-like agent from plasma obtained from patients who were maintained on semi-isynthetic diets free of ouabain for a week. Reports on multiple other candidates isolated from urine [71, 72] also suggest a dietary source.

If the primary hypothalamic inhibitor is structurally related to ouabain, a crucial question arises: Are steroids produced in the hypothalamic-pituitary region? The question is still debated. There are steroidal compounds which appear to be produced elsewhere, but are taken up, modified and activated by sites within the brain [79]. At present there is no direct evidence for an isomer of ouabain being produced or modified in the hypothalamus. Even in the eventuality that such a compound is shown to be made or modified in the hypothalamus, it will be necessary, of course, to demonstrate that the factor enters the circulation. There is the alternative possibility that these agents have a local paracrine or autocrine function [36].

3.6.2   The adrenal

Many researchers anticipated that an endogenous sodium pump inhibitor would resemble the cardioglycosides, with their steroidal 4-ring backbone. Hence, many have considered the adrenal as an attractive alternative source of production. As indicated above, many early surveys of several tissues from animals, typically using digoxin antibodies as the only probe, found high, and often the highest, levels of digitalis-like immuno-reactivity (DLI) in the adrenal. However, those studies that applied chromatography to the tissue extract have, without exception shown several regions of immunoactivity [32, 60, 62] with only a few of the immunoreactive species possessing functional [Na,K]ATPase inhibitory activity [15].

Perhaps it is this nonspecificity of the antibodies employed to assess DLI that may help to explain why the shift to high dietary sodium in most studies has not induced significantly higher adrenal DLI, despite increases in circulating DLI activity [54]. Others have administered ACTH and found that DLI increased transiently in the circulation, consistent with but by no means definitive evidence of an adrenal mediated response [30]. Adrenalectomy lowered serum DLI in several studies [6, 15] but not all [81, 82].

The discovery by Hamlyn and his coworkers of ouabain, or a close isomer of ouabain, in human plasma has focused attention on its potential source [6, 30]. Their studies found that adrenalectomy reduced levels of OLI and that the conditioned medium from cultured adrenal cells manifest OLI [6]. They also reported an adrenal tumor producing high levels of OLI [83], a finding reminiscent of two previous reports of increased DLF levels in patients with primary aldosteronism [84, 85]. However, another group found that whereas circulating levels of OLI fell after removal of the adrenals, and compensatory steroid replacement, OLI could still be increased with 2.5 weeks high-salt intake [32]. An interesting and potentially relevant observation was that administered labelled ouabain was selectively taken up by the adrenal in rats, and thereafter volume expansion resulted in its increased release from the adrenal [36]. Two more recent, extensive studies have questioned whether OLI originates in the adrenal. The first found increased circulating levels of OLI in patients with essential hypertension, primary aldosteronism, Cushing's syndrome, pheochromocytoma, acromegaly, and chronic renal failure: With surgical intervention OLI fell to normal in patients with acromegaly or primary aldosteronism, and with hemodialysis it fell in patients with chronic renal failure [31]. However, circulating OLI levels remained unchanged in patients after bilateral adrenalectomy. Moreover, when adrenal vein sampling was carried out in three patients, there was no step up in OLI concentration from the adrenal compared to the peripheral vein. The second of these studies initially took human plasma from both normal subjects and acutely ill patients and submitted it to HPLC fractionation followed by a ouabain RIA [15]. They found that most of the OLI did not coincide with true ouabain. They then studied the conditioned media from cultured bovine adrenal cells. While they found OLI in the medium, little of this activity had an HPLC retention time similar to ouabain. When they tested an inhibitor of cholesterol side-chain cleavage and subsequent steroid production, known steroids decreased but not OLI. Conversely, stimulation of steroidogenesis, which increased known steroid hormones, nevertheless failed to increase OLI [15].

At this time it is impossible to conclude whether the adrenal serves as the source of the functional sodium pump inhibitor. If the endogenous sodium pump inhibitor is structurally related to known cardioglycosides, the enzymes that participate in lactone ring formation or 14β-hydroxylation would be anticipated, but have yet to be found. However, cardioglycosides with these structural elements are known to be produced in some toads [37] and some insects [38]. Use of antibodies directed against digoxin or ouabain as the sole probe appear to be inadequate to identify this inhibitor in the adrenal, and perhaps other tissues, probably due to measurable crossreactivity with many compounds. For example while OLI is present in adrenal homogenates, the available data suggest that many different compounds contribute to the activity. Whether ouabain specifically is endogenously produced remains an unanswered question.

None of the agents currently under consideration have as yet satisfied these stringent criteria. We hope that the application of the principles discovered by Koch one hundred and thirty years ago will clarify and simplify what has become a highly contentious and confusing field.

4   Therapeutic targets

At the moment, the only therapeutic use made of this pathway involves the application of digitalis glycosides to the treatment of heart failure and some supraventricular cardiac arrhythmias. Isolation and identification of the crucial, native sodium pump inhibitors in this pathway could be the basis for a much wider range of therapeutic targets. For reasons that should be obvious from the introduction, much of the attention has focused on their potential in the areas of salt-sensitive hypertension and edema. To the extent that a circulating sodium pump inhibitor contributes to the pathogenesis of salt-sensitive hypertension, interruption of its biosynthesis or interference with its action at the receptor site could ameliorate the process.

However, the sodium pump is ubiquitous, an element of virtually every cell membrane in higher organisms, and thus one should consider a broad range of therapeutic targets.

4.1   The range of targets

The range of candidate targets is bewildering. For example, digoxin-like materials have been found in human breast cyst fluids and could contribute to their pathogenesis [89]. Changes in sodium transport occur not only in pregnancy, but also during the human menstrual cycle, and could be of interest in the pathogenesis of the premenstrual syndrome [90]. Functional bowel disorder leading to constipation and diarrhea have also been discussed in the light of intestinal transport, and the activity of [Na,K]ATPase [91–93]. Digoxin-like immunoreactive agents have been identified in patients with subarachnoid hemorrhage, and could play a role in the vasospasm that contributes to central nervous system injury in that setting [94]. There is a substantial literature on the influence of acute central nervous system ischemia on these processes [95–98]. Perhaps most impressive is the evidence to suggest that a sodium pump inhibitor could contribute to the pathogenesis of cataract formation, which merits detailed review.

4.2   The sodium pump and cataract formation

With an aging population, surgery for cataract has become the most common operation performed in the USA. The Medicare budget for this procedure exceeded three billion dollars last year despite guidelines demanding a reduction in visual acuity exceeding 50% before surgery will be paid for. Cataract remains the leading cause of blindness [99]. No pharmacological treatment is available, and indeed the pathogenesis of cataracts is sufficiently obscure that few guidelines exist on prevention.
In 1960, Nakano et al. described a strain of mice which inherit cataracts that become evident within weeks of birth [100]. About a decade later, Iwata et al. [101] demonstrated acute sodium accumulation in the lens of this strain of mice which was associated with a deficiency of the sodium pump. The Nakano mouse lens at two weeks began to show an increase in water content associated with the striking increase in local sodium content and a fall in local potassium content. They documented, further, a striking reduction in ^{86}Rb uptake, which was not associated with a change in permeability to potassium or ^{86}Rb. Thus, they concluded that an abnormality in the sodium pump was responsible. This was confirmed by a direct measurement, which revealed a reduction in [Na,K]ATPase activity, which paralleled the time course of lens opacification. In the discussion of that paper, they raised the question of a sodium pump inhibitor, but did not report an effort to identify it. Sodium pump inhibition with ouabain opacifies the lens *in vitro* [102]. Parallel lens opacification and sodium pump

deficiency have been demonstrated in a wide variety of circumstances including other genetic models in mice and rats [103,104], and rats in which lens opacification was precipitated by galactose feeding or the induction of diabetes mellitus [105, 106]. A series of studies on humans involving all forms of cataract including those primarily associated with aging, hypertension, and diabetes mellitus confirmed the parallels between sodium pump deficiency and lens opacification [106–109].

Particularly intriguing in this light is the observation that the Dahl salt-sensitive rat and other rat strains bred to develop hypertension are also prone to develop cataracts [110,111]. The cataracts in this model are associated with inhibition of lenticular sodium pump activity [113]. There are additional internal correlations that are intriguing. Rats with the largest blood pressure response to initiation of a high-salt intake were the most likely to develop cataracts [111].

In 1974, Kinoshita announced the first identification of an inhibitor of the sodium pump in Nakano mouse lens [102]. The agent was heat labile, losing activity after incubation at 100°C, and was non-dialyzable. Fukuii et al. [112] reported that the agent was a basic polypeptide sensitive to carboxypeptidase and leucine aminopeptidase with a molecular weight of approximately 6300 based on gel filtration. They concluded on the basis of these observations that the agent was a polypeptide. Russell et al. confirmed these observations and extended them by identifying an identical agent in the supernatant of lens from this strain growing in tissue culture [113]. Clearly, these cells produced something that affected sodium pump activity.

Recently Lichtstein et al. have extended this line of investigation to the human cataractous lens [114]. They found an agent in human lens extract that inhibited [Na,K]ATPase, interacted with an antibody directed against digoxin and inhibited ouabain binding. As only limited amounts of material could be obtained, the structural analysis remains tentative, but the agent(s) in the lens responsible for the digitalis-like activity resembled some bufodenolides found earlier in normal toad skin and plasma, 19-norbufalin and a peptide-conjugated 19-norbufalin.

They considered the question of whether the agents were synthesized locally in the cataractous lens or elsewhere and accumulated in the lens during cataract formation. They made an interesting speculation based on the fact that bufodienolides can be synthesized chemically from digitalis cardeneolides and that this organic synthesis requires a photo-oxidation step, raising the intriguing possibility that the endogenous digitalis-like factor when exposed to ultraviolet radiation in the lens is converted to a bufodienolide. Whether the agent thus produced the original digitalis-like factor is more active on the lens sodium pump was not determined in that study.

Taken in all, these observations raise an interesting possibility. Cataracts are a complication of a long life. With normal aging, there is a reduction in the capacity of the kidney to handle salt intake. This capacity is likely to be limited further by hypertension, diabetes mellitus, or renal failure, all factors that predispose to cataract formation. The various parallels drawn above indicate that the same forces that lead to salt-sensitive hypertension also lead to cataract formation – possibly via the same pathogenetic sequence.

Although hypertension has a wide range of treatments already available, we have many fewer options for the treatment of cataracts.

5   Summary and conclusion

One might ask, given the number of false trails that have been pursued, why we, and so many others, have continued to pursue the elusive digitalis-like factor? The answer can be found in the many review articles cited above [4–13]. In animal models of volume-dependent hypertension, evidence favoring sodium pump inhibition as at least a contributing factor, is essentially overwhelming. These observations are supported by multiple lines of less direct evidence in humans which are also compatible with a contribution of a circulating sodium pump inhibitor. Indeed, if multiple premature claims announcing the isolation of the digitalis-like factor had not appeared, this would be one of a large number of interesting scientific areas in which identification of a responsible vector was expected momentarily. The disenchantment so often expressed, we believe, reflects a response to those premature claims. We echo a recent review on the digoxin-like sodium pump inhibitor story from one of the productive groups in this area. "Now that there is little doubt that endogenous digoxin-like inhibitors of sodium transport exist…, the link between these substances, salt intake and vascular tone must be pursued with increasing vigor" [12]. That pursuit, of course, will be easier if the criteria concerning the responsible mediator are employed systematically.

Because the current situation resembles so strikingly the situation late in the nineteenth century – when efforts focused on the attempt to identify a specific microorganism as the agent responsible for specific disease – we employed Koch's Postulates as the organizing principle. The challenge faced by Robert Koch over a century ago is identical to the challenge that those of us who are interested in digitalis-like factors face today. Passionate advocacy and equally impassioned denial can be seen as a stage in the scientific process when the problem is important and has proven to be more intractable than anticipated. Substantial, but still circumstantial evidence supports strongly a role for a circulating digitalis-like factor not only in normal sodium homeostasis and in the pathogenesis of salt-sensitive hypertension, but also in the pathogenesis of a wide array of processes that have an uncertain etiology. Although supported by many lines of evidence, this intriguing concept remains controversial, in large part because the responsible factor has proven to be very elusive. Informed opinion today ranges from arguments that the agent does not exist to contrary arguments that the agent has been identified. A very large number of candidates from a wide range of chemical classes have been proposed. Indeed, the large number of candidates, none supported by absolutely definitive evidence, has contributed to the controversy. In this essay, we have attempted to define and illustrate the information that will be required before a candidate becomes widely accepted.

References

1   Hansen O.:"Do putative endogenous digitalis-like factors have a physiological role?" Letters to the Editor. Hypertension 24, 640 (1994).
2   Doris P.A.: Response #1 to Letters to the Editor: "Do putative endogenous digitalis-like factors have a physiological role?" Hypertension 24, 640–641 (1994).
3   Hamlyn J.M., Laredo J., Lu Z.-R., Hamilton B., Lighthall G.: Response #2 to Letters to the Editor: "Do putative endogenous digitalis-like factors have a physiological role?" 24, 641–643 (1994).
4   Buckalew V.M., Jr., Haddy F.J.:"Circulating natriuretic factors in hypertension". In: Brenner, B.M. and J.H. Laragh (Ed.): Hypertension: Pathophysiology, Diagnosis, and Management. Chapter 60, pp 939–954 (1990).
5   Wechter W.J., Benaksas E.J.: "Natriuretic hormones". In: Jucker E. (Ed.): Progress in Drug Research 34, 232–260, Birkhäuser Verlag Basel, Switzerland 1990.
6   Hamlyn J.M., Manunta P.: "Ouabain, digitalis-like factors and hypertension". J. Hyperten. (Suppl #7) 10, 99–111 (1992).
7   Goto A., Yamada K., Yagi N., Yoshioka M., Sugimoto T.: "Physiology and pharmacology of endogenous digitalis-like factors". Pharmacol. Rev. 44, 377–399 (1992).
8   Ruegg U.T.: "Ouabain: A link in the genesis of high blood pressure". Experientia 48, 1102–1106 (1992).
9   Blaustein M.P.: "Physiological effects of endogenous ouabain: Control of intracellular Ca^{2+} stores and cell responsiveness". Am. J. Phsiol. 264, C1367–1387 (1993).
10   MacGregor S.E., Walker J.M.: "Mini Review. Inhibitors of the Na^+, K^+-ATPase. Comp. Biochem. Physiol. 105C, 1–9 (1993).

11   Schoner W.: "Endogenous digitalis-like factors". In: Jucker E. (Ed.): Progress in Drug Research *41*, 249–281. Birkhäuser Verlag Basel, Switzerland 1993.

12   Woolfson R.G., Poston L., and De Wardener H.E.: "Digoxin-like inhibitors of active sodium transport and blood pressure: The current status". Kid. Int. *46*, 297–309 (1994).

13   Graves S.W.: "The sodium pump in hypertension". Curr. Opinion Nephrol. Hypertens. *3*, 107–111 (1994).

14   Kelly R.A. and Smith T.W.: "The search for the endogenous digitalis: an alternative hypothesis". Am. J. Physiol. *256*, C937–C950 (1989).

15   Doris P.A., Jenkins L.A., Stocco D.M.: "Is ouabain an authentic endogenous mammalian substance derived from the adrenal?" Hypertens. *23*, 632–638 (1994).

16   Lewis L.K., Yandle T.G., Lewis J.G., Richards A.M., Pidgeon G.B., Kaaja R.J., Nicholls M.G.: "Ouabain is not detectable in human plasma". Hypertens. *24*, 548-555 (1994).

17   Gomez-Sanches D.P., Foecking M.F., Sellers D., Blankenship M.S., Gomez-Sanchez C.E.: "Is the circulating ouabain-like compound ouabain?" Am. J. Hypertens. *7*, 647–650 (1994).

18   Weller T.H.: "Robert Koch and the Modern Investigator". Hospital Practice *30*, 99–101 (1995).

19   Hollenberg N.K. and Graves S.W.: "Koch's postulates and the digitalis-like factor". Hypertension Res. *18*, 1–6 (1995).

20   Nuland S.B.: Doctors: The Biography of Medicine. Alfred A. Knopf, NY 1988, pp. 238–262.

21   McGrew R.E.: Encyclopedia of Medical History. McGraw Hill Book Co., NY 1985, pp. 25–30.

22   Lyons A.S. and Petrucelli R.J.: Medicine: An Illustrated History. Harry N. Abrams Inc. Publishers, NY 1987.

23   Haber E.: The role of renin in normal and pathological cardiovascular homeostasis. Circ. *54*, 849–861 (1976).

24   Kelly R.A., O'Hara S.O., Mitch W.E., and Smith T.W.: "Identification of NaK:ATPase inhibitors in human plasma as nonesterified fatty acids and lysophospholipids". J. Biol. Chem. *261*, 11704–11711 (1986).

25   Vasdev S., Longerich L., Johnson E., Brent D., Gault M.H.: "Dehydroepiandrosterone sulfate as a digitalis-like factor in plasma of healthy human adults". Res. Comm. Chem. Pathol. Pharmacol. *49*, 387–399 (1985).

26   Graves S.W., Sharma K., and Chandler A.B.: "Methods for eliminating interferences in digoxin immunoassays caused by digoxin-like factors." Clin. Chem. *32*, 1506–1509 (1986).

27   Stewart L., Hamilton C., Ingwall J., Naomi S., Graves S., Canessa M., Williams G.H., Hollenberg N.K.: "Vascular smooth muscle response to ouabain: Relation to tissue Na^+ to the contractile response". Circ. Res. *71*, 1113–1120 (1993).

28   Hamlyn J.M., Ringel R., Schaeffer J., Levinson P.D., Hamilton B.P., Lowarski A.A., and Blaustein M.P.: "A circulating inhibitor of $[Na^+K^+]ATPase$ associated with essential hypertension". Nature *300*, 650–652 (1982).

29   Graves S.W., Soszynski P.A., Tao Q.F., Williams G.H., Hollenberg N.K.: "A labile endogenous Na-pump inhibitor in man". In: Bamberg E., Schoner W.: The Sodium Pump: Structure, Mechanism, Hormonal Control, and its Role in Disease. Darmstadt: Steinkopff; New York, Springer, 1994; pp 771–774.

30   Hamlyn J.M., Blaustein M.P., Bova S., DuCharme D.W., Harris D.W., Mandel F., Mathews W.R., and Ludens J.H.: "Identification and characterization of a ouabain-like compound from human plasma". Proc. Natl. Acad. Sci. *88*, 6259–6263 (1991).

31   Haber E., Haupert G.T., Jr.: "The search for a hypothalamic Na+,K+-ATPase inhibitor". Hypertension 9, 315–324 (1987).

32   Ludens J.H., Clark M.A., Robinson F.G., DuCharme D.W.: "Rat adrenal cortex is a source of a circulating ouabain-like compound". Hypertension 19, 721–724 (1992).

33   Xie L.Q., Markides K.E., Lee M.L., Hollenberg N.K., Williams G.H., Graves S.W.: "Bioanalytical application of multidimensional open tubular column supercritical fluid chromatography". Chromatographia 35(7/8), 363–371 (1993).

34   Naomi S., Graves S.W., Lazarus M.J., Williams G.H., Hollenberg N.K.: "Variation in apparent serum digitalis-like factor levels with different digoxin antibodies: The 'immunochemical fingerprint'." Am. J. Hypertens. 4, 795–801 (1991).

35   Graves S.W., Naomi S., Williams G.H., Hollenberg N.K.: "Digitoxin antibody cross-reactivity and evaluation of potential candidates for the circulating digitalis-like immunoreactive factor". Clin. Chem. 40, 1595–1596 (1994).

36   Leenen F.H.H., Harmsen E.E.F., Yu H., Ou C.: "Effects of dietary sodium on central and peripheral ouabain like activity in spontaneously hypertensive rats". Am. J. Physiol. 264, H2051–H2055 (1993).

37   Vinge E., Helgesen-Rosendal S., and Backstron T.: "Progesterone, some progesterone derivatives and urinary digoxin-like substances from pregnant women in radioimmuno- and 86Rb-uptake assays of digoxin". Pharmacol. Toxicol. 63, 277–280 (1988).

38   Burtis C.A., Ashwood E.R.: Tietz Textbook of Clinical Chemistry. Second edition. W.B. Saunders Co., Philadelphia, PA. 1994, pp 2203–2204.

39   Gruber K.A., Whitaker J.M., Buckalew V.M.J.: "Endogenous digitalis-like substance in plasma of volume expanded dogs". Nature 277, 743–745 (1980).

40   Glatter K.A., Graves S.W., Hollenberg N.K., Soszynski P.A., Tao Q.-F., Frem G.F., Williams G.H., and Lazarus J.M.: "Sustained volume expansion and [Na,K]ATPase inhibition in chronic renal failure". Am. J. Hyperten. 7, 1016–1025 (1994).

41   Forbush III B.: "Cardiotonic steroid binding to Na,K-ATPase". In: J.F. Hoffman and B. Forbush, III (Eds.): Structure, Mechanism, and Function of the Na/K Pump. Academic Press, New York 1983, pp. 167–201.

42   Tao Q.F., Soszynski P.A., Hollenberg N.K., Graves S.: "A sensitive assay for sodium pump inhibition". Clin. Chem. 40, 1595–1596 (1994).

43   Sekihara H., Yazaki Y., Kojima T.: "Ouabain as an amplifier of mineralocorticoid-induced hypertension". Endocrinology 131, 3077–3082 (1992).

44   Yuan C.M., Manunta P., Hamlyn J.M., Chen S., Bohen E., Yeun J., Haddy F.J., and Pamnani M.B.: "Long-term ouabain administration produces hypertension in rats". Hypertension 22, 178–187 (1993).

45   Songu-Mize E., Bealer S.L., and Caldwell R.W.: "Effect of DOCA-salt treatment duration and anteroventral third ventricular lesions on a plasma-borne sodium pump inhibitor in rats". J. Hypertens. 5, 461–467 (1987).

46   Kojima I., Yoshihara S., Ogata E.: "Involvement of endogenous digitalis-like substance in genesis of deoxycorticosterone-salt hypertension". Life Sciences 30, 1775–1781 (1982).

47   Huang C.T., Smith R.M.: "Lowering of blood pressure in chronic aortic coarctate hypertensive rats with anti-digoxin antiserum". Life Sciences 35, 115–118 (1984).

48   Zidek W., Otten E., Heckmann U.: "Transmission of hypertension in rats by cross circulation". Hypertension 14, 61–65 (1989).

49   Goodlin R.C.: "Antidogoxin antibodies in eclampsia". N. Engl. J. Med. 318, 518–519 (1988).

50   Balzan S., Montali U., Biver P., Ghione S.: "Digoxin-binding antibodies reverse the

effect of endogenous digitalis-like compounds on Na,K-ATPase in erythrocytes". J. Hypertension *9*, 304–305 (1991).

51   Mann J.F.E., Miemietz R., Ganten U., Ritz E.: "Hemodynamic effects of intact digoxin antibody and its Fab fragments in experimental hypertension". J. Hypertension *5*, 543–549 (1987).

52   Raghavan S.R.V., Gonick H.C.: "Partial purification and characterization of natriuretic fator from rat kidney". Proc. Soc. Expermintal Biol. Med. *164*, 101–104 (1980).

53   de Pover A., Castaneda-Hernandez G., Godfraind T.: "Water versus acetone-HCl extraction of digitalis-like factor from guinea-pig heart". Biochem. Pharmacol. *31*, 267–71 (1982).

54   Casteneda-Hernandez G., Godfraind T.: "Effect of high sodium intake on tissue distribution of endogenous digitalis-like material in the rat". Clin. Sci. *66*, 225–8 (1984).

55   Rauch A.L., Buckalew V.M. Jr.: "Tissue distribution of an endogenous ligand to the Na,K ATPase molecule". Biophys. Biochem. Res. Comm. *152*, 818–24 (1988).

56   Shaikh I.M., Lau B.W.C., Siegfried B.A., Valdes R. Jr.: "Isolation of digoxin-like immunoreactive factors from mammalian adrenal cortex". J. Biol. Chem. *266*, 13672–13678 (1991).

57   Fishman M.C.: "Endogenous digitalis-like activity in mammalian brain". Proc. Natl. Acad. Sci. *76*, 4661–3 (1979).

58   Haupert G.T., Sancho J.M.: "Sodium transport inhibitor from bovine hypothalamus". Proc. Natl. Acad. Sci. 76, 4658–60 (1979).

59   Tamura M., Lam T.-T., Inagami T.: "Isolation and characterization of a specific endogenous Na$^+$,K$^+$-ATPase inhibitor from bovine adrenal". Biochem. *27*, 4244–53 (1988).

60   Schreiber V., Gregorova I., Pribyl T., Stepan J.: "Digitalis-like biological activity and immunoreactivity in chromatographic fractions of rabbit adrenal extract". Endocrinologia Experimentalis *15*, 229–36 (1981).

61   Takahashi H., Makoto M., Ikegaki I., et al.: "Digitalis-like substance is produced in the hypothalamus but not in the adrenal gland in rats". J. Hypertens. *6* (Suppl 4), S345–7 (1988).

62   Doris P.A.: "Immunological evidence that the adrenal gland is a source of an endogenous digitalis-like factor". Endocrinol. *123*, 2440–44 (1988).

63   Buggy J., Fink G.D., Haywood J.R., Johnson A.K., and Brody M.J.: "Interruption of the maintenance phase of established hypertension by ablation of the anteroventral third ventricle (AV3V) in rats". Clin. Exper. Hypertens. *1*, 337–53 (1978).

64   Kaloyanides G.J., Balabanian M.B., Bowman R.L.: "Evidence that the brain participates in the humoral natriuretic mechanism of blood volume expansion in the dog". J. Clin. Invest. *62*, 1288–95 (1978).

65   Songu-Mize E., Bealer S.L., Caldwell R.W.: Effect of AV3V lesions on development of DOCA-salt hypertension and vascular Na$^+$-pump activity. Hypertens. *4*, 575–80 (1982).

66   Gruber K.A., Whitaker J.M., Buckalew V.M. Jr.: "Endogneous digitalis-like substance in plasma of volume-expanded dogs". Nature *287*, 743–5 (1980).

67   Akagawa K., Hara N., Tsukada Y.: "Partial purification and properties of the inhibitors of Na,K-ATPase and ouabain-binding in bovine central nervous system". J. Neruochem. *42*, 775–80 (1984).

68   Kramer H.J., Backer A., Schurmann J., Weiler E., and Klingmuller D.: "Further characterization of the endogenous natriuretic and digoxin-like immunoreactive activities in human urine". Regul. Pept. *4* (Suppl 4), 124–127 (1985).

69   Morgan K., Lewis M.D., Spurlock G., et al.: "Characterization and partial purifica-

tion of the sodium-potassium ATPase inhibitor released from cultured rat hypothalamic cells". J. Biol. Chem. *260*, 13595–600 (1985).

70   Halperin J.A., Riordan J.F., Tosteson D.C.: "Characteristics of an inhibitor of the Na/K pump in human cerebrospinal fluid". J. Biol. Chem. *263*, 636–51 (1988).

71   Goto A., Ishiguro T., Yamada K. et al.: "Isolation of a urinary digitalis-like factor indistinguishable from digoxin". Biochem. Biophys. Res. Comm. *173*, 1093–1101 (1990).

72   Tamura M., Harris T.M., Phillips D., et al.: "Identification of two cardiac glycosides as Na^+ pump inhibitors in rat urine and diet". J. Biol. Chem. *269*, 11972–11979 (1994).

73   Tymiak A.A., Norman J.A., Bolgar M., et al.: "Physiochemical characterization of a ouabain isomer isolated from bovine hypothalamus". Proc. Natl. Acad. Sci. USA *90*, 8189–93 (1993).

74   Ferrandi M., Minotti E., Salardi S., Florio M., Bianchi G., Ferrari P: "Ouabain-like factor in Milan hypertensive rats". Am. J. Physiol. *263*, F739–48 (1992).

75   English L.H., Epstein J., Cantley J., Housman D., Levenson R.: "Expression of an ouabain resistance gene in transfected cells. Ouabain treatment induces a K^+-transport system". J. Biol. Chem. *260*, 1114–9 (1985).

76   Yamada H., Ihara N., Sano Y.: "Morphological evidence of endogenous digitalis-like substance (EDLS) in the rat and macaque hypothalamus, using digoxin-immunohistochemistry". Endocrinol. Japon. *34*, 319–323 (1987).

77   Takahashi H., Matsuzawa M., Okabayashi H., et al.: "Evidence for a digitalis-like substance in the hypothalamopituitary axis in rats: implications in the central cardiovascular regulation associated with an excess intake of sodium". Japan. Circ. J. *51*, 1199–1207 (1987).

78   Ferrandi M., Minotti E., Florio M., Bianchi G., Ferrari P.: "Age-dependency and dietary influence on the hypothalamic ouabain-like factor (OLF) of the Milan hypertensive rats (MHS)". Biol. Chem. Hoppe-Seyler *374*, 609 (1993).

79   Jung-Testas I., Hu Y.Y., Baulieu E.E., Robel P.: "Steroid synthesis in rat brain cell cultures". J. Steroid. Biochem. *34*, 511–519 (1989).

80   Gault M.H., Vasdev S., Longerich L., et al.: "Evidence for an adrenal contribution to plasma digitalis-like factors". Clin. Physiol. Biochem. *6*, 253–261 (1988).

81   Naruse K., Naruse M., Tanabe A., et al.: "Does plasma immunoreactive ouabain originate from the adrenal gland?" Hypertension *23* (Suppl I), I102–I105 (1994).

82   Leenan F.H.H., Harmsen E., Yu H., Yuan B.: "Dietary sodium stimulates ouabain-like activity (OLA) in adrenalectomized SHR". Hypertens. *22*, 431 (1993).

83   Manunta P., Evans G., Hamilton B.P., Gann D., Resau J., Hamlyn J.M.: "A new syndrome with elevated plasma ouabain and hypertension secondary to an adrenocortical tumor". Proceedings from the 14th Scientific Meeting of the International Society of Hypertension Meeting, Madrid, Spain, June 14–19, 1992, abstract P36, pp. S27.

84   Masugi F., Ogihara T., Hasegawa T., et al.: "Circulating factor with ouabain-like immunoreactivity in patients with primary aldosteronism". Biochem. Biophys. Res. Comm. *135*, 41–45 (1986).

85   Pedrinelli R., Clerico A., Panarace G., et al.: "Does a digoxin-like substance participate in vascular and pressure control during dietary sodium changes in patients with primary aldosteronism?" J. Hypertension *9*, 457–463 (1991).

86   Kitano S., Morimoto .S, Koh E., Ogihara T.: "The adrenals release accumulated exogenous ouabain at volume expansion in reduced renal mass hypertensive rats". Hypertension *22*, 432 (1993).

87   Siperstein M.D., Murray A.W., Titrus E.: "Biosynthesis of cardiotonic steroids from cholesterol in the toad, Bufo marinus." Arch. Biochem. Biophys. *67*, 154–160 (1957).

88   Van Ockye S., Braekman J.C., Daloze D., Pasteels J.M.: "Cardenolide biosynthesis in chrysomelid beetles". Experimentia 43, 460–463 (1987).

89   Chassalow F.I., Bradlow H.L.: "Digoxin like materials in human breast cyst fluids". Ann. NY Acad. Sci. 586, 107–116 (1990).

90   Webb G.D., Ashmead G.G., al-Mahdi S., Auletta F.J., McLaughlin M.K.: "Changes in sodium transport during the human menstrual cycle and pregnancy". Clin. Sci. (Colch) 84(4), 401–405 (1993).

91   Fondacaro J.D.: "Intestinal ion transport and diarrheal disease". Am. J. Physiol. 250, G1–G8 (1986).

92   Ramakrishna B.S., Mathan V.I.: "Absorption of water and sodium and activity of adenosine triphosphatases in the rectal mucosa of troipical sprue". Gut 29, 665–668 (1988).

93   Ewe K.: "Intestinal transport in constipation and diarrhea". Pharmacology 36 (Suppl 1), S73–84 (1988).

94   Wijdicks E.F.M., Vermeulen M., van Brummelon P., den Boer N.C., van Gijn J.: "Digoxin-like immunoreactive substance in patients with aneurysmal subarachnoid hemorrhage". Br. Med. J. 294, 729–732 (1987).

95   MacMillan V.: Cerebral Na^+, K^+,-ATPase activity during exposure to and recovery from acute ischemia". J. Cereb. Blood Flow Metab. 2, 457–465 (1982).

96   Enseleit W.H., Domer F.R., Jarrott D.M., Baricos W.H.: "Cerebral phospholipid content and Na^+, K^+-ATPase activity during ischemia and postishemic reperfusion in the mongolian gerbil". J. Neruochem. 43, 320–327 (1984).

97   Schielke G.P., Moises H.C., Betz A.L.: "Blood to brain sodium transport and interstitial fluid potassium concentration during early focal ischemia in the rat". J. Cereb. Blood Flow Metab. 11, 466–471 (1991).

98   Shigeno T., Asano T., Mima T., Takakura K.: "Effect of enhanced capillary activity on the blood-brain barrier during focal cerebrous ischemia in cats". Stroke 20, 1260–1266 (1989).

99   Tielsch J.M., Javitt J.C., Coleman A., Katz J., Sommer A.: "The prevalence of blindness and visual impairment amont nursing home residents in Baltimore". N. Engl. J. Med. 332, 1205–1209 (1995).

100   Nakano K., Yamamoto S., Kutsukake G., Ogawa H., Nakajima A., and Takano E.: "Hereditary cataract in mice". Jap. J. Opthalmol. 14, 196–199 (1960).

101   Iwata S. and Kinoshita J.I.: "Mechanism of development of hereditary cataract in mice". Invest. Ophthalmol. 10, 504–512 (1971).

102   Kinoshita J.H.: "Mechanisms initiating cataract formation". Invest. Ophthalmol. 13, 713–724 (1974).

103   Unakar N.J., Tsui J.Y., Kuck J.F., and Kuck K.D.: "Sodium-potassium-dependent-ATPase activity in Emory mouse lens". Current Eye Research 5, 263–271 (1986).

104   Kamei A., Hisada T., Iwata S.: "The evaluation of therapeutic efficacy of hachimi-jio-gan (traditional Chinese medicine) to mouse hereditary cataract". J. Ocul. Pharmacol. 4, 311–319 (1988).

105   Unaker N.J., Tsui J.Y.: "Sodium-potassium-dependent ATPase I. Cytochemical localization in normal and cataractous rat lenses". Invest. Ophthalmol. Vis. Sci. 19, 630–641 (1980).

106   Ahmad S.S., Tsou K.C., Ahmad S.I., Rahman M.A., Kirmani T.H.: "Studies on cataractogeneous in human and in rats with alloxan-induced diabetes. I. Cation transport and sodium-potassium-dependent ATPase". Ophthalmic Res. 17, 1–11 (1985).

107   Kobatashi S., Roy D., Spector A.: "Sodium/potassium ATPase in normal and cataractous human lenses". Curr. Eye Res. 2, 327–334 (1982).

108   Pasino M., Maraini G.: "Cation pump activity and membrane permeability in human senile cataractous lenses". Exp. Eye Res. *34*, 887–893 (1982).

109   Garner M.H., Spector A.: "ATP hydrolysis kinetics of Na,K-ATPase in cataract." Exp. Eye Res. *42*, 339–348 (1986).

110   Rodriguez-Sargent C., Cangiano J.L., Berrios Caban G., Marrero E., Martinez-Maldonado M.: "Cataracts and hypertension in salt-sensitive rats. A possible ion transport defect." Hypertension *9*, 304–308 (1987).

111   Rodriguez-Sargent C., Estape E.S., Rodriguez-Santiago A., Ramos V.L., Irizarry J.E., and Martinez-Moldonado M.: "Lenticular rubidium uptake and plasma renin activity in weaning cataract-prone salt-sensitive rats". Hypertension *15*, 114–1148 (1990).

112   Fukuii H.N., Merola L.O., and Kinoshita J.H.: "A possible cataractogenic factor in the Nakano mouse lens". Exp. Eye Res. *26*, 477–485 (1978).

113   Russell P., Fukui H.N., and Kinoshita J.H.: "Properties of a Na^+, K^+,-ATPase inhibitor in cultured lens epithelial cells". Vision Res. *21*, 37–39 (1981).

114   Lichtstein D., Gati I., Samuelov S., Berson D., Rozenman Y., Landau L., Deutsch J.: "Identification of digitalis-like compounds in human cataractous lenses". Eur. J. Biochem. *216*, 261–268 (1993).

115   Tao Q.-F., Soszynski P.A., Hollenberg N.K., and Graves S.W.: "A sensitive [Na,K]-ATPase assay specific for inhibitors acting through the digitalis-binding site". J. Cardiovasc. Pharmacol. *25*, 859–863 (1995).

116   Krep H.H., Graves S.W., Price D.A., Lazarus M.J., Ensign A.E., Soszynski P.A., and Hollenberg N.K.: "Reversal of sodium pump inhibitor induced VSM contraction with Digibind: stoichiometry and its implications". Am. J. Hypertension *8*, 921–927 (1995).

Progress in Drug Research, Vol. 46 (E. Jucker, Ed.)
© 1996 Birkhäuser Verlag, Basel (Switzerland)

Neurotransmitters involved in the central regulation of the cardiovascular system

By Robert B. McCall

Cardiovascular Pharmacology, The Upjohn Company, Kalamazoo, MI 49001, USA

1   Introduction

Arterial blood pressure is maintained by the tonic vasomotor activity of sympathetic preganglionic neurons which are located in the intermedio-lateral cell column of the thoracic and lumbar spinal cord. Supraspinal inputs are critical in maintaining the activity of SPN. The medulla and pons have been recognized as essential for maintaining tonic sympathetic activ-ity since the late 1800's when experiments showed that transection of the brain stem caudal to the inferior colliculus failed to lower blood pressure. Transections more caudally produced increasingly greater falls in blood pressure. Reductions in blood pressure reached a maximum with tran-sections at the level of the obex (see ref [1] for historical review). A major goal of central autonomic research has been to identify the descending neuronal pathways which project to SPN and to determine the neurotrans-mitters contained within these pathways (see ref [2–6] for review). Neu-roanatomical and immunocytochemical techniques have been used to identify chemically specific pathways between areas thought to be impor-tant in central autonomic regulation. This information combined with experiments utilizing sophisticated electrophysiological and pharmaco-logical analysis have begun to elucidate the role of these pathways in cen-tral autonomic regulation and to determine the functional significance of putative neurotransmitters contained within these pathways. This review describes recent developments which have had a major influence on our understanding of the central neurotransmitters involved in the regulation of sympathetic nerve discharge.

2   General organization of central autonomic pathways

Sympathetic preganglionic neurons are located primarily in the interme-diolateral cell column of the thoracic and lumbar spinal cord but also found in the adjacent white matter of the lateral funiculus, in a band between the intermediolateral cell column and the central canal (intercalated nucleus) and in the central autonomic nucleus (see ref [7,8] for review). Neuronal tracing studies suggest that neurons in several brain stem nuclei project to the vicinity of the intermediolateral cell column [9–14]. More direct evi-dence for brain stem autonomic projections to sympathetic preganglionic neurons has been obtained using the technique of transneuronal retrograde labeling by means of viruses [15–19]. Supraspinal structures which project to the IML of the spinal cord include the rostral ventrolateral medulla, the rostral ventromedial medulla, medullary and pontine raphe nuclei

(-obscurus, pallidus and magnus), the A5 noradrenergic cell group, the Kolliker-Fuse nucleus located in the lateral portion of the parabrachial nucleus complex, the paraventricular hypothalamic nucleus and the lateral hypothalamic area. Many of these areas are interconnected and are involved in the generation of sympathetic activity. The majority of these pathways are under tonic baroreceptor-mediated inhibition which is transmitted from afferent sources through the nucleus tractus solitarius [4–6]. As discussed throughout this review, much is known regarding the neurotransmitter(s) contained within these pathways and the functional roles they play in the elaboration of central sympathetic outflow.

The areas which project to sympathetic preganglionic neurons receive a wide variety of peripheral and central autonomic inputs. Certainly the most studied and perhaps the most important of the areas which send projections to sympathetic preganglionic neurons is the rostral ventrolateral area of the medulla (see refs [3, 6] for reviews). This area is critical in the tonic and phasic discharge of sympathetic activity. The rostral ventrolateral medulla contains neurons whose discharges are correlated to sympathetic activity, are inhibited during baroreceptor reflex activation and project to the intermediolateral cell column of the spinal cord. These medullospinal sympathoexcitatory neurons receive major projections from other areas associated with autonomic control such as the nucleus tractus solitarius (NTS), the caudal ventrolateral medulla, the lateral tegmental field, medullary raphe nuclei, the Kölliker-Fuse nucleus, the periaqueductal grey area of the midbrain and from the lateral hypothalamus and the paraventricular nucleus [20–24]. The rostral ventrolateral medulla is an important site of baroreceptor mediated inhibition which is relayed via the caudal ventrolateral medulla and the lateral tegmental field [25–28]. In addition, sympathoexcitatory neurons in the rostral ventrolateral medulla are an important site of integration for chemoreceptor and somatosympathetic reflexes [29–33].

The above discussion is a brief overview of the areas of the central nervous system that are critical in the regulation of the cardiovascular system. Subsequent sections of this review will discuss these areas in greater detail. The nature and function of neurotransmitters which help to regulate activity within and between central autonomic nuclei will be emphasized.

3   Sympathetic preganglionic neurons

Sympathetic preganglionic neurons represent the final central site of integration of autonomic activity. As described above preganglionic neurons are located primarily in the intermediolateral cell column of the thoracic and lumbar spinal cord but are also found in the adjacent white matter of the lateral funiculus, in the intercalated nucleus and in the central autonomic nucleus (see ref [7] for review). Sympathetic preganglionic neurons located in several spinal segments innervate a single sympathetic ganglion and the rostrocaudal location of preganglionic neurons correspond to the rostrocaudal location of ganglia which they innervate [34]. There is evidence that sympathetic preganglionic neurons are located topographically with respect to function (e.g. vasomotor versus non-vasomotor) [35, 36]. Sympathetic preganglionic neurons are found non-uniformly in clusters throughout the thoracic and lumbar spinal cord [16, 37–39]. The dendrites of individual neurons are located in longitudinal bundles which extend between clusters of sympathetic preganglionic neurons. In addition, dendritic bundles cross to the contralateral side of the cord. This anatomic substrate theoretically allows for the synchronization of activation of multiple preganglionic neurons at different levels of the cord by medullospinal axons descending on either side of the cord [40–42].

Like other motoneurons, sympathetic preganglionic neurons utilize acetylcholine as a neurotransmitter. In addition, neuropeptides are often co-localized with acetylcholine in sympathetic preganglionic neurons. These peptides include substance P, enkephalin, neurotensin and somatostatin [43–44]. No obvious differential distribution of these neuropeptides has been noted, nor has the functional significance of their co-localization with acetylcholine been determined. The spontaneous activity of sympathetic preganglionic neurons is dependent to a large degree on descending excitatory inputs from the brainstem. Acute cervical spinal cord transection results in a loss of sympathetic activity recorded from a majority of sympathetic preganglionic nerves [45, 46]. Intracellular recordings of sympathetic preganglionic neurons confirm a lack of pacemaker potentials [47–49]. These intracellular studies indicate that preganglionic neurons receive a large amount of both excitatory and inhibitory synaptic input. A large number of putative neurotransmitters synapse directly onto sympathetic preganglionic neurons. Immunohistochemistry combined with electron microscopy reveals that axon terminals containing immunoreactive material for glutamate [50–52], GABA [40, 53, 54], glycine [55], norepinephrine [56, 57], phenylethanolamine N-methyltransferase (PNMT), the enzyme necessary to synthesize epinephrine, [58, 59], 5-HT [40, 60–62], substance P [40, 61–63], neuropeptide Y [60, 64, 65], enkephalin [62], angiotensin II [66], thyrotropin-releasing hormone [61] and somatostatin [60] synapse directly onto sympathetic preganglionic neurons. In addition, terminals containing immunoreactive material for other neuropeptides including vasoactive intestinal polypeptide, oxytocin, neurotensin, and cholecystokinin have been observed in the intermediolateral cell column. Neurons containing these neuropeptides have not yet been shown to synapse directly onto sympathetic preganglionic neurons [57, 67].

The above description serves to illustrate that sympathetic preganglionic neurons receive rich and chemically diverse inputs. This has led to a great deal of speculation regarding the nature of the neurotransmitter(s) which mediate the transfer of autonomic information from the brainstem to the spinal cord. In the last decade epinephrine, substance P and glutamate have all been considered as primary chemical mediators in the descending sympathoexcitatory pathway from the brain stem to sympathetic preganglionic neurons. Interestingly, lesions of, or antagonists to, epinephrine, substance P, glutamate and 5-HT neurons all abolish sympathetic activity and reduce blood pressure to a level similar to that in a spinal animal [4]. Clearly, not all these transmitters are primary mediators of sympathetic information carried from the brain stem to the spinal cord. It is likely that monoamines and neuropeptides act in the IML, as in other area of the central nervous system, as neuromodulators to set the level of excitability of sympathetic preganglionic neurons rather than relaying sympathetic information over a functionally specific medullospinal pathway. This conclusion is supported by the observation that midline medullary 5-HT neurons provide a tonic excitatory input to sympathetic preganglionic neurons, but receive no afferent inputs from other central sympathetic or baroreceptor pathways [68, 69, see below]. Rather, the firing of 5-HT neurons appears to relate to the state of vigilance of the animal [70]. Since 5-HT excites sympathetic preganglionic neurons, these observations suggest that 5-HT neurons may lower the threshold of sympathetic preganglionic neurons to sympathetic inputs during states of wakefulness.

Microiontophoretic application of norepinephrine and epinephrine excite sympathetic preganglionic neurons via an α_1-adrenergic receptor and inhibit via an α_2-adrenergic receptor. Intracellular recordings indicate that the effect of exogenously applied norepinephrine or epinephrine is very slow [71, 144]. As described in more detail below, slow onset, long duration EPSPs and IPSPs recorded from sympathetic preganglionic neurons are mediated by norepinephrine. The time course of these EPSPs is not consistent with a pathway mediating sympathetic activity which changes on a time frame of milliseconds rather than seconds or even minutes, but rather is consistent with a gain-setting function. Similarly, it is difficult to imagine that an agent with such a long duration of excitatory action as substance P [72, 73] could serve as the primary descending transmitter in a system where moment to moment changes in activity are essential. It is more likely that substance P functions to set the excitability of sympathetic preganglionic neurons. Pharmacologic antagonism of any of the excitatory neuromodulators might act to decrease, at least temporarily, the excitability of sympathetic preganglionic neurons to the point where primary sympathetic activity from the brain stem could not excite sympathetic preganglionic neurons. This accounts for the wide variety of pharmacologic agents that act to eliminate sympathetic activity and reduce arterial blood pressure.

The most logical candidate for a transmitter mediating primary excitatory sympathetic information from the brain stem to sympathetic preganglionic neurons would be an excitatory amino acid. Microiontophoresis of excitatory amino acids excite sympathetic preganglionic neurons [74]. Glutamate depolarization of presumed preganglionic neurons is associated with a decrease in membrane resistance and is unaffected by tetrodotoxin in a slice preparation. Focal electrical stimulation elicits a fast EPSP that is identical to the ionic mechanisms involved in glutamate depolarization and is blocked by glutamate antagonists and enhanced by a glutamate uptake inhibitor [75, 76]. In addition, excitatory amino acid antagonists markedly inhibit sympathetic activity [2, 77]. The rapid time course of glutamate effects is consistent with a system in which activity changes from moment to moment. These data suggest that glutamate is the primary fast-acting neurotransmitter responsible for transmitting sympathoexcitatory information from the brain stem.

Recent data suggests that glutamate, monoamines and some neuropeptides may operate in concert with one another. Many of the putative neurotransmitters found in the intermediolateral cell column are co-localized in the same axon terminal. Approximately 66% of all terminals which synapse onto sympathetic preganglionic neurons contain glutamate [50]. One-third of terminals in the intermediolateral cell column contain GABA [40]. However, glutamate and GABA are not co-localized in nerve terminals [50]. If these numbers are near accurate, then mathematics indicate that all other neurotransmitters must be co-localized with either glutamate or GABA. In this regard, virtually all serotonergic and catecholaminergic neurons which project to the intermediolateral cell column from the ventrolateral medulla contain phosphate-activated glutaminase which is a marker of glutamate [78]. Many 5-HT terminals also contain substance P [79]. Thus it is likely that monoamines and neuropeptides are co-released with glutamate from terminals in the intermediolateral cell column. In this circumstance a neurotransmitter may act in a fashion which is not obvious when it is studied in isolation. For example, 5-HT has no effect on the firing rate of facial and spinal motoneurons but markedly enhances the effect of excitatory inputs [80]. At the level of the sympathetic preganglionic neuron it has been demonstrated that the effect of norepinephrine is dependent in part on the concentration of excitatory amino acids. Norepinephrine inhibits cell firing in the presence of low concentrations of DL-homocysteic acid, but excites the cell if the concentration of DL-homocysteic acid is increased [81]. In contrast, our laboratory has not observed interactions between glutamate and 5-HT on sympathetic preganglionic firing similar to that observed in the facial motor nucleus [unpublished observations]. Nevertheless, the extensive co-localization of neurotransmitters in the intermediolateral cell column suggests that interactions between amino acids, monoamines and neuropeptides are important in the integration of sympathetic activity.

While glutamate appears to mediate fast EPSPs in the intermediolateral cell column, it appears that GABA and glycine may be important in mediating fast IPSPs recorded from sympathetic preganglionic neurons. In a recent slice study, electrical stimulation of the dorsolateral funiculus evoked fast EPSPs and IPSPs. The IPSPs were blocked by either the GABAA receptor antagonist bicuculline (32% of the cells) or the glycine receptor antagonist strychnine (47% of the cells). GABA and glycine applied to the bath produced hyperpolarization associated with decreased membrane resistance [82]. GABA containing terminals have been observed to make synaptic contact with dendritic processes of preganglionic neurons as well as on cell bodies in all four thoracic nuclei. Interestingly, a high density of GABA containing interneurons are found in the zona intermedia [53]. Inhibitory sympathetic interneurons which receive baroreceptor input and are presumed to project to sympathetic preganglionic neurons have been recorded in this area. These neurons also receive sympathetic afferent input from the inferior cardiac nerve [83]. The GABAergic input to sympathetic preganglionic neurons is likely to be tonically active since intrathecal or iontophoretic application of GABA antagonists increases spontaneous sympathetic nerve activity [84, 85]. Glycine containing terminals make contact with sympathetic preganglionic neurons most frequently within the central autonomic and intercalated regions of the thoracic cord. These data indicate that GABA and glycine play important roles in regulating the activity of sympathetic preganglionic neurons.

The above discussion serves to illustrate the tremendous convergence of inputs onto sympathetic preganglionic neurons. All these inputs no doubt play a role in determining the outflow of sympathetic nerve activity to the sympathetic ganglia. There is recent evidence that sympathetic preganglionic neurons themselves may influence the firing of other preganglionic neurons. Half of the thoracic sympathetic preganglionic neurons contain nitric oxide synthetase, the enzyme required for synthesis of nitric oxide [86]. Since nitric oxide is rapidly diffusible, it is thought that it may modulate synaptic transmission at some distance from its site of release. Nitric oxide has been demonstrated to facilitate catecholamine release and lead to inhibition of NMDA receptors [87, 88]. It is interesting to speculate that a descending glutaminergic excitatory volley might result not only in the generation of a sympathetic preganglionic neuron action potential but also in the release of nitric oxide in the intermediolateral cell column. This would result in a diffusional domain around the preganglionic neuron in which the sensitivity of NMDA receptors to glutamate might be reduced. In this way a functional feedback inhibitory system could be maintained and would allow a mechanism by which a large number of adjacent preganglionic neurons could be simultaneously excited and then inhibited. Indeed sympathetic activity recorded in pre- and post-ganglionic nerves takes the form of slow waves which represents the synchronous excitation and inhibition of large numbers of preganglionic neurons [1,4]. The "clustering" of sympathetic preganglionic neurons (see above) provides an anatomical basis for this hypothesis.

4   Inputs to sympathetic preganglionic neurons

4.1   Rostral ventrolateral medulla

Retrograde tracing studies indicate that a group of neurons lying in a longitudinal column located just ventral to the retrofacial nucleus and extending from the caudal pole of the facial nucleus caudally for approximately 2 mm projects to the intermediolateral cell column of the spinal cord (see ref [6] for review). Microinjection of glutamate into this area elicits robust pressor responses [89–93]. This area will be referred to as either the subretrofacial nucleus or the rostral ventrolateral medulla in this review. Attention was initially focused on the area of the rostral ventrolateral medulla by the observation that direct application of pentobarbital or glycine to the ventrolateral surface of the medulla reduced blood pressure to levels seen after spinal cord transection [94, 95]. Electrical stimulation of the rostral ventrolateral area elicits pressor responses which are accompanied by increases in sympathetic activity [89, 90, 96]. Discrete bilateral lesions in the rostral ventrolateral area of the medulla reduce blood pressure to the level observed following spinal cord transection (31, 96, 97). These initial observations led to a tremendous amount of research on the role of the subretrofacial nucleus in cardiovascular regulation. An excellent recent review by Dampney summarizes this work [6].

Sympathetic activity recorded from peripheral whole nerves takes the form of slow waves which are temporally locked to the cardiac cycle in chloralose or barbiturate anesthetized cats [98]. In baroreceptor denervated cats, sympathetic activity remains in slow waves with a frequency between 2- and 6-Hz, but is no longer locked to the cardiac cycle. This 2- to 6-Hz rhythm is thought to arise from a brain stem network oscillator (i.e. an ensemble of neurons of different types interconnected in such a way to generate the rhythm) [98]. Subretrofacial neurons whose discharges are temporally related to the cardiac cycle have been identified in the rat and cat. These neurons project to the intermediolateral cell column and are inhibited by baroreceptor reflex activation [99–105]. As such, these neurons are thought to have a sympathoexcitatory function. A second distinct rhythm with a 10-Hz oscillation is evident in sympathetic activity recorded in the cat. This 10-Hz rhythm is thought to be generated in the brain stem by an oscillator distinct from the one responsible for the generation of 2- to 6-Hz nerve activity [106–111]. The discharge of individual subretrofacial sympathoexcitatory neurons has been shown to be related to both the 2- to 6-Hz and the 10-Hz rhythm of sympathetic nerve discharge [109]. This, along with the observation that lesions of the subretrofacial nucleus eliminates both the 2- to 6-Hz and the 10-Hz rhythm [110], suggests that the subretrofacial nucleus may serve as the final brain stem site of convergence of the two network oscillators responsible for the synchronization of sympathetic activity.

Subretrofacial sympathoexcitatory neurons are also the site of convergence of inputs from a wide variety of central and peripheral sources. Electrophysiologic studies indicate that the firing of these neurons are altered by inputs from peripheral baroreceptors, chemoreceptors, cardiopulmonary receptors, somatic receptors, renal receptors, and vestibular receptors as well as from central activation of the lateral tegmental field, the hypothalamic defense area, the periaqueductal grey, the fastigial nucleus and the area postrema [26, 32, 99, 102, 111–124]. The rich convergence of inputs has led to the belief that subretrofacial sympathoexcitatory neurons represent the final brain stem site of convergence of autonomic information. This is supported by the observations that lesions of the subretrofacial nucleus blocks the effects of baroreceptors, chemoreceptors, cardiopulmonary receptors, somatic receptors as well as many central pressor pathways [29–33, 121, 125–127].

Subretrofacial sympathoexcitatory neurons can be subdivided into two groups in the rat based on axonal conduction velocity, firing characteristics and pharmacological sensitivity to the α_2-receptor agonist clonidine [25, 128–131]. The first type of neuron is similar to that found in the cat.

These neurons exhibit medullospinal axonal conduction velocities of 0.4–0.8 m/s, a slow discharge rate and an extreme sensitivity to the inhibitory effects of clonidine. Individual neurons project to both the thoracic spinal cord and the central tegmental tract in the pons [129]. The second neuronal type is characterized by axonal conduction velocities of 3.5–8.0 m/s, a maximum discharge rate of 15–35 spikes/s, and are not affected by the α_2-receptor agonist clonidine. These neurons maintain their discharge when all excitatory inputs are blocked by application of kynurenic acid and display a highly regular pacemaker-like discharge pattern under these conditions [130, 131]. The ionic conductances of these pacemaker potentials have recently been described in eloquent studies by Loewy and colleagues [132]. Both neuronal types are inhibited during baroreceptor reflex activation and both fire with a discharge related to the cardiac cycle [127–130]. Thus both types of neurons are thought to subserve a sympathoexcitatory function.

Evidence suggests that the clonidine-sensitive medullospinal sympathoexcitatory neurons recorded in the rat are C1 epinephrine containing neurons. There is a striking similarity between the location of PNMT immunoreactive neurons (i.e. putative C1 epinephrine containing neurons) which project to the intermediolateral cell column and the distribution of subretrofacial sympathoexcitatory neurons (31, 89, 133–135]. Fifty-seven percent of the neurons in the subretrofacial nucleus are immunoreactive for tyrosine hydroxylase which is a marker for catecholamine- containing neurons [136]. A very high percentage of neurons which project directly to the intermediolateral cell column are immunoreactive for PNMT [19, 34, 36, 137]. In addition to projecting to the cord, PNMT immunoreactive neurons send collaterals rostral to the central tegmental tract in the pons [129]. Non-PNMT immunoreactive neurons in the subretrofacial nucleus do not have this pattern of innervation. Haselton and Guyenet [129] demonstrated that subretrofacial neurons which could be antidromically activated from both the cord and the central tegmental tract were characterized by slow axonal conduction velocities, a slow discharge rate which was temporally related to sympathetic activity, inhibited during baroreceptor reflex activation and sensitive to the inhibitory effects of clonidine. Finally, the pacemaker neurons with high discharge rates and fast conduction velocities are not immunoreactive for PNMT [130]. These data strongly support the idea that the slow conducting neurons are C1 epinephrine-containing cells. A second group of non-catecholamine containing neurons also subserve a sympathoexcitatory function.

Two types of subretrofacial sympathoexcitatory neurons are not as obviously differentiated in the cat. Neurons with discharges related to sympathetic activity and sensitive to baroreceptor-mediated inhibition can not be differentiated on the basis of axonal conduction velocity or discharge rate. In addition, there is no evidence for the existence of sympathoexcitatory pacemaker neurons in the subretrofacial nucleus of the cat. However, it appears that two types of subretrofacial sympathoexcitatory neurons can be differentiated on the basis of sensitivity to clonidine. Indeed 50% of these neurons are inhibited by low intravenous doses of clonidine while the discharge of 50% of the neurons were unaffected by the α_2-receptor agonist. In contrast, all neurons were inhibited by the 5-HT$_{1A}$ receptor agonist 8-OH DPAT. Clonidine-sensitive and -insensitive neurons could not be differentiated on the basis of axonal conduction velocity or discharge frequency [138]. It is likely not coincidental that 50% the medullospinal subretrofacial neurons in the cat are immunoreactive for PNMT [136]. These data suggest that, like the rat, catecholaminergic and non-catecholaminergic sympathoexcitatory neurons exist in the subretrofacial nucleus of the cat. One difficulty remains. In the cat, iontophoretic clonidine fails to inhibit the firing of any subretrofacial neurons [138]. This may reflect the fact that α_2-receptors are located on distal dendrites of these neurons in the cat and therefore may not be exposed to iontophoretically applied clonidine.

The above discussion leads to the conclusion that C1 epinephrine containing neurons subserve a sympathoexcitatory function. However, a good deal of data suggests the opposite. Microiontophoretic application of epinephrine consistently inhibits the firing of sympathetic preganglionic neurons located in the intermediolateral cell column [139–141]. The epinephrine-induced inhibition of sympathetic preganglionic neuronal firing is blocked by the α_2-antagonists yohimbine and piperoxane [140, 141]. This indicates that the inhibition is mediated via an α_2-adrenergic receptor. This observation is supported by autoradiographic studies which show that α_2-adrenergic receptors are highly concentrated over clusters of SPN [142]. Ross et al. [134] suggest that the results of microiontophoretic studies must be viewed cautiously since epinephrine released from nerve terminals may act on receptors distant from those acted on by iontophoretic epinephrine. Thus, epinephrine may produce inhibition by acting on receptors located on SPN soma and excitation via receptors located on distal dendrites or antecedent interneurons. Indeed, excitatory and inhibitory effects of norepinephrine have been observed, occasionally on the same SPN [143]. More recently epinephrine has been shown to excite sympathetic preganglionic neurons via an α_1-receptor and inhibit via an α_2-receptor [81, 143]. However, microiontophoresis of α_2-antagonists fail to block the excitation of SPN elic-

ited by stimulation of pressor sites in the C1 area of the rostral ventrolateral medulla (Morrison, personal communication). In addition, selective inhibitors of central epinephrine synthesis enhanced descending
intraspinal transmission to sympathetic preganglionic neurons [144]. Similarly, inhibition of epinephrine synthesis fails to alter the pressor
response elicited by stimulation of the rostral ventrolateral medulla [145].
These data suggest that bulbospinal epinephrine neurons may depress
rather than enhance the excitability of sympathetic preganglionic neurons.

A resolution to the apparent "camps" of data described above is provided
by the work of Minson and colleagues [78]. The vast majority of medullospinal neurons in the rostral ventrolateral medulla of the rat are immunoreactive for phosphate-activated glutaminase, a glutamate-synthesiz-
ing enzyme and as such a marker for glutaminergic neurons. This includes
most if not all neurons immunoreactive for PNMT. Thus it appears that
glutamate and epinephrine are extensively co-localized in medullospinal
subretrofacial neurons. It is worth noting that epinephrine levels are less
that 0.2 pg/mg tissue in the intermediolateral cell column which is less
than 0.05% of the norepinephrine content [146]. There is ample evidence
suggesting that glutamate may be the primary excitatory neurotransmitter in the sympathoexcitatory pathway descending from the subretrofacial nucleus to sympathetic preganglionic neurons in the intermediolateral cell column. Glutamate immunoreactivity is found in axon terminals
in the intermediolateral cell column [50–52]. As described above, approximately 66% of all terminals which synapse onto sympathetic preganglionic
neurons contain glutamate [50]. Some of these terminals originate from
neurons located in the subretrofacial nucleus [374]. Stimulation of the rostral ventrolateral medulla elicits a pressor response which is associated
with a release of glutamate and aspartate from the intermediolateral cell
column [51, 52]. Intrathecal administration of the excitatory amino acid
antagonist kynurenic acid eliminates spontaneous sympathetic activity and
blocks the sympathoexcitatory effect of electrical stimulation of the rostral ventrolateral medulla [77]. Iontophoretic application of kynurenic acid
onto sympathetic preganglionic neurons blocks the excitatory effects of
rostral ventrolateral medulla stimulation [52]. These data provide strong
support for the idea that glutamate is the primary fast-acting neurotransmitter released from the terminals of subretrofacial sympathoexcitatory
neurons. As described above epinephrine acts on a slow time scale to depolarize or hyperpolarize sympathetic preganglionic neurons [81, 143]. Stimulation of the subretrofacial nucleus elicits a fast onset excitation of sympathetic nerve activity which is mediated by glutamate and a slow onset

excitation which is mediated by catecholamines [148]. The significance of co-localization of glutamate with adrenaline and other neurotransmitters (see below) is likely that monoamines and neuropeptides function to help set the level of excitability of sympathetic preganglionic neurons.

Evidence suggests that glutamate released from terminals of descending sympathoexcitatory neurons acts on both N-methyl-D-aspartate (NMDA) and non-NMDA receptors located on sympathetic preganglionic neurons. Intrathecal administration or microinjection of selective NMDA receptor antagonists into the intermediolateral cell column blocks sympathoexcitatory responses to stimulation of the rostral ventrolateral medulla [149–150]. In contrast, iontophoretic application of selective NMDA receptor antagonists failed to block the excitation recorded from the splanchnic nerve following stimulation of the rostral ventrolateral medulla. Indeed, a high density of glutamate receptors of the kainic subtype are located in the intermediolateral cell column [52]. More recently, Inokuchi et al. [76] found that focal stimulation of descending tracts excited sympathetic preganglionic neurons via activation of both NMDA and non-NMDA receptors, although the latter receptor subtype was the more dominant. Efflux data from these experiments suggest that glutamate and aspartate play an important role in the fast-acting descending sympathoexcitatory pathway.

As described above, subretrofacial sympathoexcitatory neurons represent a final site of brain stem autonomic integration and as such receive a tremendous amount of afferent inputs [151, 152]. This is reflected by the rich pharmacology of these neurons. Studies utilizing local application, microinjection or intravenous administration of pharmacological agents have demonstrated that excitatory and inhibitory amino acids, monoamines, acetylcholine, opiates and neuropeptides can influence the firing of subretrofacial sympathoexcitatory neurons and therefore affect autonomic activity. It is not surprising that excitatory amino acids excite these neurons. The non-specific excitatory amino acid antagonist kynurenic acid has been used to demonstrate a variety of inputs which utilize a glutamate-like transmitter. Thus, kynurenic acid has been shown to block the excitatory effects of stimulation of chemoreceptor [26] and vagal [153] afferents and stimulation of the hypothalamus [154]. Microdialysis experiments suggest that both glutamate and aspartate play physiological relevant roles in the rostral ventrolateral medulla [155, 156]. Recent experiments in the rat, rabbit and cat suggest that excitatory amino acids provide a tonic input to sympathoexcitatory neurons since administration of antagonists reduce arterial blood pressure. Both NMDA and non-NMDA receptors have been implicated in mediating the effects of excitatory amino acids [157, 158].

Other investigators have not been able to demonstrate changes in blood pressure following administration of excitatory amino acid antagonists into the rostral ventrolateral medulla [26, 159]. These differences may be related to the anesthetic state of the animal.

PNMT-containing sympathoexcitatory neurons receive a major input from GABAergic neurons [152]. Local application of GABA and GABA antagonists decrease and increase arterial blood pressure, respectively [160–164]. The GABA$_A$ receptor antagonist bicuculline blocks the inhibitory effects of stimulation of the area postrema [119] and hindpaw nociceptive afferents [120]. The sympathoinhibitory component of the Bezold-Jarisch reflex elicited by jugular vein injection of 5-HT is blocked by bilateral microinjections of bicuculline into the rostral ventrolateral medulla [165]. A large body of evidence suggests GABA mediates baroreceptor inhibition of subretrofacial sympathoexcitatory neurons ([161, 163, 164, see below). Microinjections of the GABA$_B$ receptor agonist baclofen into the rostral ventrolateral medulla decreases arterial blood pressure whereas administration of a selective GABA$_B$ receptor antagonist has the opposite effects [166]. More recently it has been demonstrated that iontophoretic baclofen inhibits the firing of subretrofacial sympathoexcitatory neurons [167]. Thus it appears that GABA provides a tonic inhibition of subretrofacial sympathoexcitatory neurons which is mediated via both GABA$_A$ and GABA$_B$ receptors.

Electrical stimulation of midline depressor sites inhibit the firing of sympathoexcitatory neurons in the subretrofacial nucleus. Microiontophoresis of bicuculline blocked the inhibition elicited from the midline and increases the firing rate of sympathoexcitatory neurons. In contrast, microiontophoresis of glutamate increased the firing rate of sympathoexcitatory neurons but failed to affect the midline evoked inhibition of neuronal firing. Stimulation of midline depressor sites excited a second group of spontaneously active neurons in the rostral ventrolateral medulla. These neurons were often located in the same recording field as the sympathoexcitatory neurons. The neurons were excited by midline stimulation with an onset latency of 21 ms while sympathoexcitatory neurons were inhibited with an onset of 23 ms. These data suggest that neuronal elements in medullary raphe nuclei inhibit sympathoexcitatory medullospinal neurons in the rostral ventrolateral medulla by activating closely adjacent GABAergic interneurons. This interpretation fits with the observation that the region of the rostral ventrolateral medulla containing sympathoexcitatory neurons has a high concentration of GABAergic cell bodies [169, 170]. Furthermore, this inhibition is tonically active and of non-baroreceptor origin.

The area of the rostral ventrolateral medulla receives a 5-HT input [171] and contains a high density of 5-HT_{1A} receptor binding sites [172]. However, it is unknown whether sympathoexcitatory neurons in the rostral ventrolateral medulla receive a 5-HT input or possess 5-HT_{1A} receptors. Indeed, the highest density of 5-HT_{1A} receptors in the area are found around 5-HT neurons located in the parapyramidal region [172]. Local application of 8-OH DPAT onto the ventral surface of the cat brain stem, which underlies the rostral ventrolateral medulla (i.e., Schlaefke's area), results in a decrease in arterial blood pressure and a bradycardia. The effects of 8-OH DPAT are blocked by the purported 5-HT_{1A} receptor antagonist WB 4101 [173]. Local surface application of 5-HT produces only a mild vasodepressor response, but this effect is potentiated by administration of the 5-HT_2 receptor antagonist ketanserin [173]. These data suggest that 5-HT_{1A} receptors in the rostral ventrolateral medulla mediate a vasodepressor response, while 5-HT_2 receptors mediate opposite actions of 5-HT on blood pressure.

The cardiovascular effects of 8-OH DPAT in the rostral ventrolateral medulla have been more thoroughly investigated using the microinjection technique. Microinjection of 8-OH DPAT into the subretrofacial nucleus produces a decrease in blood pressure in the rat [174, 175], cat [176, 177], and dog [178]. The decrease in blood pressure is associated with a decrease in renal sympathetic nerve activity in the dog [178] and lumbar sympathetic nerve activity in the rat [175]. Microinjection of 8-OH DPAT into the rostral ventrolateral area is also associated with an increase in hindlimb vascular conductance [174]. The cardiovascular effects of microinjected 8-OH DPAT appear to be mediated via 5-HT_{1A} receptors in that the vasodepressor effects of microinjected 8-OH DPAT are blocked by administration of the putative 5-HT_{1A} receptor antagonists spiroxatrine or spiperone [176, 177]. In the rat and cat intravenous 8-OH DPAT simultaneously inhibits the firing of subretrofacial sympathoexcitory neurons and whole sympathetic nerve activity, although the inhibition is greater in the cat [175, 179]. These data suggest that 5-HT_{1A} receptor agonists produce their vasodepressor effects, in part, by inhibiting sympathoexcitatory neurons in the subretrofacial nucleus of the rostral ventrolateral medulla.

The effect of 5-HT on rostral ventrolateral medullary neurons in the rat *in vitro* has been determined using intracellular recording techniques [180]. 5-HT evokes a slow concentration-dependent hyperpolarization in both spontaneously active and silent neurons in the slice preparation. The hyperpolarization is accompanied by a decrease in the input resistance of the cell. These data suggest that 5-HT is inhibitory to neurons in the rostral ventrolateral medulla of the rat, although the function of these neurons could not be determined. The effects of microiontophoretically applied 5-HT and 5-HT$_{1A}$ receptor agonists have been determined in the rat [181]. Iontophoretically applied 5-HT and 5-HT$_{1A}$ receptor agonists inhibit the firing of neurons located in the rostral ventrolateral medulla. Although a mixed population of neurons was studied, at least some of these cells projected to the spinal cord and some were inhibited during baroreceptor activation. This suggests that some cells were sympathoexcitatory neurons. It should be noted that most of the neurons studied were being driven by iontophoresis of an excitatory amino acid and that 5-HT$_{1A}$ receptor agonists inhibited the amino acid driven activity. This may be important since a recent study demonstrated that the inhibitory effect of 8-OH DPAT is much greater in a neuron activated by excitatory amino acids than in a spontaneously firing neuron [182]. In this regard, microiontophoretic application of 5-HT or 8-OH DPAT fails to affect the spontaneous firing of sympathoexcitatory neurons over a wide range of ejecting currents in the cat [179]. These same neurons were inhibited by subsequent intravenous administration of 8-OH DPAT. These data suggest that in the cat, at least, 5-HT$_{1A}$ receptor agonists act on central sympathetic neurons which lie antecedent to ventrolateral medulla sympathoexcitatory neurons (see below). Alternatively, 8-OH DPAT may act on distal dendrites of the rostral ventrolateral sympathoexcitatory neurons.

Application of 5-HT$_2$ receptor agonists to the ventral surface of the medulla produces an increase in arterial blood pressure and sympathetic nerve activity [177, 183]. Bilateral microinjection of the 5-HT$_2$ receptor agonists DOI or quipazine into the subretrofacial nucleus increases arterial blood pressure [183, 184]. Intravenous administration of DOI produces a marked increase in the firing of medullospinal sympathoexcitatory neurons located in the subretrofacial nucleus [185]. The increase in firing of sympathoexcitatory neurons is correlated with an increase in inferior cardiac nerve discharge following DOI administration. The increase in neuronal firing produced by DOI is reversed by the 5-HT$_2$ receptor antagonist LY 53857. These data suggest that DOI acts at the level of the medullospinal sympathoexcitatory neurons of the rostral ventrolateral medulla to produce its sympathoexcitatory effect. However, microiontophoretic application of DOI fails to affect the firing of sympathoexcitatory neurons in the rostral ventrolateral medulla even though these neurons are activated following i.v. DOI [185]. These data suggest that the sympathoexcitatory effect of DOI may result from an action on sympathetic neurons which lie antecedent to the sympathoexcitatory neurons in the rostral ventrolateral medulla. Alternatively, DOI may produce its sympathoexcitatory effect by acting on distal dendrites of the sympathoexcitatory neurons. In either case, the data indicate that sympathoexcitatory neurons in the rostral ventrolateral medulla play an important role in mediating the sympathoexcitatory response to DOI.

Cholinergic neurons have been shown to play a role in the regulation of subretrofacial sympathoexcitatory neurons. Cholinergic neurons in the pedunculopontine tegmental nucleus have been retrogradely labeled from the rostral ventrolateral medulla. Anterograde tracing of this pathway demonstrated that descending fibers from the pedunculopontine tegmental nucleus ramify and give off terminal boutons in the rostral ventrolateral medulla [186]. Cholinergic terminals form symmetric synapses (i.e. inhibitory) mainly on non-PMNT containing neurons in the rostral ventrolateral medulla [152]. Microinjection of cholinergic agonists in the subretrofacial area increases arterial blood pressure and heart rate [187–189]. The pressor effect appears to be mediated via M2 receptors in that microinjection of selective M2, but not M1, receptor agonists elicit the cardiovascular effects [190–192]. In this regard, a high density of M2 receptors has been noted in the rostral ventrolateral medulla [193]. The cholinergic input appears to be tonic in the anesthetized animal in that synthesis inhibitors or microinjection of antagonists into the rostral ventrolateral medulla produce a decrease in arterial blood pressure [187, 189, 193]. The fact that cholinergic terminals form symmetric synapses mainly on non-PMNT containing neurons suggest that the effects of cholinergic agents are mediated indirectly via inhibitory interneurons. Recently it has been observed that intravenous administration of physostigmine induces a 10-Hz rhythm in sympathetic nerve discharge that is blocked by atropine. In contrast, atropine by itself has no effect on the naturally occurring 10-Hz rhythm in sympathetic activity [194]. These data suggest that central muscarinic cholinergic transmission is not essential for generation of the 10-Hz rhythm, but rather has a facilitatory effect on this component of sympathetic activity.

Terminals immunoreactive for enkephalin form symmetric synapses directly onto C1 adrenergic neurons in the subretrofacial nucleus [152]. One source on the enkephalin innervation of the rostral ventrolateral medulla is the NTS [195]. In addition, opioid-containing neurons are intrinsic to the rostral ventrolateral medulla [152]. Microinjection of enkephalin analogues elicits a depressor response which is accompanied by a bradycardia [196, 197]. In a rat slice preparation Met-enkephalin and morphine inhibit the firing of pacemaker sympathoexcitatory pacemaker neurons in the subretrofacial nucleus [198].

Several neuropeptides have been shown to play a role in regulating the activity of sympathoexcitatory neurons in the subretrofacial nucleus. Terminals containing substance-P immunoreactive material form asymmetric synapses on C1 containing neurons [152]. Microinjection of stable substance-P agonists into rostral ventrolateral pressor sites elicits a dose-related increase in arterial blood pressure and variable effects on heart rate [199]. Application of substance P in a tissue slice preparation increases the firing of subretrofacial pacemaker neurons [198]. A similar excitatory effect in the slice preparation was noted with arginine vasopressin. The excitatory effect of arginine vasopressin was mimicked by selective V1 receptor agonists but not by V2 agonists. Selective V1 receptor antagonist, but not V2 antagonists, blocked the excitatory effect of arginine vasopressin on sympathoexcitatory pacemaker neurons [198]. Vasopressinergic neurons located diffusely in the hypothalamus project to the rostral ventrolateral medulla where they appear to make synaptic contact with dendrites of medullospinal neurons [200]. Microinjection of arginine vasopressin into the subretrofacial nucleus elicits a pressor response. This effect is blocked by microinjection of an antagonist, but the antagonist by itself failed to alter arterial blood pressure. Thus under basal conditions vasopressinergic neurons appear not to contribute to tonic sympathetic activity. However, under conditions of acute hemorrhage microinjection of the arginine vasopressin antagonist decreased arterial blood pressure [200]. These data suggest that under conditions demanding increased sympathetic drive a functional vasopressinergic mechanism operating via the rostral ventrolateral medulla may be activated in order to maintain arterial blood pressure.

The rostral ventrolateral medulla contains both angiotensin receptors [201, 202] and nerve terminals containing angiotensin immunoreactive material [203]. Most receptors appear to be the AT1 subtype [204, 205]. Microinjection of angiotensin II into the subretrofacial area elicits a dose-related increase in arterial blood pressure, iliac vascular resistance and renal sympathetic nerve activity [206, 207]. Microinjection of an angiotensin II antagonist decreased these variables [208]. The effect of angiotensin II appears specific for sympathoexcitatory neurons in the subretrofacial area since microinjections of angiotensin II increased arterial blood pressure but not phrenic nerve activity while microinjection of glutamate into the same sight increased both parameters [209]. More recently, it has been demonstrated that angiotensin III has a sympathoexcitatory function in the rostral ventrolateral medulla [208]. Interestingly, angiotensin II fails to excite pacemaker sympathoexcitatory neurons in the subretrofacial nucleus [198, 210]. This suggests that angiotensin II may act on C1 neurons in order to produce its sympathoexcitatory action. In this regard, angiotensin II excites a population of subretrofacial neurons in a slice preparation that are inhibited by α_2-receptor agonists and have firing characteristics similar to that of C1 neurons. This effect was blocked by the selective AT1 receptor antagonist losartan [210].

In summary, the subretrofacial area of the rostral ventrolateral medulla is a critical site for the integration of autonomic activity. It should be noted that the vast majority of studies have been performed in anesthetized animals. The importance of the inputs to the rostral ventrolateral medulla with regard to cardiovascular reflexes in conscious animals remains to be determined.

4.2   Rostral ventromedial medulla

Neurons in the rostral ventromedial medulla, or parapyramidal region, project to the intermediolateral cell column of the spinal cord. Neurons in this region contain 5-HT, substance P, thyrotropin releasing hormone (TRH), enkephalin and GABA. There is extensive co-localization of these putative neurotransmitters within the same neuron. The degree to which these chemicals are combined in a single neuron is extremely complex and variable [18, 211–215].

5-HT neurons of the ventromedial medulla have been postulated to play an important role in maintaining tonic vasomotor activity [215]. 5-HT neurons in this area are lateral extensions of the B_1 and B_3 cell groups and have been shown to project to the IML [12]. Chemical or electrical stimulation of this area results in a pressor response and this is attenuated by pretreatment with the 5-HT neurotoxin 5,7-dihydroxytryptamine (5,7-DHT [215]). Other studies, however, did not confirm these observations [216]. A recent study by Minson et al. [217] helps to explain these inconsistent findings. They found that glutamate microinjections into the area of the epinephrine-containing neurons evoked a pressor response which was not altered by 5,7-DHT. After ablation of the area of the epinephrine-containing neurons by electrolytic lesion, more medial microinjections of glutamate elicited a pressor response which was presumably mediated by 5-HT. These data indicate that the lateral wings of the B_1 and B_3 5-HT cell groups have a sympathoexcitatory function which is independent of the more laterally positioned sympathoexcitatory neurons in the rostral ventrolateral medulla. Interestingly, like the C1 neurons, it appears that glutamate is found in virtually all rostral ventromedial 5-HT neurons which project to the intermediolateral cell column [78]. In addition, 50% of the intermediolateral cell column terminals contain both 5-HT and substance P [218]. Some of these neurons likely contain GABA [40]. The significance of co-localization has been discussed above. The role of 5-HT in the regulation of sympathetic activity is described in more detail below. A major source of substance P input to the intermediolateral cell column of the spinal cord arises from neurons in the rostral ventromedial medulla. Unilateral electrolytic lesions of this area of the medulla bilaterally reduced the content of substance P by 40% in the intermediolateral cell column [219]. An additional substance P input to the intermediolateral cell column arises from spinal interneurons [220]. Terminals immunoreactive for substance P terminate directly onto sympathetic preganglionic neurons [40, 61–63]. Microiontophoretic application of substance P excites SPN. The onset of the excitatory response is characterized by a slow onset and continues long after the ejection current is discontinued [221–224]. Similarly, intrathecal administration of substance P or stable agonist analogs of the peptide increase blood pressure, renal sympathetic nerve activity, plasma catecholamines and total peripheral resistance [225–228].

The studies cited above have led to the widely accepted conclusion that substance P acts to excite SPN. However, the importance of the rostral ventrolateral medullary substance P neurons in the maintenance of tonic sympathetic activity is less obvious. Intrathecal administration of D-amino acid antagonists of substance P decreases arterial blood pressure in a dose-dependent fashion [229]. Microinjection of excitatory amino acids into the rostral ventrolateral medulla elicits a pressor response which is associated with an increase in the release of immunoreactive substance P from the spinal cord. Both the pressor response and the release of substance P can be prevented by intrathecal administration of a substance P antagonist [230]. Microinjection of the GABA antagonist bicuculline into the rostral ventrolateral medulla elicits a sympathetic-mediated pressor response which can be blocked by intrathecal administration of a substance P antagonist [231]. However, the significance of these observations is uncertain since D-amino acid antagonists possess neurotoxic and local anesthetic effects [232–235] and non-specifically block the sympathoexcitatory effects of intrathecal 5-HT and glutamate [228]. In summary, available evidence supports a sympathoexcitatory role of substance P in the spinal cord. The importance of this system in the tonic maintenance of sympathetic activity remains uncertain.

TRH neurons in the rostral ventromedial medulla also contain substance P, 5-HT and glutamate [78, 211, 214]. The putative neurotransmitters are also co-localized in nerve terminals which make synaptic contact with sympathetic preganglionic neurons [61, 212]. Microiontophoretically applied TRH weakly excites sympathetic preganglionic neurons suggesting that this neuropeptide may function in a sympathoexcitatory process [221,227]. Rostral ventromedial medullary 5-HT neurons also contain enkephalin [211,214] and terminals containing enkephalin immunoreactive material synapse directly onto sympathetic preganglionic neurons [62]. Enkephalin and substance P are not co-localized in rostral ventromedial medullary neurons [221]. Enkephalin depresses sympathetic activity in both an intraspinal excitatory pathway and a spinal reflex pathway [236]. Intrathecal dynorphin decreases arterial blood pressure, heart rate and sympathetic activity [237]. Finally, the opioid antagonist naloxone blocks a portion of the post excitatory depression following sympathetic preganglionic discharge [238]. These data suggest that opioids inhibit activity at the level of the sympathetic preganglionic neuron.

4.3   Medullary raphe nuclei

Neurons in the midline portions of raphe obscurus and raphe pallidus send a direct and heavy project to the intermediolateral cell column of the spinal cord [11, 17, 239]. The area appears to be heterogenous with respect to autonomic function in that electrical or chemical stimulation of the midline medulla can produce either increases or decreases in arterial blood pressure and sympathetic nerve activity [240–244]. Three types of neurons which likely play a role in autonomic regulation have been identified in the midline raphe. Two types of neurons fire spontaneously with discharges temporally related to sympathetic nerve discharge. These neurons can be differentiated on the basis of reactivity to baroreceptor reflex activation. Thus one type of neuron is inhibited (i.e. sympathoexcitatory neuron) and one is excited (i.e. sympathoinhibitory neuron) during activation of the baroreceptor reflex [68,245,246]. Sympathoinhibitory neurons project to the intermediolateral cell column, while sympathoexcitatory neurons project to the spinal cord but have not been shown to terminate in the intermediolateral cell column [68, 246]. The third cell type involved in autonomic regulation is the serotonergic neuron. These neurons project to the intermediolateral cell column and the nucleus of the solitary tract and contain neuropeptides including substance P, TRH, enkephalin and somatostatin [9, 10, 12, 14, 18, 171, 226, 247, 248]. A portion of the sympathoexcitatory response elicited by stimulation of the rostral ventrolateral medulla is mediated by collateral activation of raphe medullospinal neurons [249].

5-HT containing neurons have been differentiated electrophysiologically from sympathoexcitatory and sympathoinhibitory raphe neurons [68]. Medullospinal 5-HT neurons share several important physiological and pharmacological characteristics with identified 5-HT neurons in the dorsal raphe nucleus [250] including: 1) an extremely regular discharge rate of approximately 1 spike/s, 2) spike durations of greater than 2 ms, 3) axonal conduction velocities which are appropriate for transmission through unmyelinated axons, 4) inhibition of neuronal firing produced by microiontophoretic 5-HT and 5) sensitivity to the inhibitory effect of the 5-HT$_{1A}$ agonist 8-OH DPAT. In contrast to raphe sympathoexcitatory and sympathoinhibitory neurons, the discharges of medullary 5-HT neurons are not temporally related to sympathetic nerve activity and are not affected by baroreceptor reflex activation. However, these regularly firing 5-HT neurons can be antidromically activated by stimulation of the intermediolateral cell column [68]. The neurotransmitter content of the raphe sympathoinhibitory and sympathoexcitatory neurons is unknown.

Immunohistochemistry combined with electron microscopy reveals that axon terminals containing immunoreactive material for 5-HT synapse directly onto sympathetic preganglionic neurons [40, 60–62]. Microiontophoretically applied 5-HT typically has been found to increase the firing of sympathetic preganglionic neurons [45, 251]. This is consistent with the observation that the sympathoexcitatory response elicited from medullary raphe nuclei is blocked by 5-HT antagonists and potentiated by 5-HT uptake inhibitors [244, 249].

The effects of 5-HT on sympathetic preganglionic neurons have been studied with intracellular recording techniques in slice preparations from neonatal rats [252]. Superfusion of 5-HT causes a concentration-dependent, slow depolarization which is accompanied by an increase in synaptic activity. Similar effects are observed during superfusion with 5-carboxamidotryptamine (5-CT) and α-methyl-5-hydroxytryptamine. A comparison of the potency of these compounds suggests that the 5-HT-induced slow depolarization is mediated by a 5-HT$_2$ receptor [252]. In this regard, a high density of 5-HT$_2$ receptors exists in the intermediolateral cell column [253]. 5-HT$_{1A}$ receptors are also found in the intermediolateral cell column [253]. The 5-HT receptor subtypes on sympathetic preganglionic neurons has been explored. Iontophoretic application of 8-OH DPAT fails to alter the spontaneous firing of sympathetic preganglionic neurons. Interestingly, 8-OH DPAT antagonizes the excitatory effects of iontophoretic 5-HT on sympathetic preganglionic neurons [179]. The significance of this observation is yet to be determined but is not responsible for the sympathoinhibitory effect of the drug [69] since 8-OH DPAT alone fails to inhibit firing. Similarly, intrathecal administration of 8-OH DPAT fails to lower arterial blood pressure [254]. Microiontophoretic application of the 5-HT$_2$

receptor agonist DOI fails to alter the firing of sympathetic preganglionic neurons. In contrast, iontophoretic 5-HT increases the firing of these same neurons [185]. In addition, selective 5-HT$_2$ receptor antagonists, such as LY 53857 and ritanserin, fail to inhibit sympathetic activity and lower arterial blood pressure while other less selective 5-HT receptor antagonists block the excitatory effects of iontophoretic 5-HT and inhibit the firing of sympathetic preganglionic neurons [45, 255–259]. Selective 5-HT$_2$ receptor antagonists also fail to block the excitatory effects of iontophoretic 5-HT (unpublished observations). Thus, the receptor subtype(s) involved in mediating 5-HT effects at the level of the sympathetic preganglionic neuron remains uncertain.

5-HT neurons appear important in the tonic regulation of sympathetic activity. 5-HT antagonists methysergide and metergoline decrease the spontaneous discharge rate of sympathetic preganglionic neurons in intact cats but not in spinally transected animals [45]. Intravenous or iontophoretic administration of 8-OH DPAT markedly inhibits the firing of medullary 5-HT neurons via 5-HT$_{1A}$ receptor activation [172, 179, 259, 260]. Microinjection of 8-OH DPAT into medullary raphe nuclei produces small decreases in arterial blood pressure, heart rate, and sympathetic nerve activity [175, 261]. The hypotensive effects of 8-OH DPAT microinjected into the raphe and rostral ventromedial medulla, but not the rostral ventrolateral medulla, are prevented by prior administration of the 5-HT neurotoxin 5,7-dihydroxytryptamine [262]. The inhibition of 5-HT cell firing produced by low intravenous doses of 8-OH DPAT is accompanied by a mild inhibition of renal sympathetic nerve activity [263, 264]. These observations suggest that a small portion of spontaneous sympathetic discharge is maintained by tonic 5-HT activity. Recently, it has been demonstrated that the 10-Hz rhythm in SND is dependent upon serotonergic activity. Extremely low doses of 8-OH DPAT which inhibit the firing of 5-HT neurons but lack activity in postsynaptic areas innervated by 5-HT, abolishes the 10-Hz rhythm in sympathetic nerve activity. The 5-HT receptor antagonist methysergide has a similar inhibitory action. In contrast, stimulation of the midline medulla or administration of DOI markedly potentiates the 10-Hz rhythm [265]. Thus, 5-HT may play a role in determining the pattern as well as the power of sympathetic activity.

4.4   A5 Noradrenergic cell group

The major noradrenergic input to the SPN in the intermediolateral cell column of the spinal cord arises from the A5 cell group of the ventrolateral pons [266, 267]. Over 90% of the neurons in the A5 area project to the thoracic spinal cord. At least 90% of the spinally projecting neurons in the A5 area contain norepinephrine [267]. The A5 noradrenergic cell group also sends projections to the central nucleus of the amygdala, perifornical area of the hypothalamus, midbrain periaqueductal gray, parabrachial nucleus, the ventrolateral medulla and the nucleus tractus solitarius [267]. Thus the pattern of A5 noradrenergic innervation is similar to that of the C1 epinephrine-containing cell group [268]. The A5 area receives inputs from the paraventricular nucleus, the Kolliker-Fuse nucleus, the parabrachial nucleus, the intermediate and caudal portion of the nucleus of the solitary tract and the A1 area [267–269]. Thus, virtually all areas which project to, or receive inputs from, the A5 area are involved in cardiovascular regulation.

Anatomically it has been established that the only type of neuron in the ventrolateral pons which projects to the spinal cord is the A5 noradrenergic neuron. Thus, cells in this region which can be antidromically activated from the spinal cord are noradrenergic neurons [266, 270]. A5 noradrenergic neurons discharge in a slow regular firing pattern and are characterized by extreme sensitivity to the inhibitory effects of clonidine. The inhibition of firing by clonidine is mediated via α_{2A}-receptors [271, 272] and may reflect inhibitory input from either A5 collaterals [273] or from C1 adrenergic neurons [274]. Baroreceptor reflex activation inhibits the firing of many but not all A5 neurons [246, 275, 276]. Finally, the discharge of approximately 40% of the A5 noradrenergic neurons is related temporally to activity recorded from the splanchnic sympathetic nerve [246]. Thus these neurons likely have a sympathoexcitatory function. In addition, the extensive A5 projections to virtually all areas involved in cardiovascular regulation suggest that these neurons may be important in the integration of cardiovascular responses [267]. For example, A5 neurons are thought to facilitate the carotid sympathetic chemoreflex [277].

Electrical and glutamate stimulation of the A5 area results in increases and decreases in blood pressure, respectively [278–281]. Intraventricular administration of the noradrenergic neurotoxin 6-OHDA abolishes the depressor response to chemical stimulation [282]. There is disagreement as to whether the pressor response to electrical stimulation remains intact following 6-OHDA [278, 281, 282]. The decrease in arterial blood pressure following chemical stimulation of the A5 area is associated with a decrease in cardiac output, decreases in vascular resistance in skeletal muscle and increases in mesenteric and skin vascular resistance [282]. The hemodynamic effects associated with glutamate stimulation of the A5 area are prevented by pretreatment with 6-OHDA [282]. Loewy et al. [280]

found that individual A5 catecholamine neurons project to both the IML and the nucleus tractus solitarius. Microinjection of 6-OHDA into either of these areas blunt the A5 depressor response. This suggests that both areas contribute to the decrease in blood pressure following chemical stimulation of A5 norepinephrine neurons. More recently, microinjection of the excitatory amino acid NMDA into the A5 area has been shown to increase splanchnic and renal sympathetic nerve discharge. The sympathoexcitatory effect was blocked by microinjection of 6-OHDA into the A5 area or by intrathecal injection of the a1-receptor antagonist prazosin [283]. Microinjection of 6-OHDA directly into the A5 area produces extensive destruction of norepinephrine neurons but fails to alter arterial blood pressure in conscious animals [284]. This observation likely reflects the redundancy of central pathways involved in the maintenance of blood pressure and suggests a modulatory role of A5 neurons in cardiovascular regulation.

Microiontophoretic application of norepinephrine consistently inhibits the firing rate of sympathetic preganglionic neurons [139–141, 285]. The inhibitory effects of microiontophoretically applied norepinephrine are blocked by α_2-adrenergic antagonists (i.e., yohimbine and piperoxane) but not by the α_1-receptor antagonist prazosin or by β-receptor antagonists [139, 141]. This indicates that the inhibitory effects of norepinephrine are mediated by α_2-adrenergic receptors. Consistent with this view is the observations that microiontophoretic application of the α_2-agonist clonidine inhibits the firing rate of sympathetic preganglionic neurons while the α_1-agonist phenylephrine has no effect [139]. In addition, α_2-adrenergic receptors are highly concentrated over clusters of sympathetic preganglionic neurons in the IML [42].

Although the above data suggest that noradrenergic neurons inhibit the firing of sympathetic preganglionic neurons, there is evidence suggesting the opposite. Administration of α_1-adrenergic receptor antagonists (i.e., prazosin, WB-4101 or ketanserin) inhibit spontaneous sympathetic nerve discharge via an action in the spinal cord [286, 287]. Since α_1-receptors are thought to mediate excitatory effects of norepinephrine in the central nervous system [288], these data indirectly support a sympathoexcitatory role of norepinephrine in the spinal cord. Intrathecal administration of norepinephrine results in an inhibition followed by an excitation of renal sympathetic activity. The inhibitory response is blocked by α_2-receptor antagonists while the excitatory response is blocked by α_1-receptor antagonists [289]. Administration of the catecholamine precursor L-dopa increases excitability in spinal sympathetic pathways [290]. More direct evidence for an excitatory function of norepinephrine at the level of sympathetic preganglionic neurons comes from work done in spinal cord slice preparations. Superfusion of a spinal slice with norepinephrine causes a membrane depolarization in antidromically identified sympa-.thetic preganglionic neurons and results in repetitive cell discharges [71, 75, 291–294]. Pretreating the slices with α_1-receptor antagonists but not α_2- or β-receptor antagonists prevent the depolarizing effect of norepinephrine [75].

Nishi and coworkers [71, 75, 76, 292] found that sympathetic preganglionic neurons in a slice preparation exhibit a fast excitatory postsynaptic potential (EPSP) [or rarely a fast inhibitory postsynaptic potential (IPSP)] in response to single focal stimulation. Trains of repetitive stimuli produced a slow EPSP which was occasionally accompanied by a slow IPSP. The slow EPSP was always associated with an increased input resistance, disappeared at levels of anodal hyperpolarization exceeding –80 mV and was specifically blocked by the α_1-receptor antagonist prazosin. Norepinephrine superfusion produced a depolarization that shared the same characteristics of the slow EPSP. The slow IPSP was not normally observed until the slow EPSP was eliminated by prazosin. Following the use of prazosin, norepinephrine produced a hyperpolarization. Both the slow IPSP and the norepinephrine-induced hyperpolarization were accompanied by a decreased input resistance, reversed at –90 mV and abolished by the α_2-adrenergic receptor antagonist yohimbine. This data supports the hypothesis that noradrenergic neurons can both excite and inhibit sympathetic preganglionic neurons. The inhibitory interaction is mediated by α_2-receptors located on or near the soma. The excitatory interaction occurs through α_1-receptors located on distal dendrites. Since the recording electrode of large multibarreled pipettes used in microiontophoretic experiments must be near the soma to record action potentials, iontophoresis of norepinephrine appears to have only an inhibitory effect. In contrast, norepinephrine reaches the excitatory receptors located on dendritic trees in a superfused slice preparation. Although the above hypothesis is attractive and fits well with present data, it will be difficult to prove. Alternatively, the effects of noradrenergic neurons are mediated via one subtype of α-receptor, while epinephrine-containing neurons selectively interact with the other subclass of α-receptor. In this case, microiontophoretic application of a catecholamine might not give an accurate idea of the physiologic function of the neurotransmitter.

In summary, evidence exists for both an excitatory and an inhibitory role of norepinephrine in the regulation of the sympathetic nervous system. It seems likely that A5 neurons are not part of the central circuitry which transmits specific autonomic information from the brain stem to the spinal cord. Indeed, α-receptor antagonist fail to block cardiovascular reflexes and have relatively minor effects on spontaneous sympathetic activity [2]. Rather it seems likely that A5 neurons modulate sympathetic activity which might include both excitation of some neurons and inhibition of others in order to distribute blood flow to appropriate beds. More recently, it has been demonstrated that clonidine and prazosin both preferentially inhibit the 10-Hz rhythm of sympathetic nerve discharge [295]. Thus, like 5-HT, noradrenergic neurons might play an important role in determining the pattern of sympathetic activity.

4.5   Paraventricular nucleus

In addition to the neurosecretory pathways to the posterior pituitary, paraventricular neurons project to nuclei that are involved in central autonomic regulation. These neurons are located in the parvocellular subdivision of the paraventricular nucleus and send descending projections to the medulla and spinal cord [296–299]. Approximately 15% of these neurons send axon collaterals to both the dorsal medulla (i.e., nucleus tractus solitarius (NTS) and dorsal motor nucleus of the vagus) and to the spinal cord [300]. The remaining neurons appear to project solely to either the dorsal medulla or the spinal cord. Immunohistochemistry has been used to demonstrate that a portion of the descending neurons contain AVP or oxytocin and neurophysin [296, 300, 301]. However, the majority of the fibers has not been characterized as to neurotransmitter content [302]. Electrophysiology studies confirm the existence of PVN pathways to the NTS, the ventrolateral medulla and the spinal cord [303–306]. Descending PVN neurons have been shown to receive baroreceptor inputs [305]. Ascending inputs from brain stem catecholamine cell groups are discussed below. The PVN is under tonic GABAergic inhibition [307–309]. Thus, the PVN receives afferent input from medullary cardiovascular sites and exerts regulatory effects on the cardiovascular system through release of vasopressin into the peripheral circulation and through efferent signals to the medulla and to the spinal cord.

The cardiovascular control by PVN neurons is not well understood. Electrical [310–312] or chemical [312–315] stimulation of the PVN elicits both pressor and depressor responses. Immunohistochemical studies show that spinally projecting neurons from the PVN contain oxytocin and vasopressin. These two putative neurotransmitters are contained in the IML [287, 300, 316, 317]. An early study reported that microiontophoresis of AVP and oxytocin, as well as electrical stimulation of the PVN, inhibits the firing of sympathetic preganglionic neurons [310]. More recent studies fail to support these observations. Electrical stimulation of the parvocellular subdivision of the PVN elicits a pressor response which is accompanied by an increase in sympathetic activity and vaso-constriction in the mesenteric, renal and skeletal muscle vascular beds [302, 317]. Backman and Henry [318] found that microiontophoretic application of AVP increased the firing of sympathetic preganglionic neu-rons. Superfusion of AVP depolarizes putative sympathetic preganglionic neurons in a slice preparation [319]. Vasopressin$_1$ antagonists block the depolarizing effect of AVP while a vasopressin$_2$ agonist has little effect. AVP-induced depolarizations are partially reduced, but never elimi-nated, by a low Ca/high Mg solution or by tetrodotoxin. This suggests that AVP excites sympathetic preganglionic neurons by a direct depo-larization and by an indirect effect via the release of an excitatory trans-mitter [319]. Based on these data, it seems likely that a non-AVP con-taining pathway mediates depressor responses elicited by stimulation of the PVN (see above).

The role of AVP in mediating the pressor response to PVN stimulation has been investigated. Intrathecal administration of as little as 1 pmole of AVP elicits a pressor response which is accompanied by vasoconstric-tion in renal, mesenteric and hindquarter vascular beds [302, 320]. The effect is due to an action of vasopressin within the spinal cord since block-ade of peripheral vasopressin receptors had no effect on the response. Intrathecal administration of a vasopressin antagonist at doses which had no non-specific depressant effects blocked the pressor response to intra-thecal AVP. The same dose of the AVP antagonist failed to block the pres-sor response to stimulation of the PVN. Assuming the antagonist had access to the same group of receptors affected by neurally released AVP, these data suggest that the cardiovascular effects produced by stimula-tion of the PVN do not depend on the release of vasopressin from spinal cord nerve terminals [302]. Support for this conclusion is found in stud-ies performed using Brattleboro rats which lack hypothalamic and spinal AVP. Stimulation of the PVN in Brattleboro rats elicits a pressor response which is identical to that observed in Long Evans control rats [302]. Thus, although AVP appears to depolarize sympathetic preganglionic neurons, the role that this transmitter plays in regulating the firing of sympathetic preganglionic neurons remains unclear. In addition, the identity of other spinal transmitters arising in the PVN is unknown. The role of AVP in modulating baroreceptor reflexes at the level of the NTS is described below.

5   Pathways involved in the baroreceptor reflex

5.1   Baroreceptor afferent input

The central neuronal networks involved in cardiovascular regulation receive a large array of afferent information which arises from arterial baroreceptors located in the aortic arch and carotid sinus, cardiac baroreceptors located in the atria and ventricles of the heart and arterial chemoreceptors found primarily in the carotid and aortic bodies [321]. The cell bodies of these viscerosensory afferent neurons are located in the petrosal and nodose ganglia. Baroreceptor afferent fibers enter the central nervous system in the IX and X cranial nerves and terminate in the NTS. The basic function of the baroreceptor reflex in buffering against acute changes in arterial blood pressure is reviewed elsewhere [322, 323]. In addition to vagal and glossopharyngeal afferents, a large amount of afferent information enters the central nervous system via the dorsal roots of the spinal cord. This information arises from somatic and visceral receptors and is transmitted to multiple levels of the spinal cord as well as to brain stem nuclei including the NTS (for review see [324, 325]). It is interesting to note that the discharge of NTS and spinal sympathoinhibitory baroreceptor interneurons is temporally related to at least five parts of the cardiac cycle suggesting input from five or more cardiac locked afferent sources [83].

The site of termination of baroreceptor afferents in the NTS has been determined using anatomical and electrophysiological techniques. Baroreceptor afferents in the aortic depressor nerve terminate rostral to the obex in the dorsomedial and lateral subnuclei of the NTS [324–329]. Chemoreceptor afferents arising in the carotid body terminate caudal to the obex in the commissural subnucleus of the NTS [327, 328, 330]. Afferents in the carotid sinus nerve subserve both chemoreceptor and baroreceptor function and terminate in both these areas [331, 332]. Electrophysiological data suggest that little if any convergence occurs between chemoreceptor and baroreceptor afferent input on NTS neurons [333].

Afferent terminals which terminate in the NTS contain a wide variety of putative neurotransmitters including excitatory amino acids, neuropeptides and monoamines [334, 335]. Several years ago a debate raged as to whether substance P or glutamate represented the primary neurotransmitter in baroreceptor afferents [4]. This discussion has quieted and it is generally believed that glutamate is the primary neurotransmitter of baroreceptor afferent fibers. Microinjection of L-glutamate into the NTS mimics baroreceptor reflex activation by eliciting a dose-dependent hypotension, bradycardia and apnea [336]. Biochemical studies indicate that the intermediate area of the NTS contains a high-affinity uptake system for inactivation of L-glutamate and a high concentration of this excitatory amino acid. These data are consistent with this area being richly innervated by glutaminergic neurons [337]. Unilateral removal of the nodose ganglion results in a 50% reduction in the uptake of L-glutamate bilaterally into homogenates of NTS and a reduction in the content of glutamate in the NTS [337]. Electrical stimulation of baroreceptor afferent nerves elicits hypotension and bradycardia which is associated with an increase in release of L-glutamate from the NTS [338, 339]. Microinjection of the excitatory amino acid antagonist kynurenic acid abolishes baroreceptor reflexes elicited by electrical stimulation of the aortic depressor nerve [340, 341]. Microinjection of the glutamate antagonist glutamic acid diethylester (GDEE) into the NTS results in increases in arterial blood pressure and heart rate and blocks the baroreceptor-mediated bradycardia produced by intravenous injection of phenylephrine [340]. NTS microinjections of GDEE or a second glutamate antagonist, HA-966, but not saline, block baroreceptor reflexes as judged by 1) inhibition of sympathetic activity elicited by stimulation of baroreceptor afferent nerves, 2) the baroreceptor-mediated locking of sympathetic slow waves to the cardiac cycle and 3) the inhibition of sympathetic activity associated with an intravenous pressor dose of phenylephrine [341]. Collectively, these data suggest that an excitatory amino acid functions as a neurotransmitter released by baroreceptor afferents in the NTS.

Antagonists of the N-methyl-D-aspartate, kainate and quisqualate receptors reduce the effects of solitary tract afferent stimulation in a slice preparation [342]. Microinjection of selective NMDA receptor antagonists into the NTS reduces but does not abolish the baroreceptor activation produced by stimulation of the aortic depressor nerve [147]. In contrast, non-NMDA receptor antagonists completely block the effects of baroreceptor afferent stimulation [343, 344]. More recently, it has been suggested that both NMDA and non-NMDA receptors play a partial role in mediating the effects of baroreceptor afferent excitatory amino acids [345]. Similarly, both NMDA and non-NMDA receptors appear to be involved in the vasodepressor response to stimulation of cardio-pulmonary vagal afferent C fibers [346]. The effects of excitatory amino acids contained within chemoreceptor afferents also appear to be mediated by both NMDA and non-NMDA receptors in the NTS [347]. Although the above data provide strong support for the idea that glutamate functions as the primary fast-acting neurotransmitter released from baroreceptor afferents in the NTS it should be noted for completeness that at least three recent papers question portions of this assumption [348–350].

5.2   Neurotransmitters within the NTS

The NTS is richly innervated by monoamine, amino acid and peptidergic containing neurons. A large body of work has attempted to identify putative neurotransmitters which modulate baroreceptor reflexes within the NTS. One of the most thoroughly investigated neurochemicals in this regard is GABA. GABA neurons are intrinsic to the NTS. GABA containing terminals synapse primarily onto dendritic spines and shafts throughout the NTS [351–353]. Studies indicate that NTS neurons involved in cardiovascular regulation are tonically inhibited by GABA. Microinjection of GABA or the GABA agonists muscimol and baclofen into the NTS elicits an increase in arterial blood pressure and hyperpolarizes NTS neurons [354–357]. The increase in arterial blood pressure results from an increase in sympathetic nerve activity and an elevation of plasma AVP levels [354]. Similar results are observed following microinjection of the GABA uptake inhibitor nipecotic acid into the NTS [354, 355, 358]. These effects may be mediated by both $GABA_A$ and $GABA_B$ receptors [354–356, 358]. In contrast, microinjection of the $GABA_A$ antagonist bicuculline or the $GABA_B$ antagonist CGP-35348 results in a decrease in arterial blood pressure [354, 355, 359]. Microiontophoretically applied bicuculline increases the firing rate of NTS neurons which receive afferent input from the carotid sinus nerve [360]. Finally, microinjections of muscimol or nipecotic acid into the NTS reduce the depressor response to aortic nerve stimulation [361]. These data are consistent with the hypothesis that NTS neurons involved in baroreceptor pathways are under tonic GABAergic inhibition.

Electrical stimulation of the hypothalamus elicits a "defense reaction" which is accompanied by increases in arterial blood pressure and heart rate. The defense reaction is also associated with a central mediated inhibition of the baroreceptor reflex [362]. Intracellular recordings from NTS neurons receiving a baroreceptor input indicate hypothalamic stimulation elicits IPSPs in these cells and made them unresponsive to baroreceptor afferent input [363]. The inhibitory effect of hypothalamic stimulation can be antagonized by bicuculline but not by strychnine suggesting the involvement of $GABA_A$ receptors in the response. However, descending fibers from the hypothalamus are not GABAergic. This suggests that hypothalamic neurons project to GABAergic neurons intrinsic to the NTS and these interneurons inhibit neurons in the baroreceptor reflex [364]. Similarly, GABAergic modulation of the baroreceptor reflex at the level of the NTS has been observed to occur during the pressor response associated with stimulation of the uvula cortex of the posterior cerebellar vermis [321, 365] and during exercise [366].

The NTS is heavily innervated by catecholamine containing neurons [367]. Microinjection of either norepinephrine or epinephrine into the NTS consistently produces a decrease in arterial blood pressure and heart rate [368]. Microiontophoretic application of norepinephrine or epinephrine inhibits the firing of NTS neurons regardless of the response of these neurons to baroreceptor reflex activation [369]. The firing of NTS neurons is also inhibited by microiontophoretic application of the α_1-receptor agonist methoxamine and the α_2-receptor agonist clonidine. Furthermore the inhibitory effects on iontophoretic catecholamines are reduced by both α_1- and α_2-receptor antagonists [369, 370]. These data suggest that the inhibitory effect of catecholamines in the NTS is mediated by both α_1- and α_2-receptors. Microinjections of the α_2-receptor antagonists yohimbine or idazoxan into the NTS increase arterial blood pressure and completely inhibit the depressor and bradycardic responses to electrical stimulation of the aortic depressor nerve [371]. Destruction of the catecholamine innervation of the NTS by microinjection of 6-OHDA results in a permanent lability of arterial blood pressure, despite preservation of reflex bradycardia [372]. These data suggest that catecholamines modulate baroreceptor reflexes.

The NTS is heavily innervated by 5-HT-containing neurons arising in raphe obscurus, raphe pallidus, raphe magnus and the rostral ventromedial medulla [373]. Microinjection of 5-HT into the NTS produces either pressor [374, 375] or depressor [376, 377] responses. Both the pressor and depressor effects of microinjected 5-HT can be blocked by the 5-HT antagonist metergoline [374, 376, 377]. The magnitude of the 5-HT-induced pressor response is potentiated by microinjection of the 5-HT uptake inhibitor fluoxetine [374]. These observations suggest that different 5-HT receptor subtypes may mediate excitation and inhibition in the NTS. The hypotension and bradycardia produced by 5-HT is blocked by NTS microinjection of the $5-HT_2$ receptor antagonist ketanserin. Bilateral NTS microinjections of ketanserin produce an increase in the level and the variability of arterial blood pressure but do not block the baroreceptor reflex arc [377]. Similarly, metergoline does not affect baroreceptor reflexes [376]. These data suggest that $5-HT_2$ receptors facilitate baroreceptor activity in the NTS. Microinjection of $5-HT_1$ agonists such as 8-OH DPAT and RU-24969 have no cardiovascular effects [377]. This is somewhat surprising since $5-HT_{1A}$ receptors are densely distributed in areas of the NTS associated with cardiovascular control [378]. The vast majority of NTS neurons recorded in a slice preparation were depolarized in the presence of 5-HT and the 5-HT$_3$ receptor agonist 2-methyl-5-HT. This response was resistant to tetrodotoxin and Co^{++} application. In addition, 2-methyl-5-HT increased the amplitude and frequency of both excitatory and inhibitory spontaneous synaptic potentials. Selective 5-HT$_3$ receptor antagonists blocked the effects of 2-methyl-5-HT [379]. These data suggest that 5-HT via 5-HT$_3$ receptors can modulate baroreceptor activity through both pre- and postsynaptic mechanisms.

Acetylcholine is also found in the NTS. Microinjections of acetylcholine into the NTS elicit a baroreceptor reflex-like response which includes a decrease in arterial blood pressure and a bradycardia [337, 380]. The vasodepressor effects of acetylcholine are mediated via M2 receptors [381]. Microinjections of cholinergic antagonists into the NTS fail to block the baroreceptor reflex or alter blood pressure at doses which block the vasodepressor effects of acetylcholine [337, 382]. These data suggest that cholinergic mechanisms in the NTS are not involved in the tonic regulation of cardiovascular function or the baroreceptor reflex. Microinjections of glycine into the NTS decrease arterial blood pressure and heart rate [383]. Anatomically, glycine containing terminals are located in an area of the NTS which is rich in cholinergic neurons [384]. The depressor response to microinjections of glycine are blocked by muscarinic antagonists and potentiated by physostigmine [385]. These data suggest that glycine may act via cholinergic neurons to produce vasodepressor responses in the NTS.

The NTS contains many neuropeptides which may act to modulate baroreceptor afferent processing. Microinjections of AVP into the NTS consistently increase arterial blood pressure and spontaneous sympathetic nerve discharge [386, 387]. Pretreatment with microinjected AVP antagonists block the pressor effect of AVP [386]. Microinjection of an AVP antagonist into the NTS reduces the increase in arterial blood pressure elicited by electrical stimulation of the PVN [388]. Microinjections of AVP antagonists alone have no cardiovascular effects [387], suggesting that the AVP innervation of the NTS is not tonically active.

The NTS is richly innervated by NPY containing neurons [389, 390]. Microinjection of NPY into the NTS was originally report to produce a dose-related decrease in arterial blood pressure and heart rate [391]. More recently it has been observed that a long lasting pressor response follows the depressor response associated with NPY microinjections. During the pressor period produced by NPY, the depressor effects of microinjected glutamate are blocked and the baroreceptor reflex is blunted [392, 393].

These data suggest that NPY may serve as a long-term regulator of baroreceptor reflex activity.

Microinjection of angiotensin II (Ang) into the NTS has been reported .to produce both pressor and depressor effects [394–396]. The action of Ang may be a function of the microinjected dose since at least three investigators now report that low doses of microinjected Ang produce depressor responses while higher doses elicit pressor responses [395–397]. Microinjection of low doses of the amino terminal angiotensin heptapeptide (Ang 1-7) similarly reduced arterial blood pressure [397]. This is significant since Ang 1-7 lacks a direct vascular action. These data suggest that the Ang receptors in the NTS are distinct from those found in the vasculature. Microinjection of the Ang antagonist saralasin has been reported to produce a small increase in arterial blood pressure [396] but also has been shown to enhance baroreceptor reflexes [397]. Thus the role of Ang in the NTS remains unclear.

Microinjection of Met- or Leu-enkephalin into the NTS produces an increase in blood pressure and heart rate. The opioid antagonist naloxone blocks these actions [398]. Microinjection of β-endorphin into the NTS has been reported to produce a depressor response [399]. Microinjection of either TRH or somatostatin into the NTS results in a decrease in arterial blood pressure and a bradycardia [375, 400]. Low doses of calcitonin gene-related peptide decreased blood pressure and heart rate when microinjected into the NTS and potentiated the depressor response to microinjection of norepinephrine [401].

5.3 Caudal ventrolateral medulla

The caudal ventrolateral medulla corresponds to the external formation of the nucleus ambiguus at the level of the obex and overlaps at its most rostral extent with the sympathoexcitatory neurons of the rostral ventrolateral medulla. This area contains the A1 noradrenergic cell group [402]. Electrical or chemical stimulation of this area produces cardiovascular effects opposite those observed in more rostral portions of the ventrolateral medulla. Microinjection of glutamate into the caudal ventrolateral medulla results in decreases in arterial blood pressure and sympathetic nerve discharge [402–404]. Conversely, microinjection of hyperpolarizing agents such as GABA or the GABA agonist muscimol results in increases in blood pressure, heart rate and sympathetic activity [405, 406].

There is a good deal of evidence in the rat and rabbit that the caudal ventrolateral medulla plays a crucial role in the baroreceptor reflex, receiving input from the NTS and sending efferents to the rostral ventrolateral medulla. The ventrolateral medulla is heavily innervated by neurons arising in the NTS [23, 77, 89]. The NTS areas projecting to the ventrolateral medulla correspond to the zones in which baroreceptor afferents contained within the IXth and Xth cranial nerves terminate [89, 407]. Indeed, electrophysiology studies indicate that medullospinal sympathoexcitatory neurons in the rostral ventrolateral medulla receive a baroreceptor input [98–105]. Microinjections of tetrodotoxin into the rostral ventrolateral medulla prevent the increases in arterial blood pressure and sympathetic nerve activity observed following lesions of the caudal ventrolateral medulla [133]. Microinjection of the GABA agonist muscimol into the caudal ventrolateral medulla hyperpolarizes the area (i.e., silences neurons without interfering with axonal conduction), increases arterial blood pressure and blocks baroreceptor reflexes [405, 406]. Similarly, microinjection of the glutamate antagonist kynurenic acid into the caudal ventrolateral medulla blocks baroreceptor but not chemoreceptor reflexes [26]. Microinjections of NMDA receptor antagonists into the caudal ventrolateral medulla have been shown to block baroreceptor inhibition of sympathetic activity [147, 408–410]. Electrophysiological studies reveal neurons in the caudal ventrolateral medulla which can be antidromically activated from the subretrofacial area and which receive afferent input from the NTS [411–415]. At least some of these neurons are likely to be C1 epinephrine-containing sympathoexcitatory cells [416]. Neurons in subretrofacial nucleus inhibited during baroreceptor reflex activation are also inhibited by glutamate and excited by GABA microinjected into the caudal ventrolateral medulla [415]. Finally, baroreceptor activation increases c-fos mRNA in caudal ventrolateral medulla neurons [417]. These data are compatible with the hypothesis that second-order baroreceptor neurons arising in the NTS project to the caudal ventrolateral medulla. These neurons utilize a glutamate-like transmitter to excite inhibitory neurons which project to the rostral ventrolateral medulla. NMDA receptors may mediate the glutamate-induced excitation of inhibitory interneurons.

Present evidence suggests that GABA mediates baroreceptor-induced inhibition of sympathoexcitatory neurons in the rostral ventrolateral medulla in the rat and rabbit. It was originally proposed that the GABAergic input to the subretrofacial nucleus originated in the NTS. However this is not the case [169]. It is not known if GABAergic neurons involved in baroreceptor inhibition are intrinsic to the rostral ventrolateral medulla or if they project to this area from the caudal ventrolateral medulla. The distribution of GABA neurons in the ventrolateral medulla has been described [169, 170]. Microinjection of the GABA antagonist bicuculline into the rostral ventrolateral medulla increases arterial blood pressure and produces a 48% reduction in the baroreceptor-mediated depressor response to aortic depressor nerve stimulation [164]. Bicuculline applied to the ventral surface of the medulla oblongata in the area of the rostral medulla reduces the inhibition of renal sympathetic nerve activity produced by baroreceptor reflex activation [418]. However, neither of these studies controlled for the large increase in sympathetic activity produced by bicuculline. More recently, Sun and Guyenet found that microiontophoresis of bicuculline blocked the baroreceptor-induced inhibition of medullospinal sympathoexcitatory neurons in the rostral ventrolateral medulla [163]. Microiontophoretically applied glutamate produced an increase in neuronal firing comparable to that observed with bicuculline, but did not significantly alter the baroreceptor mediated inhibition of the sympathoexcitatory neurons. These data suggest that GABA mediates the baroreceptor inhibition of rostral ventrolateral sympathoexcitatory neurons.

The story is not as clear in the cat. GABA antagonists given intravenously or microinjected into the rostral ventrolateral medulla failed to block the baroreceptor mediated inhibition of inferior cardiac sympathetic nerve discharge [103]. GABA antagonists also did not block baroreceptor-mediated temporal locking of sympathetic slow waves to the cardiac cycle [419]. Intravenous picrotoxin failed to block the baroreceptor mediated inhibition of medullospinal sympathoexcitatory neurons recorded in the rostral ventrolateral medulla. In contrast, picrotoxin antagonized the GABA-mediated inhibition of sympathoexcitatory neurons produced by stimulation of the midline medulla and the inhibitory effect of microiontophoretically applied GABA [103]. Thus, picrotoxin was present in sufficient concentration to antagonize the inhibition produced by GABA. An interesting ancillary observation made in this study was that midcollicular transection of the brain stem did not alter sympathetic activity but prevented the increase in sympathetic activity produced by intravenous picrotoxin. These data suggest that forebrain GABAergic neurons tonically inhibit excitatory pathways projecting to sympathetic neurons in the brain stem [103]. The caudal ventrolateral medulla should not be thought of as simply a relay in the baroreceptor reflex pathway. Evidence indicates that the caudal ventrolateral medulla is the source of tonic inhibition of non-baroreceptor origin. Disruption of caudal ventrolateral medullary neuronal activity results in an increase in arterial blood pressure which surpasses that observed following baroreceptor afferent denervation [159, 420]. Microinjection of muscimol increases arterial blood pressure even when blood pressure is maintained below the threshold for arterial baroreceptor activation [406]. In baroreceptor denervated rats, lesions of the caudal ventrolateral medulla produced a sustained increase in arterial blood pressure and splanchnic sympathetic nerve discharge [421]. Microinjections of the excitotoxic agent kainic acid into the rostral portion of the caudal ventrolateral medulla produced a pressor response due to increased sympathetic nerve activity and prevented baroreceptor-mediated inhibition of sympathetic activity. Microinjections into more caudal portions of the caudal ventrolateral medulla elicited similar increases in arterial blood pressure and sympathetic activity but actually enhanced baroreceptor reflex function [414]. These data indicate that the caudal ventrolateral plays an important role in tonic non-baroreceptor inhibition of sympathetic activity. In addition, the caudal ventrolateral medulla has been shown to be critical in the generation of the 10-Hz component of sympathetic nerve discharge [108–110].

The A1 noradrenergic cell group lies in the caudal ventrolateral medulla at, and caudal, to the level of the obex. Early studies suggested that many of the depressor effects of caudal ventrolateral medullary stimulation resulted from activation of A1 neurons. This is not likely the case (see [268] for review). In addition, A1 neurons do not transmit baroreceptor inhibition to sympathoexcitatory neurons in the subretrofacial area. For example, A1 neurons do not project to the vicinity of subretrofacial sympathoexcitatory neurons [422]. In addition, adrenergic receptor blockade in the rostral ventrolateral medulla fails to affect baroreceptor-mediated sympathoinhibition [423].

A1 noradrenergic neurons have been characterized using electrophysiologic methods. Two types of neurons in the A1 area of the caudal ventrolateral medulla can be distinguished on the basis of axonal conduction velocities following antidromic activation of the lateral hypothalamus. Neurons with slow conduction velocities (i.e. 0.3 m/s) fire spontaneously with action potentials similar in appearance to those recorded from other catecholamine neurons and 50% of these neurons are sensitive to the neurotoxic effects of 6-OHDA. These neurons are likely to be noradrenergic A1 neurons [424, 425]. 6-OHDA insensitive neurons have been postulated to be caudally positioned C1 epinephrine-containing neurons [425]. C1 neurons are sensitive to baroreceptor inhibition (see above). Approximately 50% of the A1 area neurons antidromically activated from the hypothalamus are sensitive to baroreceptor inhibition [426, 427]. Indeed, only 50% of the A1 area neurons projecting to the hypothalamus contain norepinephrine [3, 268]. These data suggest that A1 norepinephrine-containing neurons may not be sensitive to baroreceptor inhibition although confirmation awaits more definitive experiments. Less ambiguous is the observation that the vast majority of A1 area neurons antidromically activated from the hypothalamus and inhibited by clonidine are excited by vagal afferent nerve stimulation [3, 268]. Severe hemorrhage activates A1 norepinephrine neurons [428, 429] apparently as a result of vagal afferent activation [430].

Neurons in the caudal ventrolateral medulla project to the supraoptic and paraventricular nuclei of the hypothalamus. These nuclei contain the arginine-vasopressin (AVP) neurosecretory cells. Double-labeling experiments show that over 80% of these ascending neurons are A1 norepinephrine-containing neurons [431, 432]. Electrical stimulation of the A1 area produces an increase in the release of AVP [433]. Topical application of GABA antagonists on the ventrolateral surface of the medulla results in an increase in AVP secretion which is not attributable to changes in arterial blood pressure [434]. These data suggest that neurons in the caudal ventrolateral medulla are involved in the ascending control of AVP release. More recent studies indicate that microinjection of muscimol into the caudal ventrolateral medulla inhibits the release of AVP in response to hemorrhage and constriction of the inferior vena cava [435, 436]. Microinjections of L-glutamate or the GABA antagonist bicuculline cause dose dependent increases in plasma AVP [437]. Finally, microinjection of norepinephrine into the paraventricular nucleus enhances AVP release [438]. These studies suggest that A1 norepinephrine neurons stimulate the release of AVP.

Electrophysiology studies provide more support for this hypothesis. Electrical stimulation of the A1 region elicits an increase in firing of AVP-containing neurons in the paraventricular nucleus and in the supraoptic nucleus. The excitatory effect of A1 stimulation is abolished by local administration of 6-OHDA [439, 440]. Interestingly, pretreatment with 6-OHDA fails to alter basal levels of plasma AVP [441]. The excitatory effect of A1 stimulation on AVP secretory neurons in the paraventricular nucleus is blocked by microiontophoretic application of the α-adrenergic antagonist phentolamine [442]. Norepinephrine enhances the excitability and promotes bursting activity in supraoptic nucleus neurosecretory neurons via an α_1-receptor mechanism *in vitro* [443]. Taken together, these data support the concept that ascending noradrenergic neurons facilitate the release of AVP. Since 6-OHDA pretreatment fails to alter basal levels of AVP, norepinephrine may act as a modulator to maintain the sensitivity of neurosecretory neurons to stimuli that normally elicit AVP release [441].

The role of the caudal ventrolateral medulla in regulating AVP release is likely more complicated than is indicated by the above discussion. For example, the data presented above suggest that lesions of the caudal ventrolateral medulla would result in a decrease or no change in the release of AVP. In fact, however, lesion of the caudal ventrolateral medulla results in large increases in plasma AVP [444–446]. Moreover, microiontophoretic application of norepinephrine onto AVP secretory neurons inhibits rather than excites the discharges of these neurons. More recently, it has been demonstrated that the majority of PVN neurons antidromically activated by stimulation of the posterior pituitary are excited by microiontophoretic norepinephrine. In contrast, PVN neurons antidromically activated from the caudal ventrolateral medulla are consistently inhibited by norepinephrine [447]. Superfusion of norepinephrine in a hypothalamic slice preparation excites AVP secretory neurons in the supraoptic and paraventricular nuclei. The excitatory response is mediated via an α_1-receptor since the response can be blocked by prazosin. Following prazosin, norepinephrine inhibits rather than excites AVP neurons [448]. These data suggest that norepinephrine has a dual action on AVP secretory neurons. Similarly, norepinephrine produces both excitation and inhibition of the firing of SPN (see above). The differences between the effects of iontophoretically applied norepinephrine *in vivo* and superfused norepinephrine *in vitro* may be explained if the different techniques expose different populations of receptors to norepinephrine. The story is further complicated by the fact that norepinephrine neurons innervate both AVP-positive and closely adjacent AVP-negative neurons [449]. Electrical stimulation of the A1 area inhibits non-AVP neurons in the paraventricular nucleus via a β-receptor [442]. Thus, the actual role of the A1 norepinephrine neurons in regulating AVP release requires additional studies.

5.4   Lateral tegmental field

The lateral tegmental field of the medulla is located dorsomedial and caudal to the subretrofacial area of the ventrolateral area and corresponds to the nucleus reticularis parvocellularis and nucleus reticularis ventralis. The area was originally described as a pressor area in the cat by Wang and Ranson [240]. The pressor response to electrical stimulation has been at least partially attributed to activation of rostral ventrolateral medulla axons which pass through the area prior to descending to the spinal cord [451, 452]. The additional observation that chemical stimulation of the lateral tegmental field produced only minor changes in arterial blood pressure [451] would seem to diminish the importance of the area in the regulation of the cardiovascular system.

More recent experiments suggest that the lateral tegmental field may play a greater role in blood pressure regulation than originally appreciated. Microinjection of glutamate or NMDA into the lateral tegmental field increases arterial blood pressure by 50–75 mmgHg and is accompanied by an increase in sympathetic activity [453–454]. Electrophysiological recordings have identified two types of neurons (i.e. excited and inhibited during baroreceptor activation) with discharges related to sympathetic nerve activity [109, 455, 456]. Thus, neurons involved in both sympathoexcitatory and inhibitory functions are found in the lateral tegmental field. Electrical stimulation of the lateral tegmental field elicits a discharge in inferior cardiac sympathetic activity which can be distinguished from that elicited from the rostral ventrolateral medulla by a longer onset latency. Characterization of sympathetic neurons has likewise revealed a longer duration from unit discharge to the peak of inferior cardiac nerve activity than the similarly observed temporal relationship between subretrofacial sympathoexcitatory neurons and inferior cardiac nerve discharge [109]. These data have led to the proposal that the lateral tegmental field is an important site in the generation of basal sympathetic discharge in the cat. Since lateral tegmental sympathoexcitatory neurons project to the subretrofacial area [109, 456] it is possible that the lateral tegmental field influences sympathetic activity via the rostral ventrolateral medulla. In support of this hypothesis, the pressor response to microinjections of glutamate into the lateral tegmental field is prevented by subretrofacial injection of the excitatory amino acid antagonist kynurenic acid [457].

The observation that the firing of lateral tegmental field sympathetic neurons is altered during baroreceptor reflex activation suggests that this area may play a role in the baroreceptor reflex. Direct evidence for this suggestion has recently been obtained from two different laboratories. Microinjection of the neurotoxin kainic acid destroys cell bodies while leaving fibers of passage intact [458]. Kainic acid lesions of the lateral tegmental field in the cat disrupts baroreceptor function as judged by the reflex sympathoinhibition during pressor responses, the temporal locking of sympathetic slow waves to the cardiac cycle and the shift to higher frequencies in the power spectra of sympathetic activity [28, 459]. The kainic acid lesion was localized to the lateral tegmental field as determined by diffusion of dye spots, diffusion of excitability as judged by 2-deoxyglucose autoradiography and demonstration of the functional integrity of the rostral ventrolateral medulla [28, 459]. These data suggest that destruction of LTF neurons produce a severe impairment of baroreceptor reflexes and illustrate the importance of the lateral tegmental field in central autonomic regulation. It is interesting to note that a role of baroreceptor function has not been described for the rat or rabbit. Other differences regarding the role of GABA in baroreceptor function between rat, rabbit and cat are described above.

The lateral tegmental field appears to be critical in mediating the central sympatholytic actions of 5-HT$_{1A}$ receptor agonists such as 8-OH DPAT. 8-OH DPAT produces a parallel inhibition of subretrofacial sympathoexcitatory unit firing and sympathetic nerve activity. However, in the cat iontophoretic 8-OH DPAT has little effect on cell firing [179]. These data suggest that 8-OH DPAT acts on antecedent neurons in the lateral tegmental field which provide a tonic excitatory input to subretrofacial sympathoexcitatory neurons. 8-OH DPAT inhibits the firing of lateral tegmental field neurons [455, 459]. The inhibition of neuronal firing exactly parallels the inhibition of inferior cardiac sympathetic nerve activity [455] and renal sympathetic nerve activity [459]. Microiontophoresis of either 5-HT or 8-OH DPAT directly inhibits the firing of lateral tegmental field sympathoexcitatory neurons [455].

The data described above suggests that the lateral tegmental field plays an important role in the sympathoinhibitory action of 5-HT$_{1A}$ receptor agonists. This is confirmed in experiments in which the lateral tegmental field was lesioned using the excitatory amino acid kainic acid. 8-OH DPAT fails to lower arterial blood pressure, heart rate, inferior cardiac sympathetic nerve activity, or renal nerve activity in animals with histologically verified lateral tegmental field kainic acid lesion. In contrast, the α_2-receptor agonist clonidine decreases blood pressure and sympathetic activity in the kainic lesioned animal [28, 459, 460]. Interestingly, kainic acid lesions of the lateral tegmental field attenuate the hypotensive effects of 8-OH DPAT applied to the ventral surface of the medulla [461]. Activity of drugs applied to the ventral surface has been used as evidence for an action in the ventrolateral medulla. However, at least in this case, the integrity of the lateral tegmental field is needed for the expression of the sympatholytic effects of 8-OH DPAT applied onto the ventral surface of the medulla.

5.5   Nucleus ambiguus

The nucleus ambiguus is the site of origin of most vagal motoneurons which innervate the heart, although some cardiac vagal motoneurons are located in the dorsal motor nucleus of the vagus [462–466]. The nucleus ambiguus lies in the ventrolateral medulla medial to the subretrofacial area described above. Electrophysiological studies indicate that cardiac vagal motoneurons fire with both a cardiac and respiratory rhythm (see ref [321] for review). The baroreceptor input to cardiac vagal motoneurons in nucleus ambiguus comes directly from the NTS [467–469]. In an analogous manner with the sympathetic arm of the reflex, it appears that the pathway from the NTS to nucleus ambiguus vagal motoneurons is mediated by a excitatory amino acid. In this regard, microinjection of kynurenic acid into the nucleus ambiguus blocks the vagal component of the baroreceptor reflex [159]. The respiratory rhythmicity observed in these neurons is a consequence of inhibition during inspiration. This inhibitory effect may be mediated by acetylcholine since it is abolished by atropine [470]. A number of other neurotransmitters likely are involved in regulating the firing of vagal motoneurons. Perhaps the best studied of these is 5-HT. The nucleus ambiguus and the dorsal vagal motor nucleus receive a dense input from 5-HT containing neurons [171]. Neuronal perikarya and the dendrites of cardiac vagal motoneurons are often found to be ensheathed in 5-HT-immunoreactive axonal boutons, and synaptic specializations exist between these boutons and cardiac vagal motoneurons [464]. Finally, a dense concentration of $5-HT_{1A}$ receptors are located in both the nucleus ambiguus and the dorsal motor vagal nucleus [471–473].

$5-HT_{1A}$ receptor agonists inhibit sympathetic activity and stimulate vagal activity (for review see ref [69]). The bradycardic effect of $5-HT_{1A}$ receptor agonists is blocked by atropine or vagotomy, indicating these drugs stimulate the vagus [474–476]. A great deal of evidence indicates that the vagal stimulatory effect of $5-HT_{1A}$ receptor agonists results from a direct effect on vagal motoneurons located in the nucleus ambiguus and in the dorsal vagal motor nucleus. Microinjection of 5-HT into nucleus ambiguus of the cat produces a vagal bradycardia [477]. This effect is mimicked by microinjection of 8-OH DPAT [478]. In the rat i.c.v. administration of 5-HT elicits a vagal bradycardia [479]. Microinjections of 8-OH DPAT or flesinoxan into the dorsal vagal motor nucleus decreased heart rate in the rat [480]. Similarly, microinjection of 8-OH DPAT into the rat nucleus ambiguus elicits a vagal-mediated bradycardia (Calaresu, personal communication). Interestingly, tolerance develops rapidly to the vagal bradycardic effects of $5-HT_{1A}$ receptor agonists in cats and man [481–482]. Taken together, these data suggest that $5-HT_{1A}$ agonists elicit a vagal-mediated bradycardia via a direct action on vagal preganglionic motoneurons. 5-HT in the nucleus ambiguus plays an important role in the bradycardia elicited during the von Bezold-Jarisch reflex and during upper airway exposure with smoke [483–484].

6   Conclusions

It is apparent that a tremendous leap in our knowledge of the anatomy and functional importance of central pathways involved in autonomic regulation has occurred in the last decade. The neuronal innervation of sympathetic preganglionic neurons is well understood as is the role of neurotransmitters which regulate the activity of these neurons. It has become apparent that as a general rule excitatory amino acids function as the primary fast-acting excitatory neurotransmitter while GABA keeps the system in check by providing a tonic inhibitory input. For example, excitatory amino acids function as the "output" neurotransmitter in critical autonomic nuclei such as the subretrofacial nucleus and the NTS. GABA tonically inhibits neurons in these nuclei. Other neurotransmitters including neuropeptides and monoamines likely play a modulatory role. To take one example, 5-HT has been shown to innervate and alter the firing of neurons in virtually all nuclei described in this review. However, 5-HT neurons which innervate autonomic nuclei discharge in a regular manner and receive no known cardiovascular afferent inputs. Thus, it is reasonable to assume that 5-HT, along with other monoamines and neuropeptides, function to set the excitability of target autonomic neurons located in areas such as the subretrofacial nucleus and the intermediolateral cell column. The long time course of action of monoamines and neuropeptides support the view that these neurotransmitters function to regulate excitability over a long period of time and allow neurons involved in autonomic regulation to function in accordance with the state of vigilance of the animal. In this regard, virtually all the studies described in this review were performed in anesthetized animals. The relative contributions of specific neurotransmitters to autonomic control in conscious functioning animals is virtually unknown.

I will finish on a speculative note. Early in my scientific career I always viewed "species variation" as an easy way to explain inexplicable results. Over the years I have softened this view considerably. While writing this review I had the pleasure of having dinner with Gerry Gebber, Sue Barman and Patrice Guyenet. Needless to say this group provided an entertaining and stimulating discussion. Conversation turned to sympathetic rhythms. Sympathetic nerve activity is characterized by a 2- to 6-Hz and a 10-Hz rhythm in the cat. In the rat a 10-Hz rhythm has not been described and apparently does not exist. We have noted that spontaneous shifts in the frequency of sympathetic activity from a 2- to 6-Hz to a 10-Hz rhythm produces profound increases in arterial blood pressure without increasing the total power in sympathetic activity (unpublished observation). This suggests that the 10-Hz rhythm may be a more effective means to ultimately produce vasoconstriction than slower rhythms of sympathetic activity. Small animals such as the rat may not require such a high frequency rhythm generator since the rapid heart rate in a small animal would result in a high frequency rhythm in sympathetic activity due to the waxing and waning of baroreceptor-mediated inhibition. Thus no organized oscillating network of neurons may be required in small animals. In this regard, no organized oscillator was noted in baroreceptor denervated rats (G.L. Gebber, personal communication). If correct, it is likely that the neural circuitry involved in cardiovascular regulation is considerably different in small and large animals. In this regard several important differences in neuronal organization have been noted between the cat and the rat.

References

1   G. L. Gebber: Brainstem systems involved in cardiovascular regulation. In: W.C. Randall (Ed.): Nervous control of cardiovascular function. Oxford: Oxford University Press, 1984: 346–368.
2   R.B. McCall: Effects of putative neurotransmitters on sympathetic preganglionic neurons. In: R.M. Berne (Ed.): Annual Reviews of Physiology, vol. 50. Palo Alto: Annual Reviews Inc., 1988: 553–564.
3   P.G. Guyenet: Role of the ventral medulla oblongata in blood pressure regulation. In: A.D. Loewy and K.M. Spyer (Eds.): Central Regulation of Autonomic Functions, Oxford: Oxford Univ. Press, 1990, 145–167.
4   R.B. McCall: Role of neurotransmitters in the central regulation of the cardiovascular system. In: E. Jucker (Ed.): Prog. Drug Res. Basel: Birkhäuser Verlag, 1990; 25–84.
5   R.A.L. Dampney: Functional organization of central pathways regulating the cardiovascular system. Physiol. Rev. 1994: 74, 323–364.
6   R.A.L. Dampney: The subretrofacial vasomotor nucleus: anatomical, chemical and pharmacological properties and role in cardiovascular regulation. Prog. in Neurobiol. 1994; 42: 197–227.
7   J.B. Cabot: Sympathetic preganglionic neurons: cytoarchitecture, ultrastructure, and biophysical properties. In: A.D. Loewy and K.M. Spyer (Eds.): Central Regulation of Autonomic Functions, Oxford: Oxford Univ. Press, 1990, 22–34.
8   J.H. Coote: The organization of cardiovascular neurons in the spinal cord. Rev. Physiol Biochem. Pharmacol. 1988; 160: 13–35.
9   C.G. Charlton and C.J. Helke: Substance P-containing medullary projections to the intermediolateral cell column: Identification with retrogradely transported rhodamine-labeled latex microspheres and immunohistochemistry. Brain Res. 1987; 418: 245–254.
10   C.J. Helke, S.C. Sayson, J.R. Keeler and C.G. Charlton: Thyrotropin-releasing hormone-immunoreactive neurons project from the ventral medulla to the intermediolateral cell column: partial coexistence with serotonin. Brain Res. 1986; 381: 1–7.
11   A.D. Loewy: Raphe pallidus and raphe obscurus projections to the intermediolateral cell column in the rat. Brain Res. 1981; 222: 129–133.
12   A.D. Loewy and S. McKellar: Serotonergic projections from the ventral medulla to the intermediolateral cell column in the rat. Brain Res. 1981; 211: 146–152.
13   M. Miura, T. Onai and K. Takayama: Projections of the upper structure to the spinal cardioacceleratory center in cats: an HRP study using a new microinjection method. J. Auton. Nerv. Syst. 1983; 7: 119–140.

14   C.A. Sasek and C.J. Helke: Enkephalin-immunoreactive neuronal projections from the medulla oblongata to the intermediolateral cell column-relationship to substance P-immunoreactive neurons. J. Comp. Neurol. 1989; 287: 484–494.

15   Z.Q. Ding, Y.-W. Li, S.L. Wesselingh and W.W. Blessing: Transneuronal labelling of neurons in rabbit brain after injection of Herpes simplex virus type 1 into the renal nerve. J. Auton. Nerv. Syst. 1993; 42: 23–31.

16   A.S. Jansen, D.G. Farwell and A.D. Loewy: Specificity of pseudorabies virus as a retrograde marker of sympathetic preganglionic neurons: implications for transneuronal labeling studies. Brain Res. 1993; 617: 103–112.

17   A.M. Strack, W.B. Sawyer, J.H. Hughes, K.B. Platt and A.D. Loewy: A general pattern of CNS innervation of the sympathetic outflow demonstrated by transneuronal pseudorabies viral infections. Brain Res. 1989; 491: 156–162.

18   A.M. Strack, W.B. Sawyer, K.B. Platt and A.D. Loewy: CNS cell groups regulating the sympathetic outflow to adrenal gland as revealed by transneuronal cell body labeling with pseudorabies virus. Brain Res. 1989; 491: 274–296.

19   S.L. Wesselingh, Y.W. Li and W.W. Blessing: PNMT-containing neurons in the rostral medulla oblongata (C1, C3 groups are transneuronally labelled after injection of herpes simplex virus type 1 into the adrenal gland. Neurosci. Lett. 1989; 106: 99–104.

20   P. Carrive, R. Bandler and R.A.L. Dampney: Anatomical evidence that hypertension associated with the defence reaction in the cat is mediated by a direct projection from a restricted portion of the midbrain periaqueductal grey to the subretrofacial nucleus of the medulla. Brain Res. 1988; 460: 339–345.

21   R.A.L. Dampney, J. Czachurski, K. Dembowsky, A.K. Goodchild and H. Seller: Afferent connections and spinal projections of the vasopressor region in the rostral ventrolateral medulla of the cat. J. Auton. Nerv. Syst. 1987; 20: 73–86.

22   R.A.L. Dampney, A.K. Goodchild, L.G. Robertson and W. Montgomery: Role of ventrolateral medulla in vasomotor regulation: a correlative anatomical and physiological study. Brain Res. 1982; 249: 223–235.

23   C.A. Ross, D.A. Ruggiero and D.J. Reis: Projections from the nucleus tractus solitarii to the rostral ventrolateral medulla. J. Comp. Neurol. 1985; 242: 511–534.

24   K. Takayama, J. Okada and M. Muira: Evidence that neurons of the central amygdaloid nucleus directly project to the site concerned with circulatory and respiratory regulation in the ventrolateral nucleus of the cat – a WGA-HRP study. Neurosci. Lett. 1990; 109: 241–246.

25   A.M. Allen and P.G. Guyenet: Alpha 2-adrenoceptor-mediated inhibition of bulbospinal barosensitive cells of rat rostral medulla. Am. J. Physiol. 1993; 265: R1065–R1075.

26   N. Koshiya, D.H. Huangfu and P.G. Guyenet: Ventrolateral medulla and sympathetic chemoreflex in the rat. Brain Res. 1993; 609: 174–184.

27   S.K. Agarwal and F.R. Calaresu: Monosynaptic connection from caudal to rostral ventrolateral medulla in the baroreceptor reflex pathway. Brain Res. 1991; 555: 70–74.

28   M.E. Clement and R.B. McCall: Impairment of baroreceptor reflexes following kainic acid lesions of the lateral tegmental field. Brain Res. 1993; 618: 328–332.

29   C. Dean and J.H. Coote: A ventromedullary relay involved in the hypothalamic and chemoreceptor activation of sympathetic postganglionic neurones to skeletal muscle, kidney and splanchnic area. Brain Res. 1986; 377: 279–285.

30   A.R. Granata, D.A. Ruggiero, D.H. Park, T.H. Joh and D.J. Reis: Lesions of epinephrine neurons in the rostral ventrolateral medulla abolish the vasodepressor components of baroreflex and cardiopulmonary reflex. Hypertension 1983; 5: V80–V84.

31   A.R. Granata, D.A. Ruggiero, D.H. Park, T.H. Joh and D.J. Reis: Brain stem area with C1 epinephrine neurons mediates baroreflex vasodepressor responses. Am. J. Physiol. 1985; *248*: H547–H567.

32   R.M. McAllen: Mediation of fastigial pressor response and a somatosympathetic reflex by ventral medullary neurones in the cat. J. Physiol. 1985; *368*: 423–433.

33   R.L. Stornetta, S.F. Morrison, D.A. Ruggiero and D.J. Reis: Neurons of rostral ventrolateral medulla mediate somatic pressor reflex. Am. J. Physiol. 1989; *256*: R448–R462.

34   A.M. Strack, W.B. Sawyer, L.M. Marubio and A.D. Loewy: Spinal origin of sympathetic preganglionic neurons in the rat. Brain Res. 1988; *455*: 187–191.

35   M.B. Hancock: Separate populations of lumbar preganglionic neurons identified with the retrograde transport of HRP and 4,6-diamidine-phenylindole (DAPI). J. Auton. Nerv. Syst. 1982; *5*: 135–143.

36   Y.-W. Li, Z.Q. Ding, S.I. Wesselingh and W.W. Blessing: Renal and adrenal sympathetic preganglionic neurons in rabbit spinal cord-tracing with herpes simplex virus. Brain Res. 1992; *573*: 147–152.

37   J.L. Henry and F.R. Calaresu: Topography and numerical distribution of neurons of the thoraco-lumbar intermediolateral nucleus. J. Comp. Neurol. 1972; *144*: 205–214.

38   B.J. Oldfield and E.M. McLachlan: An analysis of the sympathetic preganglionic neurons projecting from the upper thoracic spinal roots of the cat. J. Comp. Neurol. 1981; *196*: 329–346.

39   T.A. Rando, C.W. Bowers and R.E. Zigmond: Localization of neurons in the rat spinal cord which project to the superior cervical ganglion. J. Comp. Neurol. 1981; *196*: 73–83.

40   S.J. Bacon and A.D. Smith: Preganglionic sympathetic neurones innervating the rat adrenal medulla: immunocytochemical evidence of synaptic input from nerve terminals containing substance P, GABA or 5-hydroxytryptamine. J. Auton. Nerv. Syst. 1988; *24*: 97-122.

41   C.J. Forehand: Morphology of sympathetic preganglionic neurons in the neonatal rat spinal cord-an intracellular horseradish peroxidase study. J. Comp. Neurol. 1990; *298*: 334–342.

42   P.L. Vera, B.E. Hurwitz and N. Schneiderman: Sympathoadrenal preganglionic neurons in the adult rabbit send their dendrites into the contralateral hemicord. J. Auton. Nerv. Syst. 1990; *30*: 193–198.

43   T.L. Krukoff: Coexistence of neuropeptides in sympathetic preganglionic neurons of the cat. Peptides 1987; *8*: 109-112.

44   T.L. Krukoff, J. Ciriello and F.R. Calaresu: Segmental distribution of peptide- and 5-HT-like immunoreactivity in nerve terminals and fibers of the thoracolumbar sympathetic nuclei of the cat. J. Comp. Neurol. 1985; *240*: 103–116.

45   R.B. McCall: Serotonergic excitation of sympathetic preganglionic neurons: a microiontophoretic study. Brain Res. 1983; *289*: 121–127.

46   L.C. Weaver and R.D. Stein: Effects of spinal cord transection on sympathetic discharge in decerebrate-unanesthetized cats. Am. J. Physiol. 1989; *257*: R1506–1511.

47   J.H. Coote and D.R. Westbury: Intracellular recordings from sympathetic preganglionic neurones. Neurosci. Lett. 1979; *15*: 171–176.

48   K. Dembowsky, J. Czachurski and H. Seller: An intracellular study of the synaptic input to sympathetic preganglionic neurones of the third thoracic segment of the cat. J. Auton. Nerv. Syst. 1985; *13*: 201–244.

49   E.M. McLachlan and G.D.S. Hirst: Some properties of preganglionic neurons in upper thoracic spinal cord of the cat. J. Neurophysiol. 1980; *43*: 1251–1265.

50   I.J. Llewellyn-Smith, K.D. Phend, J.B. Minson, P.M. Pilowsky and J.P. Chalmers: Glutamate-immunoreactive synapses on retrogradely-labelled sympathetic preganglionic neurons in rat thoracic spinal cord. Brain Res. 1992; *581*: 67–80.

51   S.F. Morrison, J. Callaway, T.A. Milner and D.J. Reis: Glutamate in the spinal sympathetic intermediolateral nucleus: localization by light and electron microscopy. Brain Res. 1989; *503*: 5–15.

52   S.F. Morrison, P. Ernsberger, T.A. Milner, J.Callaway, A.Gong and D.J. Reis: A glutamate mechanism in the intermediolateral nucleus mediates sympathoexcitatory responses to stimulation of the rostral ventrolateral medulla. In: J. Ciriello, M. M. Caverson and C. Polosa (Eds.): Central Neural Organization of Cardiovascular Control. Progress in Brain Research. Amsterdam: Elsevier, 1989: vol. 81, 159–169.

53   N. Bogan, A. Mennone and J.B. Cabot: Light microscopic and ultrastructural localization of GABA-like immunoreactive input to retrogradely labeled sympathetic preganglionic neurons. Brain Res. 1989; *505*: 257–270.

54   T. Chiba and R. Semba: Immuno-electron microscopic studies on the gamma-aminobutyric acid and glycine receptor in the intermediolateral nucleus of the thoracic spinal cord of rats and guinea pigs. J. Auton. Nerv. Syst. 1991; *36*: 173–182.

55   J.B. Cabot, V. Alessi and A. Bushnell: Glycine-like immunoreactive input to sympathetic preganglionic neurons. Brain Res. 1992; *571*: 1–18.

56   T. Chiba and S. Masuko: Direct synaptic contacts of catecholamine axons on the preganglionic sympathetic neurons in the rat thoracic spinal cord. Brain Res. 1986; *380*: 405–408.

57   T. Chiba and S. Masuko: Synaptic structure of the monoamine and peptide nerve terminals in the intermediolateral nucleus of the guinea pig thoracic spinal cord. J. Comp. Neurol. 1987; *262*: 242–255.

58   H. Bernstein-Goral and M.C. Bohn: Phenylethanolamine N-methyltransferase-immunoreactive terminals synapse on adrenal preganglionic neurons in the rat spinal cord. Neuroscience 1989; *32*: 521–537.

59   T.A. Milner, S.F. Morrison, C. Aboate and D.J. Reis: Phenylethanolamine N-methyl-transferase-containing terminals synapse directly on sympathetic preganglionic neurons in the rat. Brain Res. 1988; *448*: 205–222.

60   T. Chiba: Direct synaptic contacts of 5-hydroxytryptamine-, neuropeptide Y-, and somatostatin-immunoreactive nerve terminals on the preganglionic sympathetic neurons of the guinea pig. Neurosci. Lett. 1989; *105*: 281–286.

61   P. Poulat, L. Marlier, N. Rajaofetra and A. Privat: 5-hydroxytryptamine, substance P and thyrotropin-releasing hormone synapses in the intermediolateral cell column of the rat thoracic spinal cord. Neurosci. Lett. 1992; *136*: 19–22.

62   P.L. Vera, V.R. Holets and K.E. Miller: Ultrastructural evidence of synaptic contacts between substance-P-immunoreactive, enkephalin-immunoreactive, and serotonin-immunoreactive terminals and retrogradely labeled sympathetic preganglionic neurons in the rat-a study using a double-peroxidase procedure. Synapse 1990; *6*: 221–229.

63   P. Pilowsky, I.J. Llewellyn-Smith, J. Lipski and J. Chalmers: Substance P immunoreactive boutons form synapses with feline sympathetic preganglionic neurons. J. Comp. Neurol. 1992; *320*: 121–135.

64   I.J. Llewellyn-Smith, J.B. Minson, D.A. Morilak, J.R. Oliver and J.P. Chalmers: Neuropeptide Y-immunoreactive synapses in the intermediolateral cell column of rat and rabbit thoracic spinal cord. Neurosci. Lett. 1990; *108*: 243–248.

65 Y.-W. Li, Z.Q. Ding, S.L. Wesselingh and W.W. Blessing: Renal sympathetic preganglionic neurons demonstrated by herpes simplex virus transneuronal labelling in the rabbit: close apposition of neuropeptide Y-immunoreactive terminals. Neuroscience 1993; *53*: 1143–1152.

66 P.G. Galabov: Ultrastructural localization of angiotensin II-like immunoreactivity in the vegetative networks of the spinal cord of the guinea pig. J. Auton. Nerv. Syst. 1992; *40*: 215–222.

67 N.M. Appel and R.P. Elde: The intermediolateral cell column of the thoracic spinal cord is comprised of target-specific subnuclei: evidence from retrograde transport studies and immunohistochemistry. J. Neurosci. 1988; *8*: 1767–1775.

68 R.B. McCall and M.E. Clement: Identification of serotonergic and sympathetic neurons in medullary raphe nuclei. Brain Res. 1989; *477*: 172–182.

69 R.B. McCall and M.E. Clement: Role of serotonin$_{1A}$ and serotonin$_2$ receptors in the central regulation of the cardiovascular system. Pharmacol. Rev. 1994; *46*: 231–243.

70 C.A. Fornal and B.L. Jacobs: Physiological and behavioral correlates of serotonergic single-unit activity. In: N.N. Osborne and M. Hamon (Eds.): Neuronal serotonin, Chichester: John Wiley and Sons Ltd., 1988.

71 H. Inokuchi, M. Yoshimura, C. Polosa and S. Nishi: Adrenergic receptors (α_1 and α_2) modulate different potassium conductances in sympathetic preganglionic neurons. Can. J. Physiol. Pharmacol. 1992; *70*: S92–S97.

72 S.B. Backman and J.L. Henry: Effects of substance P and thyrotropin-releasing hormone on sympathetic preganglionic neurones in the thoracic intermediolateral nucleus of the cat. Can J Physiol Pharmacol. 1983; *62*: 248–251.

73 M.P. Gilbey, K.E. McKenna and L.P. Schramm: Effects of substance P on sympathetic preganglionic neurones. Neurosci Lett. 1983; *41*: 157–159.

74 R.B. McCall: Serotonergic excitation of sympathetic preganglionic neurons: a microiontophoretic study. Brain Res. 1983; *289*: 121–127.

75 S. Nishi, M. Yoshimura and C. Polosa: Synaptic potentials and putative transmitter actions in sympathetic preganglionic neurons. In: J. Ciriello, F.R. Calaresu, L.P. Renaud and C. Polosa (Eds.): Organization of the autonomic nervous system: central and peripheral mechanisms. New York: Alan Liss Inc. 1987; 15–26.

76 H. Inokuchi, M. Yoshimura, S. Yamada, C. Polosa and S. Nishi: Fast excitatory postsynaptic potentials and the responses to excitant amino acids of sympathetic preganglionic neurons in the slice of the cat spinal cord. Neuroscience 1992; *46*: 657–667.

77 P.G. Guyenet, M.-K. Sun and D.L. Brown: Role of GABA and excitatory aminoacids in medullary baroreflex pathway. In: J. Ciriello, F.R. Calaresu, L.P. Renaud, and C. Polosa (Eds.): Organization of the autonomic nervous system: central and peripheral mechanisms. New York: Alan Liss Inc. 1987; 215–225.

78 J. Minson, P. Pilowsky, I.J. LLewellyn-Smith, T. Kaneko, V. Kapoor and J.P. Chalmers: Glutamate in spinally projecting neurons of the rostral ventral medulla. Brain Res. 1991; *555*: 326–331.

79 O. Johansson, T. Hokfelt and B. Pernow et al.: Immunohistochemical support for three putative transmitters in one neuron: co-existence of 5-hydroxytryptamine, substance P and thyrotropin releasing hormone-like immunoreactivity in medullary neurons projecting to the spinal cord. J. Neurosci. 1981; *6*: 1857–1881.

80 R.B. McCall and G.K. Aghajanian: Serotonergic facilitation of facial motoneuron excitation. Brain Res. 1979; *169*: 11–27.

81 D.I. Lewis and J.H. Coote: Excitation and inhibition of rat sympathetic preganglionic neurones by catecholamines. Brain Res. 1990; *530*: 229–234.

82   H. Inokuchi, M. Yoshimura, A. Trzebski, C. Polosa and S. Nishi: Fast inhibitory post-synaptic potentials and responses to inhibitory amino acids of sympathetic preganglionic neurons in the adult cat. J. Auton. Nerv. Syst. 1992; *41*: 53–60.

83   R.B. McCall, G.L. Gebber and S.M. Barman: Spinal interneurons in the baroreceptor reflex arc. Am. J. Physiol. 1977; *232*: H657–H665.

84   S.B. Backman and J.L. Henry: Effects of GABA and glycine on sympathetic preganglionic neurons in the upper thoracic intermediolateral nucleus of the cat. Brain Res. 1983; *277*: 365–369.

85   F.J. Gordon: Spinal GABA receptors and central cardiovascular control. Brain Res. 1985; *328*: 165–169.

86   D. Blottner and H.G. Baumgarten: Nitric oxide synthetase (NOS)-containing sympathoadrenal cholinergic neurons of the rat IML cell column: evidence from histochemistry, immunohistochemistry, and retrograde labeling. J. Comp. Neurol. 1992; *316*: 45–55.

87   J.A. Gally, P.R. Montague, G.N. Reeke and G.M. Edelman: The NO hypothesis: possible effects of a short-lived, rapidly diffusible signal in the development and function of the nervous system. Proc. Natl. Acad. Sci. 1990; *87*: 3547–3551.

88   J. Garthwaite: Glutamate, nitric oxide and cell-cell signalling in the nervous system. Trends Neurosci. 1991; *14*: 60–67.

89   C.A. Ross, D.A. Ruggerio, D.H. Park, et al.: Tonic vasomotor control by the rostral ventrolateral medulla: effect of electrical or chemical stimulation of the area containing C1 adrenaline neurons on arterial pressure, heart rate and plasma catecholamines and vasopressin. J. Neurosci. 1984; *4*: 474–494.

90   R.A.L. Dampney, A.K. Goodchild, L.G. Robertson and W. Montgomery: Role of ventrolateral medulla in vasomotor regulation: a correlative anatomical and physiological study. Brain Res. 1982; *249*: 223–235.

91   P.J. Gad, W.P. Norman, A.M.T. Da Salve and R.A. Gills: Cardiorespiratory effects produced by microinjecting L-glutamic acid into medullary nuclei associated with the ventral surface of the feline medulla. Brain Res. 1986; *381*: 281–288.

92   R.N. Willette, P.P. Barcas, A.J. Krieger and H.N. Sapru: Vasopressor and depressor areas in the rat medulla: identification by microinjection of L-glutamate. Neuropharmacol. 1983; *22*: 1071–1079.

93   R.N. Willette, S. Punnen-Grandy, A.J. Krieger, H.N. Sapru: Differential regulation of regional vascular resistance by the rostral and caudal ventrolateral medulla in the rat. J. Auton. Nerv. Syst. 1987; *18*: 143–151.

94   W. Feldberg and P.G. Guertzenstein: A vasodepressor effect of pentobarbitone sodium. J. Physiol. 1972; *224*: 83–103.

95   P.G. Guertzenstein and A. Silver: Fall in blood pressure from discrete regions of the ventral surface of the medulla by glycine and lesions. J. Physiol. 1974; *242*: 489–503.

96   R.A. Dampney and E.A. Moon: Role of ventrolateral medulla in vasomotor response to cerebral ischemia. Am. J. Physiol. 1980; *239*: H349–H358.

97   E.E. Benarroch, A.R. Granata, D. Ruggiero, D.H. Park and D.J. Reis: Neurons of the C1 area mediate cardiovascular responses initiated form the ventral medullary surface. Am J Physiol. 1986; *250*: R932-R945.

98   S.M. Barman and G.L. Gebber: Basis for the naturally occurring activity of rostral ventrolateral medullary sympathoexcitatory neurons. In: J. Ciriello, M.M. Caverson and C. Polosa (Eds.): Central Neuronal Organization of Cardiovascular Control. Progress in Brain Research. Amsterdam: Elsevier, 1989: vol. 81, 117–129.

99   S.M. Barman and G.L. Gebber: Axonal projection patterns of ventrolateral medullospinal sympathoexcitatory neurons. J. Neurophysiol. 1985; *53*: 1551–1566.

100   D.L. Brown and P.G. Guyenet: Cardiovascular neurons of brainstem with projections to spinal cord. Am. J. Physiol. 1984; *247*: R1009–R1016.

101   P.G. Guyenet and D.L. Brown: Nucleus paragigantocellularis lateralis and lumbar sympathetic discharge in the rat. Am. J. Physiol. 1986; *250*: R1081–R1094.

102   R.M. McAllen: Identification and properties of subretrofacial bulbospinal neurones: a descending cardiovascular pathway in the cat. J. Auton. Nerv. Syst. 1986; *17*: 151–164.

103   R.B. McCall: Lack of involvement of GABA in baroreceptor-mediated sympathoinhibition. Am. J. Physiol. 1986; *253*: R1065–R1073.

104   R.B. McCall: GABA-mediated inhibition of sympathoexcitatory neurons by midline medullary stimulation. Am. J. Physiol. 1988; *255*: R605-R615.

105   M.-K. Sun and P.G. Guyenet: GABA-mediated baroreceptor inhibition of reticulospinal neurons. Am. J. Physiol. 1985; *249*: R672-R680.

106   S.M. Barman and G.L. Gebber: Lateral tegmental field neurons play a permissive role in governing the 10-Hz rhythm in sympathetic nerve discharge. Am. J. Physiol. 1993; *265*: R1006–R1013.

107   S.M. Barman, G.L. Gebber and S. Zhong: The 10-Hz rhythm in sympathetic nerve discharge. Am. J. Physiol. 1992; *262*: R1006–1014.

108   S.M. Barman, H.S. Orer and G.L. Gebber: Caudal ventrolateral medullary neuron are elements of the network responsible for 10-Hz rhythm in sympathetic nerve discharge. J. Neurophysiol. 1994; *72*: 106–120.

109   S.M. Barman and G.L. Gebber: Rostral ventrolateral medullary and caudal medullary raphe neurons with activity correlated to the 10-Hz rhythm in sympathetic nerve discharge. J. Neurophysiol. 1992; *68*: 1535–1547.

110   S. Zhong, S.M. Barman and G.L. Gebber: Effects of brain stem lesions on 10-Hz and 2- to 6-Hz rhythms in sympathetic nerve discharge. Am. J. Physiol. 1992; *262*: R1015–R1024.

111   S.M. Barman and G.L. Gebber: Lateral tegmental field neurons of cat medulla: a source of basal activity of ventrolateral medullospinal sympathoexcitatory neurons. J. Neurophysiol. 1987; *57*: 1410–1424.

112   D.L. Brown and P.G. Guyenet: Electrophysiological study of cardiovascular neurons in the rostral ventrolateral medulla in rats. Circ. Res. 1985; *56*: 359–369.

113   R.M. McAllen: Actions of carotid chemoreceptors on subretrofacial bulbospinal neurons in the cat. J. Auton. Nerv. Syst. 1992; *40*: 181–188.

114   S.F. Morrison and D.J. Reis: Reticulospinal vasomotor neurons in the RVL mediate the somatosympathetic reflex. Am. J. Physiol. 1989; *256*: R1084–R1097.

115   Y. Saeki, N. Terui and M. Kumada: Participation of ventrolateral medullary neurons in the renal-sympathetic reflex in rabbits. Jpn. J. Physiol. 1988; *38*: 267–281.

116   L. Salve-Carvalho, J.F.R. Paton, G.E. Goldsmith and K.M. Spyer: The effects of electrical stimulation of lobule IXb of the posterior cerebellar vermis on neurones within the rostral ventrolateral medulla in the anaesthetized cat. J. Auton. Nerv. Syst. 1991; *36*: 97–106.

117   M.-K. Sun: Medullospinal vasomotor neurones mediate hypotension from stimulation of prefrontal cortex. J. Auton. Nerv. Syst. 1992; *38*: 209–218.

118   M.-K. Sun and K.M. Spyer: Responses of rostroventrolateral medulla spinal vasomotor neurones to chemoreceptor stimulation in rats. J. Auton. Nerv. Syst. 1991; *33*: 79–84.

119   M.-K. Sun and K.M. Spyer: GABA-mediated inhibition of medullary vasomotor neurones by area postrema stimulation in rats. J. Physiol. 1991; *436*: 669–684.

120   M.-K. Sun and K.M. Spyer: Nociceptive inputs into rostral ventrolateral medulla spinal vasomotor neurones in rats. J. Physiol. 1991; *436*: 685–700.

121   A.J.M. Verberne and P.G. Guyenet: Midbrain central gray-influence on medullary sympathoexcitatory neurons and the baroreflex in rats. Am J. Physiol. 1992; *263*: R24–R33.

122   M.A. Vizzard, A. Standish and W.S. Ammons: Renal afferent input to the ventrolateral medulla of the cat. Am J. Physiol. 1992; *263*: R412–R422.

123   B.J. Yates, Y. Yamagata and P.S. Bolton: The ventrolateral medulla of the cat mediates vestibulosympathetic reflexes. Brain Res. 1991; *552*: 265–272.

124   B.J. Yates, Y. Goto and P.S. Bolton: Responses of neurons in the rostral ventrolateral medulla of the cat to natural vestibular stimulation. Brain Res. 1993; *601*: 255–264.

125   D.F. Cechetto and S.J. Chen: Hypothalamic and cortical sympathetic responses relay in the medulla of the rat. Am. J. Physiol. 1992; *263*: R544–R552.

126   R.A.L. Dampney: Brain stem mechanisms in the control of arterial pressure. Clin Exp. Hypertens. 1981; *3*: 379–393.

127   A.F. Sved, D.L. Mancini, J.C. Graham, A.M. Schreihofer and G.E. Hoffman: PNMT-containing neurons of the C1 cell group express c-fos in response to changes in baroreceptor input. Am. J. Physiol. 1994; *266*: R361–R367.

128   S.F. Morrison, T. A. Milner and D.J. Reis: Reticulospinal vasomotor neurons of the rat rostral ventrolateral medulla: relationship to sympathetic nerve activity and the C1 adrenergic cell group. J. Neurosci. 1988; *8*: 1286–1301.

129   J.R. Haselton and P.G. Guyenet: Electrophysiological characterization of putative C1 adrenergic neurons in the rat. Neuroscience 1989; *30*: 199–214.

130   M.-K. Sun, J.T. Hackett and P.G. Guyenet: Sympathoexcitatory neurons of rostral ventrolateral medulla exhibit pacemaker properties in the presence of a glutamate-receptor antagonist. Brain Res. 1988; *438*: 23–40.

131   M.-K. Sun, B.S. Young, J.T. Hackett and P.G. Guyenet: Rostral ventrolateral medullary neurons with intrinsic pacemaker properties are not catecholaminergic. Brain Res. 1988; *451*: 345–349.

132   I. M. Kangraga and A.D. Loewy: Whole-cell patch-clamp recordings from visualized bulbospinal neurons in the brainstem slices. Brain Res. 1994; *641*: 181–190.

133   D.J. Reis, C. Ross, A. R. Granata and D.A. Ruggiero: Role of C1 area of rostroventrolateral medulla in cardiovascular control. In: J.P. Buckley and D.M. Ferrario (Eds.): Brain peptides and catecholamines in cardiovascular regulation. New York: Raven Press, 1987; 1–14.

134   C.A. Ross, D.A. Ruggiero, T.H. Joh, D.H. Park and D.J. Reis: Rostral ventrolateral medulla: selective projections to the thoracic autonomic cell column from the region containing C1 adrenaline neurons. J. Comp. Neurol. 1984; *228*: 168–185.

135   D.C. Tucker, C.B. Saper, D.A. Ruggiero and D.J. Reis: Organization of central adrenergic pathways: I. Relationships of ventrolateral medullary projections to the hypothalamus and spinal cord. J. Comp. Neurol. 1987; *259*: 591–603.

136   J.W. Polson, G.M. Halliday, R.M. McAllen, M.J. Coleman and R.A.L. Dampney: Rostrocaudal differences in morphology and neurotransmitter content of cells in the subretrofacial vasomotor nucleus. J. Auton. Nerv. Syst. 1992; *38*: 117–138.

137   D.A. Ruggiero, S.L. Cravo, V. Arango and D.J. Reis: Central control of the circulation by the rostral ventrolateral reticular nucleus-anatomical substrates. In: J. Ciriello, M.M. Caverson and C. Polosa (Eds.): Central Neural Organization of Cardiovascular Control. Progress in Brain Research. Amsterdam: Elsevier, 1989: vol. 81, 49–79.

138   M.E. Clement and R.B. McCall: Effects of clonidine on sympathoexcitatory neurons in the rostral ventrolateral medulla. Brain Res. 1991; *550*: 353–357.

139   P.G. Guyenet and J.B. Cabot: Inhibition of sympathetic preganglionic neurons by catecholamines and clonidine: mediation by an adrenergic receptor. J. Neurosci. 1981; *1*: 908–917.

140   P.G. Guyenet and R.L. Stornetta: Inhibition of sympathetic preganglionic discharges by epinephrine and α-methylepinephrine. Brain Res. 1982; *235*: 271–283.

141   K. Kadzielawa: Inhibition of the activity of sympathetic preganglionic neurones and neurones activated by visceral afferents, by alpha-methylnoradrenaline and endogenous catecholamines. Neuropharmacol. 1983; *22*: 3–17.

142   A.V. Seybold and R.P. Elde: Receptor autoradiography in thoracic spinal cord: correlation of neurotransmitter binding sites with sympathoadrenal neurons. J. Neurosci. 1984; *4*: 2533–2542.

143   T. Miyazaki, J.H. Coote and N.J. Dun: Excitatory and inhibitory effects of epinephrine on neonatal rat sympathetic preganglionic neurons *in vitro*. Brain Res. 1989; *497*: 108–116.

144   C. Sangdee and D.N. Franz: Evidence for inhibition of sympathetic preganglionic neurons by bulbospinal epinephrine pathways. Neurosci. Lett. 1983; *37*: 167–173.

145   G.A. Head and P.R.C. Howe: Effects of 6-hydroxydopamine and the PNMT inhibitor LY134046 on pressor responses to stimulation of the subretrofacial nucleus in anaesthetized stroke-prone spontaneously hypertensive rats. J. Auton. Nerv. Syst. 1987; *18*: 213–224.

146   A.F. Sved: PNMT-containing catecholaminergic neurons are not necessarily adrenergic. Brain Res. 1989; *481*: 113–118.

147   T. Kubo and M. Kihara: Evidence of N-methyl-D-aspartate receptor-mediated modulation of the aortic baroreceptor reflex in the rat nucleus tractus solitarii. Neurosci. Lett. 1988; *87*: 69–74.

148   D. Haungfu, L.J. Hwang, T. A. Riley and P.G. Guyenet: Role of serotonin and catecholamines in sympathetic responses evoked by stimulation of rostral medulla. Am. J. Physiol. 1994; *266*: R338–R352.

149   M.K. Bazil and F.J. Gordon: Effect of blockade of spinal NMDA receptors on sympathoexcitation and cardiovascular responses produced by cerebral ischemia. Brain Res. 1991; *555*: 149–152.

150   K. Sundara and H. Sapru: NMDA receptors in the intermediolateral column of the spinal cord mediate sympathoexcitatory cardiac responses elicited from the ventrolateral medullary pressor area. Brain Res. 1991; *544*: 33–41.

151   A.R. Granata and H.T. Chang: Relationship of calbindin D–28k with afferent neurons to the rostral ventrolateral medulla in the rat. Brain Res. 1994; *645*: 265–277.

152   T.A. Milner, V.M. Pickel, S.F. Morrison and D.J. Reis: Adrenergic neurons in the rostral ventrolateral medulla: ultrastructure and synaptic relations with other transmitter-identified neurons. In: J. Ciriello, M.M. Caverson and C. Polosa (Eds.): Central Neural Organization of Cardiovascular Control. Progress in Brain Research. Amsterdam: Elsevier, 1989: vol. 81, 29–47.

153   M.-K. Sun and P.G. Guyenet: Arterial baroreceptor and vagal inputs to sympathoexcitatory neurons in rat medulla. Am. J. Physiol. 1986; *252*: R699–R709.

154   M.-K. Sun and P.G. Guyenet: Hypothalamic glutamatergic input to medullary sympathoexcitatory neurons in rats. Am. J. Physiol. 1986; *251*: R798–810.

155 V. Kapoor, D. Nakahara, R.J. Blood and J.P. Chalmers: Preferential release of neuroactive amino acids from the ventrolateral medulla of the rat *in vivo* as measured by microdialysis. Neuroscience 1990; *37*: 187–191.

156 V. Kapoor, V.J. Minson and J.P. Chalmers: Ventral medulla stimulation increases blood pressure and spinal cord amino acid release. NeuroReport 1992; *3*: 55–58.

157 T.P. Abrahams, P.J. Hornby, K.Chen, A.M. daSilva and R.A. Gills: The non-NMDA subtype of excitatory amino acid receptor plays the major role in control of cardiovascular function by the subretrofacial nucleus in cats. J. Pharmacol. Exp. Therap. 1994; *270*: 424–432.

158 Z.J. Gieroba and W.W. Blessing: Blockade of excitatory amino acid receptors in the ventrolateral medulla does not abolish the cardiovascular actions of L-glutamate. Naunyn Schmied. Arch. Pharmacol. 1993; *347*: 66–72.

159 P.G. Guyenet, T.M. Filtz and S.R. Donaldson: Role of excitatory amino acids in rat vagal and sympathetic baroreflexes. Brain Res. 1987; *407*: 272–284.

160 R.A. Gills, I.J. Namath, C. Easington, T.P. Abrahams, A. Guidotti, J.A. Quest, P. - Hamosh and A.M. Taveira-daSilva: Drug interaction with gamma-aminobutyric acid/benzodiazepine receptors at the ventral surface of the medulla results in pronounced changes in cardiorespiratory activity. J. Pharmacol. Exp. Therap. 1989; *248*: 863–870.

161 R.A.L. Dampney, W.W. Blessing and E. Tan: Origin of tonic GABAergic inputs to vasopressor neurons in the subretrofacial nucleus of the rabbit. J. Auton. Nerv. Syst. 1988; *24*: 227–239.

162 T. Kubo and M. Kihara: Studies on GABAergic mechanisms responsible for cardiovascular regulation in the rostral ventrolateral medulla of the rat. Arch. Int. Pharmacodyn. Ther. 1987; *285*: 277–287.

163 M.-K. Sun and P.G. Guyenet: GABA-mediated baroreceptor inhibition of reticulospinal neurons. Am. J. Physiol. 1985; *249*: R672–R680.

164 R.N. Willette, P.P. Barcas, A.J. Krieger and H.N. Sapru: Endogenous GABAergic mechanisms in the medulla and the regulation of blood pressure. J. Pharmacol. Exp. Therap. 1984; 230: 34–39.

165 A.J.M. Verberne and P.G. Guyenet: Medullary pathway of the Bezold-Jarisch reflex in the rat. Am. J. Physiol. 1992; *263*: R1190–R1202.

166 M. Amano and T. Kubo: Involvement of both $GABA_A$ and $GABA_B$ receptors in tonic inhibitory control of blood pressure at the rostral ventrolateral medulla of the rat. Naunyn Schmied. Arch. Pharmacol. 1993; *348*: 146–153.

167 Y.-W. Li and P.G. Guyenet: Neuronal inhibition by a $GABA_B$ receptor agonist in the rostral ventrolateral medulla of the rat. Am. J. Physiol. 1995; *268*: R428–R437.

168 R.B. McCall and S.J. Humphrey: Evidence for GABA mediation of sympathetic inhibition evoked from midline medullary depressor sites. Brain Res. 1985; *339*: 356–361.

169 D.A. Ruggiero, M.P. Meeley, M. Anwar and D.J. Reis: Newly identified GABAergic neurons in regions of the ventrolateral medulla which regulate blood pressure. Brain Res. 1985; *339*: 171–177.

170 M. Kihara and T. Kubo: Immunocytochemical localization of GABA containing neurons in the ventrolateral medulla oblongata of the rat. Histochem. 1989; *91*: 309–314.

171 H.W.M. Steinbusch: Distribution of serotonin-immunoreactivity in the central nervous system of the rat-cell bodies and terminals. Neuroscience 1981; *6*: 557–618.

172 K.B. Thor, A. Blitz-Siebert and C.J. Helke: Discrete localization of high-density 5-HT_{1A} binding sites in the midline raphe and parapyramidal region of the ventral medulla oblongata of the rat. Neurosci. Lett. 1990; *108*: 249–254.

173 R.A. Gills, K.J. Hill, J.S. Kirby, J.A. Quest, P. Hamosh, W.P. Norman and K.J. Kellar: Effect of activation of central nervous system serotonin$_{1A}$ receptors on cardiorespiratory function. J. Pharmacol. Exp. Therap. 1989; *248*: 851–857.

174 T.A. Lovick: Systemic and regional haemodynamic responses to microinjection of 5-HT agonists in the rostral ventrolateral medulla in the rat. Neurosci. Lett. 1989; *107*: 157–161.

175 A. Nosjean and P.G. Guyenet: Role of the ventrolateral medulla in the sympatholytic effect of 8-OH DPAT in rats. Am. J. Physiol. 1991; *260*: R600–R609.

176 A.K. Mandal, K.J. Kellar, and R.A. Gills: The subretrofacial nucleus: a major site of action for the cardiovascular effects of 5-HT$_{1A}$ and 5-HT$_2$ agonist drugs. In: J.R. Fozard and P.R. Saxena (Eds.): Serotonin: Molecular Biology, Receptors and Functional Effects, Birkhäuser Verlag, Basel, 1991; 289–299.

177 K.A. King and J.R. Holtman: Characterization of the effects of activation of ventral medullary serotonin receptor subtypes on cardiovascular activity and respiratory motor outflow to the diaphragm and larynx. J. Pharmacol. Exp Therap. 1990; *252*: 665–674.

178 M. Laubie, M. Drouillat, H. Dabire, C. Cherqui and H. Schmitt: Ventrolateral medullary pressor area: site of hypotensive and sympatho-inhibitory effects of 8-OH DPAT in anesthetized dogs. Eur. J. Pharmacol. 1989; *160*: 385–394.

179 M.E. Clement and R.B. McCall: Studies on the site and mechanism of the sympatholytic action of 8-OH DPAT. Brain Research 1990; *525*: 232–241.

180 D.I. Lewis and J.H. Coote: The actions of 5-hydroxytryptamine on the membrane of putative sympatho-excitatory neurones in the rostral ventrolateral medulla of the adult rat *in vitro*. Brain Research 1993; *609*: 103–109.

181 W.H. Wang and T.A. Lovick: Inhibitory serotonergic effects on rostral ventrolateral medullary neurons. Pflugers Arch. 1992; *422*: 93–97.

182 E.J. Mah and K.A. Cunningham: Electrophysiological studies of the serotonergic (5-HT) modulation of glutamate-evoked activity in amygdala neurons. Neurosci. Abst. 1993; *19*: 1554.

183 A.K. Mandal K.J. Kellar, W.P. Norman and R.A. Gills: Stimulation of serotonin$_2$ receptors in the ventrolateral medulla of the cat results in nonuniform increases in sympathetic outflow. Circ. Res. 1990; *67*: 1267–1280.

184 C. Vayssettes-Courchay, F. Bouysset, T.J. Verbeuren, M. Laubie and H. Schmitt: Quipazine-induced hypotension in anaesthetized cats is mediated by central and peripheral 5-HT$_2$ receptors: role of the ventrolateral pressor area. Europ. J. Pharmacol. 1991; *192*: 389–395.

185 M.E. Clement and R.B. McCall: Studies on the site and mechanism of the sympathoexcitatory action of 5-HT$_2$ agonists. Brain Res. 1990; *515*: 299–302.

186 Y. Yasui, D.F. Cechetto and C.B. Saper: Evidence for a cholinergic projection from the pedunculopontine tegmental nucleus to the rostral ventrolateral medulla in the rat. Brain Res. 1990; *517*: 19–24.

187 S.B. Lee, S.Y. Kim and K.W. Sung: Cardiovascular regulation by cholinergic mechanisms in rostral ventrolateral medulla of spontaneously hypertensive rats. Eur. J. Pharmacol. 1991; *205*: 117–123.

188 K. Sundaram and J. Sapru: Cholinergic nerve terminals in the ventrolateral medullary pressor area: pharmacological evidence. J. Auton. Nerv. Syst. 1988; *22*: 221–228.

189 R.N. Willette, S. Punnen, A.J. Krieger and H.N. Sapru: Cardiovascular control by cholinergic mechanisms in the rostral ventrolateral medulla. J. Pharmacol. Exp. Therap. 1984; *231*: 457–463.

190 R. Giuliano, D.A. Ruggiero, S.F. Morrison, P. Ernsberger and D.J. Reis: Cholinergic regulation of arterial pressure by the C1 area of the rostral ventrolateral medulla. J. Neurosci. 1989; 9: 923–942.

191 K. Sundaram and H. Sapru: Cholinergic nerve terminals in the ventrolateral medullary pressor area: pharmacological evidence. J. Auton. Nerv. Syst. 1988; 22: 221–228.

192 H. Sapru: Cholinergic mechanisms subserving cardiovascular function in the medulla and spinal cord. Prog. Brain Res. 1989; 81: 171–179.

193 S.P. Arneric, R. Giuliano, P. Ernsberger, M.D. Underwood and D.J. Reis: Synthesis, release and receptor binding of acetylcholine in the C1 area of the rostral ventrolateral medulla: contributions in regulating arterial pressure. Brain Res. 1990; 511: 98–112.

194 H.S. Orer, S.M. Barman, S. Zhong and G.L. Gebber: A modulatory role of central cholinergic transmission in control of the 10-Hz rhythm in sympathetic nerve discharge. Brain Res. 1994; 661: 283–288.

195 D.A. Morilak, P. Somogyi, R.A.J. McIlhinney and J.P. Chalmers: An enkephalin-containing pathway from nucleus tractus solitarius to the pressor area of the rostral ventrolateral medulla of the rabbit. Neuroscience 1989; 31: 187–194.

196 S. Punnen, R. Willette, A.J. Krieger and H.N. Sapru: Cardiovascular response to injections of enkephalin in the pressor area of the ventrolateral medulla. Neuropharmacol. 1984, 23: 939–946.

197 H.N. Sapru, S. Punnen and R.N. Willette: Role of enkephalins in ventrolateral medullary control of blood pressure. In: J.P. Buckley and C.M. Ferrario (Eds.): Brain Peptides and Catecholamines in Cardiovascular Regulation. New York: Raven, 1987; 153–167.

198 M.-K. Sun and P.G. Guyenet: Effects of vasopressin and other neuropeptides on rostral medullary sympathoexcitatory neurons in vitro. Brain Res. 1989; 492: 261–270.

199 R.W. Urbanski, J. Murugaian, A. Krieger and H.N. Sapru: Cardiovascular effects of substance P receptor stimulation in the ventrolateral medullary pressor and depressor areas. Brain. Res. 1989; 491: 383–389.

200 R.E. Gomez, M.A. Cannata, T.A. Milner, M. Anwar, D.J. Reis and D.A. Ruggiero: Vasopressinergic mechanisms in the nucleus reticularis lateralis in blood pressure control. Brain Res. 1993; 604: 90–105.

201 A.M. Allen, S.Y. Chai, P.M. Sexton, S.J. Lewis, A.J.M. Verberne, B. Jarrott, W.J. Louis, J. Clevers, M.J. McKinley, G. Paxinos and F.A.O. Mendelsohn: Angiotensin II receptors and angiotensin converting enzyme in the medulla oblongata. Hypertension 1987; 9 Suppl.: III198–III205.

202 A.M. Allen, R.A.L. Dampney and F.A.O. Mendelsohn: Angiotensin receptor binding and pressor effects in cat subretrofacial nucleus. Am J. Physiol. 1988; 255: H1011–H1017.

203 R.W. Lind, L.W. Swanson and D. Ganten: Organization of angiotensin immunoreactive cells and fibers in the rat central nervous system. Neuroendocrinology 1985; 40: 2–24.

204 G.P. Aldred, S.Y. Chai, K.-F. Song, J.-L Zhuo, D. MacGregor and F.A.O. Mendelsohn: Distribution of angiotensin receptor subtypes in the rabbit brain. Regul. Peptides 1993; 21: 119–130.

205 K.-F. Song, A.M. Allen, G. Paxinos and F.A.O. Mendelsohn: Mapping of angiotensin receptor subtype heterogeneity in rat brain. J. Comp. Neurol. 1992; 316: 467–484.

206 S. Sasaki and R.A. Dampney: Tonic cardiovascular effects of angiotensin II in the ventrolateral medulla. Hypertension 1990; 15: 274–283.

207   H. Muratani, C.M. Ferrario and D.B. Averill: Ventrolateral medulla in spontaneously hypertensive rats-role of angiotensin II. Am J. Physiol. 1993; *264*: R388–R395.

208   S. Sasaki, Y.W. Li and R.A. Dampney: Comparison of the pressor effects of angiotensin II and III in the rostral ventrolateral medulla. Brain Res. 1993; *600*: 335–338.

·209 Y.-W. Li, J.W. Polson and R.A. Dampney: Angiotensin II excites vasomotor neurons but not respiratory neurons in the rostral and caudal ventrolateral medulla. Brain Res. 1992; *577*: 161–164.

210   Y.-W. Li and P.G. Guyenet: Neuronal excitation by angiotensin II in the rostral ventrolateral medulla of the rat *in vitro*. Am J. Physiol. 1995; *268*: R272–R277.

211   R.M. Bowker, K.N. Westlund, M.C. Sullivan, J.F. Wilber and J.D. Coulter: Descending serotonergic, peptidergic and cholinergic pathways from the raphe nuclei: a multiple transmitter complex. Brain Res. 1983; *288*: 33–48.

212   N.M. Appel, M.W. Wessendorf and R.P. Elde: Thyrotropin-releasing hormone in spinal cord: coexistence with serotonin and with substance P in fibers and terminals apposing identified preganglionic sympathetic neurons. Brain Res. 1987; *415*: 137–143.

213   D.E. Millhorn, T. Hokfelt, K. Serogy, W. Oertel, A.A.J. Verhofstad and J.-Y. Wu: Immunohistochemical evidence for colocalization of g-aminobutyric acid and serotonin in neurons of the ventral medulla oblongata projecting to the spinal cord. Brain Res. 1987; *410*: 179–185.

214   C.J. Helke, K.B. Thor and D.A. Sasek: Chemical neuroanatomy of the parapyramidal region of the ventral medulla in the rat. In: J. Ciriello, M.M. Caverson and C. Polosa (Eds.): Central Neural Organization of Cardiovascular Control. Progress in Brain Research. Amsterdam: Elsevier, 1989: vol. 81, 177–188.

215   P.R.C. Howe, D.M. Kuhn, J.B. Minson, B.H. Stead and J.P. Chalmers: Evidence for a bulbospinal serotonergic pressor pathway in the rat brain. Brain Res. 1983; *270*: 29–36.

216   G.A Head and P.R.C. Howe: Effects of 6-hydroxydopamine and the PNMT inhibitor LY134046 on pressor responses to stimulation of the subretrofacial nucleus in anaesthetized stroke-prone spontaneously hypertensive rats. J. Auton. Nerv. Syst. 1987; *18*: 213–224.

217   J.B. Minson, J.P. Chalmers, A.C. Caon and B. Renaud: Separate areas of rat medulla oblongata with populations of serotonin-and adrenaline-containing neurons alter blood pressure after L-glutamate stimulation. J. Auton. Nerv. Syst. 1987; *19*: 39–50.

218   M.W. Wessendorf and R. Elde: The coexistence of serotonin- and substance P-like immunoreactivity in the spinal cord of the rat as shown by immunofluorescent double labeling. J. Neurosci. 1987; *7*: 3252–3263.

219   C.J. Helke, J.J. Neil, V.J. Massari and A.D. Loewy: Substance P neurons project from the ventral medulla to the intermediolateral cell column in the rat. Brain Res. 1982; *243*: 147–152.

220   B.M. Davis, J.E. Krause, J.F. McKelry and J.B. Cabot: Effects of spinal lesions on substance P levels in the rat sympathetic preganglionic cell column: evidence for local spinal regulation. Neurosci. 1984; *13*: 1311–1326.

221   S.B. Backman and J.L. Henry: Effects of substance P and thyrotropin-releasing hormone on sympathetic preganglionic neurones in the thoracic intermediolateral nucleus of the cat. Can. J. Physiol. Pharmacol. 1983; *62*: 248–251.

222   M.P. Gilbey, K.E. McKenna and L.P. Schramm: Effects of substance P on sympathetic preganglionic neurones. Neurosci Lett. 1983; *41*: 157–159.

223   S.B. Backman, H. Sequeiramartinho and J.L. Henry: Adrenal versus nonadrenal sympathetic preganglionic neurones in the lower thoracic intermediolateral nucleus of

the cat: effects of serotonin, substance P, and thyrotropin-releasing hormone. Can. J. Physiol. Pharmacol. 1990; 68: 1108–1118.

224   N.J. Dun and N. Mo: *In vitro* effects of substance P on neonatal rat sympathetic preganglionic neurones. J. Physiol. 1988; 399: 321–334.

225   C.J. Helke, E.T. Phillip and J.T. ONeil: Regional peripheral and CNS hemodynamic effects of intrathecal administration of a substance P receptor agonist. J. Auton. Nerv. Syst. 1987; 21: 1–7.

226   A.P.M. Yusof and J.H. Coote: The action of a substance P antagonist on sympathetic nerve activity in the rat. Neurosci Lett. 1987; 75: 329–333.

227   J.R. Keeler, C.G. Charlton and C.J. Helke: Cardiovascular effects of spinal cord substance P: studies with a stable receptor agonist. J. Pharmacol. Exp. Therap. 1985; 233: 755–760.

228   K. Yashpal, S. Gauthier and J.L. Henry: Substance P given intrathecally at the spinal T_9 level increases arterial pressure and heart rate in the rat. J. Auton. Nerv. Syst. 1987; 18: 93–103.

229   A.D. Loewy and W.B. Sawyer: Substance P antagonist inhibit vasomotor responses elicited from ventral medulla in rat. Brain Res. 1982; 245: 379–383.

230   Y. Takano, J.E. Martin, S.E. Leeman and A.D. Loewy: Substance P immunoreactivity released from spinal cord after kainic acid excitation of the ventral medulla oblongata: a correlation with increases in blood pressure. Brain Res. 1984; 291: 168–172.

231   J.R. Keeler and C.J. Helke: Spinal cord substance P mediates bicuculline-induced activation of cardiovascular responses from the ventral medulla. J. Auton. Nerv. Syst. 1985; 13: 19–33.

232   T. Hokfelt, S. Vincent, L. Hellsten, et al.: Immunohistochemical evidence for a "neurotoxic" action of (D-Pro², D-Trp⁷·⁹) substance P, an analogue with substance P antagonistic activity. Acta Physiol. Scand. 9181; 113: 571–573.

233   C. Post, J.-A. Karlsson, F.G. Butterworth, C.G.A. Persson and G.R. Strichartz: Local anaesthetic effects of substance P (SP) analogues *in vitro*. In: C.C. Jordan and P. Oehme (Eds.): Substance P: metabolism and biological activity. London, Taylor and Francis, 1985; 227–241.

234   B.F. Cox, R.L. Schelper, F.M. Faraci and M.J. Brody: Autonomic, sensory, and motor dysfunction following intrathecal administration of three substance P antagonists. Exp. Brain Res. 1988; 70: 61–72.

235   C.J. Helke and E.T. Phillips: Substance P antagonist-induced spinal cord vasoconstriction: effects of thyrotropin-releasing hormone and substance P agonists. Peptides 1988; 9: 1307–1315.

236   D.N. Franz, B.D. Hare and K.L. McCloskey: Spinal sympathetic neurons: possible sites of opiate-withdrawal suppression by clonidine. Science 1982; 215: 11643–1645.

237   C.W. Xie, J. Tang and J.S. Han: Clonidine stimulates the release of dynorphin in the spinal cord of the rat: a possible mechanism for its depressor effects. Neurosci Lett. 1986; 65: 224–228.

238   K.E. McKenna and L.P. Schramm: Mechanisms mediating the silent period. Studies in the isolated spinal cord of the neonatal rat. Brain Res. 1985; 329: 233–240.

239   K. Amendt, J. Czachurski, K. Dembowsky and H. Seller: Bulbospinal projections to the intermediolateral cell column: a neuroanatomical study. J. Auton. Nerv. Syst. 1979; 1: 103–117.

240   S.C. Wang and S.W. Ranson: Autonomic responses to electrical stimulation of the lower brain stem. J Comp Neurol. 1939; 71: 437–455.

241   R.B. McCall and L.T. Harris: Role of serotonin and serotonin receptor subtypes in

100   Robert B. McCall

the central regulation of blood pressure. In: R.H. Rech and G.A. Gudelsky (Eds.): 5-HT agonists as psychoactive drugs, Ann Arbor: NPP Books, 1988; 1433–162.

242   R.B. McCall: Role of serotonin in the regulation of sympathetic nerve discharge. In P. Saxena, D.I. Wallis, W. Wouters and P. Bevan (Eds.): Cardiovascular Pharmacology of 5-hydroxytryptamine: prospective therapeutic applications. Dordrecht: Kluwer Academic Publishers, 1990, 271–283.

243   J.R. Adair, B.L. Hamilton, K.A. Scappaticci, C.J. Helke and R.A. Gills: Cardiovascular responses to electrical stimulation of the medullary raphe area of the cat. Brain Res. 1977; 128: 141–145.

244   R.B. McCall: Evidence for a serotonergically mediated sympathoexcitatory response to stimulation of medullary raphe nuclei. Brain Res. 1984; 311: 131–139.

245   S.F. Morrison and G.L. Gebber: Classification of raphe neurons with cardiac-related activity. Am. J. Physiol. 1982; 243: R49–R59.

246   S.F. Morrison and G.L. Gebber: Raphe neurons with sympathetic-related activity: baroreceptor responses and spinal connections. Am. J. Physiol. 1984; 246: R338–R348.

247   M.D. Hirsch and C.J. Helke: Bulbospinal thyrotropin-releasing hormone projections to the intermediolateral cell column: a double fluorescence immunohistochemical-retrograde tracing study in the rat. Neuroscience 1988; 25: 625–638.

248   R.B. Lynn, M.S. Kreider and R.R. Miselis: Thyrotropin-releasing hormone-immunoreactive projections to the dorsal motor nucleus and the nucleus of the solitary tract of the rat. J. Comp. Neurol. 1991; 311: 271–288.

248   S.F. Morrison: Raphe pallidus excites a unique class of sympathetic preganglionic neurons. Am. J. Physiol. 1993; 265: R82–R89.

250   G.K. Aghajanian and R.Y. Wang: Physiology and pharmacology of central serotonergic neurons. In: M.A. Lipton, A. DiMascio and K.F. Killam (Eds.): Psychopharmacology: A generation of progress, Raven Press, New York, 1978; 171–183.

251   W.C. DeGroat and R.W. Ryall: An excitatory action of 5-hydroxytryptamine on sympathetic preganglionic neurons. Exp Brain Research 1967; 3: 299–305.

252   D.I. Lewis, E. Sermasi and J.H. Coote: Excitatory and indirect inhibitory actions of 5-hydroxytryptamine on sympathetic preganglionic neurones in the neonate rat spinal cord in vitro. Brain Res. 1993; 610: 267–275.

253   K.B. Thor, S. Mickolaus and C.J. Helke: Autoradiographic localization of 5-hydroxytryptamine$_{1A}$, 5-hydroxytryptamine$_{1B}$, and 5-hydroxytryptamine$_{1C/2}$ binding sites in the rat spinal cord. Neuroscience 1993; 55: 235–252.

254   A.P.M. Yusoff and J.H. Coote: Excitatory and inhibitory actions of intrathecally administered 5-hydroxytryptamine on sympathetic nerve activity in the rat. J. Auton. Nerv. Syst. 1988; 222: 229–236.

255   R.B. McCall and S.J. Humphrey: Involvement of serotonin in the central regulation of blood pressure: evidence for a facilitating effect on sympathetic nerve activity. J. Pharmacol. Exp. Therap. 1982; 222: 94–102.

256   R.B. McCall and L.T. Harris: Characterization of the central sympathoinhibitory action of ketanserin. J. Pharmacol. Exp. Therap. 1987; 241: 736–740.

257   A.G. Ramage: The effects of ketanserin, methysergide and LY 53857 on sympathetic nerve activity. Eur. J. Pharmacol. 1985; 113: 295–303.

258   A.G. Ramage: Are drugs that act both on serotonin receptors and α_1-adrenoceptors more potent hypotensive agents than those that act only on α_1-adrenoceptors? J. Cardiovasc. Pharmacol. 1988; 11: S30–S34.

259   R.B. McCall, M.E. Clement and L.T. Harris: Studies on the mechanism of the sympatholytic effect of 8-OH DPAT: lack of correlation between inhibition of seroto-

nin neuronal firing and sympathetic activity. Brain Res. 1989; *501*: 73–83.

260   K.B. Thor, A. Blitz-Siebert and C.J. Helke: Autoradiographic localization of 5-HT1 binding sites in the medulla oblongata of the rat. Synapse 1992; *10*: 185–205.

261   B. Valenta and E. Singer: Hypotensive effects of 8-hydroxy–2-(di-n-propyl-amino) tetralin and 5-methylurapidil following stereotaxic microinjection into the ventral medulla of the rat. Br. J. Pharmacol. 1990; *99*: 713–720.

262   C.J. Helke, C.H. McDonald and E.T. Philips: Hypotensive effects of 5-HT(1A) receptor activation-ventral medullary sites and mechanisms of action in the rat. J. Auton. Nerv. Syst. 1993; *42*: 177–188.

263   A.G. Ramage and S.J. Wilkinson: Evidence that different regional sympathetic outflows vary in their sensitivity to the sympathoinhibitory actions of putative 5-HT$_{1A}$ and α_2 adrenoceptor agonists in anaesthetized cats. Br. J. Pharmacol. 1989; *98*: 1157–164.

264   A.G. Ramage, M.E. Clement and R.B. McCall: 8-OH DPAT-induced inhibition of renal sympathetic nerve activity and serotonin neuronal firing. Eur. J. Pharmacol. 1992; *219*: 165–167.

265   H.S. Orer, M.E. Clement, S.M. Barman, S. Zhong, G.L. Gebber and R.B. McCall: The role of serotonergic neurons in the maintenance of the 10-Hz rhythm in sympathetic nerve discharge. Am. J. Physiol. 1995; in press.

266   C.E. Byrum, R. Stornetta and P.G. Guyenet: Electrophysiological properties of spinally-projecting A5 noradrenergic neurons. Brain Res. 1984; *303*: 15–29.

267   C.E. Byrum and P.G. Guyenet: Afferent and efferent connections of the A5 noradrenergic cell group in the rat. J. Comp. Neurol. 1987; *261*: 529–542.

268   P.G. Guyenet: Central noradrenergic neurons: the autonomic connection. Prog. Brain Res. 1991; *88*: 365–380.

269   M.L. Woodruff, R.H. Baisden, D.L. Whittington and J.E. Kelly. Inputs to the pontine A5 noradrenergic cell group: a horseradish peroxidase study. Exp. Neurol. 1986; *94*: 762–778.

270   D. Huangfu, N. Koshiya and P.G. Guyenet: A5 noradrenergic unit activity and sympathetic nerve discharge in rats. Am J. Physiol. 1991; *261*: R393–R402.

271   D.L. Rosin, D. Zheng, R.L. Stornetta, F.R. Norton, T. Riley, M.D. Okusa, P.G. Guyenet and K.R. Lynch: Immunohistochemical localization of alpha 2A-adrenergic receptors in catecholaminergic and other brainstem neurons in the rat. Neuroscience 1993; *56*: 139–155.

272   P.G. Guyenet, R.L. Stornetta, T. Riley, F.R. Norton, D.L. Rosin and K.R. Lynch: Alpha 2A-adrenergic receptors are present in lower brainstem catecholaminergic and serotonergic neurons innervating spinal cord. Brain Res. 1994; *638*: 285–294.

273   G.K. Aghajanian, J.M. Cedarbaum and R.Y. Wang: Evidence for norepinephrine-mediated collateral inhibition of locus coeruleus neurons. Brain Res. 1977; *136*: 570–577.

274   B. Astier and G. Aston-Jones: Electrophysiological evidence for medullary adrenergic inhibition of rat locus coeruleus neurons. Soc. Neurosci. Abstr. 1989, *15*: 1012.

275   R. Andrade and G.K. Aghajanian: Single cell activity in the noradrenergic A5 region: Response to drugs and peripheral manipulations of blood pressure. Brain Res. 1982; *242*: 125–135.

276   P.G. Guyenet: Baroreceptor-mediated inhibition of A5 noradrenergic neurons. Brain Res. 1984; *303*: 31–40.

277   N. Koshiya and P.G. Guyenet: A5 noradrenergic neurons and the carotid sympathetic chemoreflex. Am. J. Physiol. 1994; *267*: R519–R526.

278   A.D. Loewy et al.: Electrophysiological evidence that the A5 catecholaminergic cell group is a vasomotor center. Brain Res. 1979; *178*: 196–200.

279   J.J. Neil and A.D. Loewy: Decreases in blood pressure in response to L-glutamate microinjections in the A5 catecholamine cell group. Brain Res. 1982; *241*: 271–278.

280   A.D. Loewy, L. Marson, D. Parkinson, M.A. Perry and W.B. Sawyer: Descending noradrenergic pathways involved in the A5 depressor response. Brain Res. 1986; *386*: 313–324.

281   M.L. Woodruff, R.H. Baisden and D.L. Whittington: Effects of electrical stimulation of the pontine A5 cell group on blood pressure and heart rate in the rabbit. Brain Res. 1986; *379*: 10–23.

282   K.A. Stanek, J.J. Neil, W.B. Sawyer and A.D. Loewy: Changes in regional blood flow and cardiac output after L-glutamate stimulation of A5 cell group. Am. J. Physiol. 1984; *246*: H44–H51.

283   D. Huangfu, L.J. Hwang, T.A. Riley and P.G. Guyenet: Splanchnic nerve response to A5 area stimulation in rats. Am. J. Physiol. 1992; *263*: R437–R446.

284   R.L. Stornetta, P.G. Guyenet and R. McCarty: Modulation of autonomic outflow by pontine A5 noradrenergic neurons. In: K. Nakamura (Ed.): Brain and blood pressure control, Utrecht, Elsevier Science Publishers, 1986; 23–28.

285   J.H. Coote, V.H. Macleod, S. Fleetwood-Walker and M.P. Gilbey: The response of individual sympathetic preganglionic neurones of microelectrophoretically applied endogenous monoamines. Brain Res. 1981; *215*: 1135–145.

286   R.B. McCall and M.R. Schuette: Evidence for an alpha–1 receptor-mediated central sympathoinhibitory action of ketanserin. J. Pharmacol. Exp. Therap. 1984; *228*: 704–710.

287   R.B. McCall and S.J. Humphrey: Evidence for a central depressor action of postsynaptic alpha–1 adrenergic antagonists. J. Auton. Nerv. Syst. 1981; *3*: 9–23.

288   G.K. Aghajanian and M.A. Rogawski: The physiological role of a-adrenoceptors in the CNS: new concepts from single-cell studies. Trends in Pharmacol. Sciences 1983; *4*: 315–317.

289   H. Shi, D.I. Lewis and J.H. Coote: Effects of activating spinal alpha-adrenoreceptors on sympathetic nerve activity in the rat. J. Auton. Nerv. Syst. 1988; *23*: 69–78.

290   B.D. Hare, R.J. Neuymayr and D.N. Franz: Opposite effects of L-dopa and 5-HTP on spinal sympathetic reflexes. Nature 1972; *239*: 336–337.

291   R.C. Ma and N.J. Dun: Norepinephrine depolarizes lateral horn cells of neonatal rat spinal cord *in vitro*. Neurosci Lett. 1985; *60*: 163–168.

292   M. Yoshimura, C. Polosa and S. Nishi: Noradrenaline modifies sympathetic preganglionic neuron spike and afterpotential. Brain Res. 1986; *362*: 370–374.

293   M. Yoshimura, C. Polosa and S. Nishi: Noradrenaline induces rhythmic bursting in sympathetic preganglionic neurons. Brain Res. 1987; *420*: 147–151.

294   M. Yoshimura, C. Polosa and S. Nishi: Slow IPSP and the noradrenaline-induced inhibition of the cat sympathetic preganglionic neuron *in vitro*. Brain Res. 1987; *419*: 383–386.

295   H.S. Orer, S. Zhong, S.M. Barman and G.L. Gebber: Differential control of 10-Hz and 2- to 6-Hz sympathetic nerve discharge by central adrenergic neurons. Am. J. Physiol., 1995; in press.

296   L.W. Swanson: Immunohistochemical evidence for a neurophysin-containing autonomic pathway arising in the paraventricular nucleus of hypothalamus. Brain Res. 1977; *128*: 346–353.

297   L.W. Swanson and S. McKellar: The distribution of oxytocin- and neurophysin-stained

fibers in the spinal cord of the rat and monkey. J. Comp. Neurol. 1979; *188*: 87–106.

298   W.E. Armstrong, S. Warach, G.I. Hatton and T.H. McNeil: Subnuclei in the rat hypo-
      thalamic paraventricular nucleus: a cytoarchitectural, horseradish peroxidase and
      immunocytochemical analysis. Neuroscience 1980; *5*: 1931–1958.

299   Y. Hosoya, Y. Sugiura, N. Okado, A.D. Loewy and K. Kohno: Descending input from
      the hypothalamic paraventricular nucleus to sympathetic preganglionic neurons in
      the rat. Exp. Brain Res. 1991; *85*: 10–20.

300   L.W. Swanson and H.G.J.M. Kuypers: The paraventricular nucleus of the hypothal-
      amus: cytoarchitectonic subdivisions and organization of projections to the pitui-
      tary, dorsal vagal complex, and spinal cord as demonstrated by retrograde fluores-
      cence double-labeling methods. J. Comp. Neurol. 1980; *194*: 555–570.

301   M.V. Sofroniew: Vasopressin and oxytocin in the mammalian brain and spinal cord.
      Trends in Neurosci. 1983; *5*: 467–472.

302   M.J. Brody, T.P. O'Neill and J.P. Porter: Role of paraventricular and arcuate nuclei
      in cardiovascular regulation. In: Magro A., Oswald W., Reis D., Vanhoutte P. (Eds.):
      Central and peripheral mechanisms of cardiovascular regulation, New York: Ple-
      num Press, 1986; 443–464.

303   H. Kannan and H. Yamashita: Connections of neurons in the region of the nucleus
      tractus solitarius with the hypothalamic paraventricular nucleus: their possible
      involvement in neural control of the cardiovascular system. Brain Res. 1985; *329*:
      205–212.

304   M.M. Caverson, J. Ciriello and F.R. Calaresu: Paraventricular nucleus of the hypo-
      thalamus: an electrophysiological investigation of neurons projecting directly to inter-
      mediolateral nucleus in the cat. Brain Res. 1984; *305*: 380–383.

305   T.A. Lovick and J.H. Coote: Electrophysiological properties of paraventriculo-spi-
      nal neurones in the rat. Brain Res. 1988; *454*: 123–130.

306   H. Yamashita, K. Inenaga and K. Koizumi: Possible projections from regions of par-
      aventricular and supraoptic nuclei to the spinal cord: electrophysiological studies.
      Brain Research 1984; *296*: 373–378.

307   T. Segura, E.M. Hasser, R.E. Shade and J.R. Haywood: Evidence of an endogenous
      forebrain GABAergic system capable of inhibiting baroreceptor-mediated vasopres-
      sin release. Brain Res. 1989; *499*: 53–62.

308   D.S. Martin, T. Segura and J.R. Haywood: Cardiovascular responses to bicuculline
      in the paraventricular nucleus of the rat. Hypertension 1991; *18*: 48–55.

309   D.S. Martin and J.R. Haywood: Hemodynamic responses to paraventricular nucleus
      disinhibition with bicuculline in conscious rats. Am J. Physiol. 1993; *265*: H1727–H1733.

310   M.P. Gilbey, J.H. Coote, S. Fleetwood-Walker and D.F. Peterson: The influence of
      the paraventriculo-spinal pathway, and oxytocin and vasopressin on sympathetic pre-
      ganglionic neurones. Brain Res. 1982; *251*: 283–290.

311   J.P. Porter and M.J. Brody: Neural projections from paraventricular nucleus that sub-
      serve vasomotor functions. Am. J. Physiol. 1985; *248*: R271–R281.

312   H. Yamashita, H. Kannan, M. Kasal and T. Osaka: Decrease in blood pressure by
      stimulation of the rat hypothalamic paraventricular nucleus with L-glutamate or
      weak current. J. Auton. Nerv. Syst. 1987; *19*: 229–234.

313   A.J. Gelsema, M.J. Roe and F.R. Calaresu: Neurally mediated cardiovascular
      responses to stimulation of cell bodies in the hypothalamus of the rat. Brain Res.
      1989; *482*: 67–77.

314   H. Kannan, Y. Hayashida and H. Yamashita: Increase in sympathetic outflow by par-
      aventricular nucleus stimulation in awake rats. Am J. Physiol. 1989; *256*: R1325–R1330.

315   T. Katafuchi, Y. Omura and M. Kurosawa: Effects of chemical stimulation of paraventricular nucleus on adrenal and renal nerve activity in rats. Neurosci. Lett. 1988;
86: 195–200.

316   V. Holets and R. Elde: The differential distribution and relationship of serotonergic and peptidergic fibers to sympathoadrenal neurons in the intermediolateral cell
column of the rat: a combined retrograde axonal transport and immunofluorescence
study. Neuroscience 1982; *7*: 1155–1174.

317   J. Ciriello and F.R. Calaresu: Role of paraventricular and supraoptic nuclei in central cardiovascular regulation in the cat. Am. J. Physiol. 1980; *239*: R137–R142.

318   S.B. Backman and J.L. Henry: Effects of oxytocin and vasopressin on thoracic sympathetic preganglionic neurons in the cat. Brain Res. Bull. 1984; *13*: 679–684.

319   R.C. Ma and N.J. Dun: Vasopressin depolarizes lateral horn cells of the neonatal rat
spinal cord *in vitro*. Brain Res. 1985; *348*: 36–43.

320   J.P. Porter and M.J. Brody: The paraventricular nucleus and cardiovascular regulation: role of spinal vasopressinergic mechanisms. J. Hyperten. 1986; *4* (suppl. 3):
S181–S184.

321   K.M. Spyer: Central nervous mechanisms contributing to cardiovascular control. J.
Physiol. 1994; *474*: 1–19.

322   M.J. Brody: Central nervous system mechanisms of arterial pressure regulation. Fed-
eration Proc. 1986; *45*: 2700–2706.

323   P. Sleight: Arterial baroreceptors and hypertension, Oxford: Oxford Univ. Press, 1980.

324   A. Malliani: Cardiovascular sympathetic afferent fibres. Rev. Physiol. Biochem. Pharmacol. 1982; *94*: 11–75.

325   A. Sato and R.F. Schmidt: Somatosympathetic reflexes: afferent fibres, central pathways, discharge characteristics. Physiol. Rev. 1973; *53*: 916–947.

326   J. Ciriello: Brainstem projections of aortic baroreceptor afferent fibers in the rat.
Neurosci. Lett. 1983; *36*: 37–42.

327   S. Donoghue, R.B. Fielder, D. Jordan and K.M. Spyer: The central projections of
carotid baroreceptors and chemoreceptors in the cat: a neurophysiological study. J.
Physiol. 1984; *347*: 397–411.

328   S. Donoghue, M. Garcia, D. Jordan and K.M. Spyer: Identification and brainstem
projections of aortic baroreceptor afferent neurones in nodose ganglia of cats and
rabbits. J. Physiol. 1982; *322*: 337–352.

329   J.H. Wallach and A.D. Loewy: Projections of the aortic nerve to the nucleus tractus
solitarius in the rabbit. Brain Res. 1980; *188*: 247–251.

330   J.C.W. Finley and D.M. Katz: The central organization of carotid body afferent projections to the brainstem of the rat. Brain Res. 1992; *572*: 108–116.

331   J. Ciriello, A.W. Hrycyshyn and F.R. Calaresu: Horseradish peroxidase study of brain
stem projections of carotid sinus and aortic depressor nerves in the cat. J. Auton.
Nerv. Syst. 1981; *4*: 43–61.

332   G.D. Housley, R.L. Martin-Body, N.J. Dawson and J.D. Sinclair: Brain stem projections of the glossopharyngeal nerve and its carotid sinus branch in the rat. Neuroscience 1987; *22*: 237–250.

333   S. Donoghue, R.B. Felder, M.P. Gilbey, D. Jordan and K.M. Spyer: Post-synaptic activity evoked in the nucleus tractus solitarius by carotid sinus and aortic nerve afferents in the cat. J. Physiol. 1985; *360*: 261–273.

334   H. Ichikawa, A. Rabchevsky and C.J. Helke: Presence and coexistence of putative
neurotransmitters in carotid sinus baro- and chemoreceptor afferent neurons. Brain
Res. 1993; *611*: 67–74.

335   R.M. Sykes, K.M. Spyer and P. N. Izzo: Central distribution of substance P, calcito-
      nin gene-related peptide and 5-hydroxytryptamine in vagal sensory afferents in the
      rat dorsal medulla. Neuroscience 1994; *59*: 195–210.

336   W.T. Talman, M.H. Perrone and D.J. Reis: Evidence for L-glutamate as the neuro-
      transmitter of baroreceptor afferent nerve fibers. Science 1980; *209*: 813–815.

337   W.T. Talman, A.R. Granata and D.J. Reis: Glutamatergic mechanisms in the nucleus
      tractus solitarius in blood pressure control. Fed Proc. 1984; *43*: 39–44.

338   A.R. Granata and D.J. Reis: Release of [3H]L-glutamine acid (L-Glu) and [3H]D-
      aspartic acid (D-Asp) in the area of nucleus tractus solitarius *in vivo* produced by
      stimulation of the vagus nerve. Brain Res. 1983; *259*: 77–93.

339   M.P. Meeley, M.D. Underwood, W.T. Talman and D.J. Reis: Content and *in vitro*
      release of endogenous amino acids in the area of the nucleus of the solitary tract of
      the rat. J. Neurochem. 1989; *53*: 1807–1817.

340   W.T. Talman, M.H. Perrone, P. Scher, S. Kwo and D.J. Reis: Antagonism of the baro-
      receptor reflex by glutamate diethyl ester, an antagonist to L-glutamate. Brain Res.
      1981; *217*: 186–191.

341   S.J. Humphrey and R.B. McCall: Evidence that L-glutamic acid mediates barore-
      ceptor function in the cat. Clin exp Hyperten. 1984; *6*: 1311–1329.

342   B.D. Miller and R.B. Felder: Excitatory amino acid receptors intrinsic to synaptic
      transmission in nucleus tractus solitarii. Brain Res. 1988; *456*: 333–343.

343   F.J. Gordon and C. Leone: Non-NMDA receptors in the nucleus of the tractus sol-
      itarius play the predominant role in mediating aortic baroreceptor reflexes. Brain
      Res. 1991; *568*: 319–322.

344   M.C. Andersen and M.Y. Yang: Non-NMDA receptors mediate sensory afferent syn-
      aptic transmission in medial nucleus tractus solitarius. Am. J. Physiol. 1990; *259*:
      H1307–H1311.

345   H. Ohta and W.T. Talman: Both NMDA and non-NMDA receptors in the NTS par-
      ticipate in the baroreceptor reflex in rats. Am. J. Physiol. 1994; *267*: R1065–R1070.

346   A. Vardhan, A. Kachroo and H.N. Sapru: Excitatory amino acid receptors in the
      nucleus tractus solitarius mediate the responses to the stimulation of cardio-pul-
      monary vagal afferent C fiber endings. Brain Res. 1993; *618*: 23–31.

347   A. Vardhan, A. Kachroo and H.N. Sapru: Excitatory amino acid receptors in com-
      missural nucleus of the NTS mediate carotid chemoreceptor responses. Am J. Phys-
      iol. 1993; *264*: R41–R50.

348   W.T. Talman: Kynurenic acid microinjected into the nucleus tractus solitarius of rat
      blocks the arterial baroreflex but not responses to glutamate. Neurosci. Lett. 1989;
      102: 247–252.

349   A.F. Sved and M.G. Backes: Neuroanatomical evidence that vagal afferent nerves
      do not possess a high affinity uptake system for glutamate. J. Auton. Nerv. Syst. 1992;
      38: 219–229.

350   A.F. Sved and J.T. Curtis: Amino acid neurotransmitters in nucleus tractus solitar-
      ius: an *in vivo* microdialysis study. J. Neurochem. 1993; *61*: 2089–2098.

351   V.M. Pickel, J. Chan and T.A. Milner: Cellular substrates for interactions between
      neurons containing phenylethanolamine N-methyltransferase and GABA in the
      nuclei of the solitary tracts. J. Comp. Neurol. 1989; *286*: 243–259.

352   W.W. Blessing: Distribution of glutamate decarboxylase-containing neurons in rab-
      bit medulla oblongata with attention to intramedullary and spinal projections. Neu-
      roscience 1990; *37*: 171–185.

353   P.N. Izzo, R.M. Sykes and K.M. Spyer: gamma-Aminobutyric acid immunoreactive

structures in the nucleus tractus solitarius: a light and electron microscopic study. Brain Res. 1992; *591*: 69–78.

354   J.M. Catelli, W.J. Giakas and A.F. Sved: GABAergic mechanisms in nucleus tractus solitarius alter blood pressure and vasopressin release. Brain Res. 1987; *403*: 279–289.

355   T. Kubo and M. Kihara: Evidence for gamma-aminobutyric acid receptor-mediated modulation of the aortic baroreceptor reflex in the nucleus tractus solitarii of the rat. Neurosci Lett. 1988; *89*: 156–160.

356   J.C. Sved and A.F. Sved: Cardiovascular responses elicited by gamma-aminobutyric acid in the nucleus tractus solitarius: evidence for action at the GABAB receptor. Neuropharmacol. 1989; *28*: 515–520.

357   P.A. Brooks, S.R. Glaum, R.J. Miller and K.M. Spyer: The actions of baclofen on neurones and synaptic transmission in the nucleus tractus solitarii of the rat *in vitro*. J. Physiol. 1992; *457*: 115–129.

358   A.F. Sved and J.C. Sved: Endogenous GABA acts on GABAB receptors in nucleus tractus solitarius to increase blood pressure. Brain Res. 1990; *526*: 235–240

359   A.F. Sved and K. Tsukamoto: Tonic stimulation of GABAB receptors in the nucleus tractus solitarius modulates the baroreceptor reflex. Brain Res. 1992; *592*: 37–43.

360   P.N. McWilliam and S.L. Shepheard: A GABA-mediated inhibition of neurones in the nucleus tractus solitarius of the cat that respond to electrical stimulation of the carotid sinus nerve. Neurosci. Lett. 1988; *94*: 321–326.

361   T. Kubo and M. Kihara: Evidence for the presence of GABAergic and glycine-like systems responsible for cardiovascular control in the nucleus tractus solitarii of the rat. Neurosci Lett. 1987; *74*: 331–336.

362   J.H. Coote, S.M. Hilton and A.W. Zbrozyna: The pontomedullary area integrating the defence reaction in the cat and its influence on muscle blood flow. J. Physiol. 1973; *229*: 257–274.

363   S.W. Mifflin, K.M. Spyer and D.J. Withington-Wray: Baroreceptor inputs to the nucleus tractus solitarius in the cat; modulation by the hypothalamus. J. Physiol. 1988; *399*: 369–387.

364   P.N. Izzo, R.M. Sykes and K.M. Spyer: γ-aminobutyric acid immunoreactive structures in the nucleus tractus solitarius: A light and electron microscopic study. Brain Res. 1992; *591*: 69–79.

365   J.F.R. Paton and K.M. Spyer: Cerebellar cortical regulation of circulation. News in Physiol. Sci. 1992; *7*: 124–129.

366   P.M. McWilliam, T. Yang and L.X. Chen: Changes in the baroreceptor reflex at the start of muscle contraction in the decerebrate cat. J. Physiol. 1991; *436*: 549–558.

367   D. Riche, J. De Pommery and D. Menetrey: Neuropeptides and catecholamines in efferent projections of the nuclei of the solitary tract in the rat. J. Comp. Neurol. 1990; *293*: 399–424.

368   P.R.C. Howe: Blood pressure control by neurotransmitters in the medulla oblongata and spinal corD.J. Auton. Nerv. Syst. 1985; *12*: 95–115.

369   P.D. Feldman and H.C. Moises: Adrenergic responses of baroreceptive cells in the nucleus tractus solitarii of the rat: a microiontophoretic study. Brain Res. 1987; *420*: 351–361.

370   P.D. Feldman and H.C. Moises: Electrophysiological evidence for alpha 1- and alpha 2-adrenoceptors in solitary tract nucleus. Am. J. Physiol. 1988; *254*: H756–762.

371   A.F. Sved, K. Tsukamoto and A.M. Schreihofer: Stimulation of alpha 2-adrenergic receptors in nucleus tractus solitarius is required for the baroreceptor reflex. Brain Res. 1992; *576*: 297–303.

372 D.J. Reis,T.H. Joh, M.A. Nathan, B. Renaud, D.W. Snyder and W.T.Talman: Nucleus tractus solitarii: catecholaminergic innervation in normal and abnormal control of arterial pressure. In: P. Myer and H. Schmitt (Eds.): Nervous system and hypertension, Toronto: Wiley-Flammarion, 1979; 147–164.

373 K.B. Thor and C.J. Helke: Serotonin and substance P colocalization in medullary projections to the nucleus tractus solitarius: dual color immunohistochemistry combined with retrograde tracing. J. Chem. Neuroanat. 1989; 2: 139–148.

374 W. A. Wolf, D.M. Kuhn and W. Lovenberg: Blood pressure responses to local application of serotonergic agents in the nucleus tractus solitarii. Europ. J. Pharmacol. 1981; 69: 291–299.

375 D.A. Carter and S.L. Lightman: Cardio-respiratory actions of substance P, TRH and 5-HT in the nucleus tractus solitarius of rats: evidence for functional interactions of neuropeptides and amine neurotransmitters. Neuropeptides 1985; 6: 425–436.

376 R. Laguzzi, D.J. Reis and W.T. Talman: Modulation of cardiovascular and electrocortical activity through serotonergic mechanisms in the nucleus tractus solitarius of the rat. Brain Research 1984; 304: 321–328.

377 A. Shvaloff and R. Laguzzi: Serotonin receptors in the rat nucleus tractus solitarii and cardiovascular regulation. Eur. J. Pharmacol. 1986; 132: 283–288.

378 K.B. Thor, A. Blitz-Siebert and C.J. Helke: Autoradiographic localization of 5HT1 binding sites in autonomic areas of the rat dorsomedial medulla oblongata. Synapse 192; 10: 217–227.

379 S.R. Glaum, P.A. Brooks, K.M. Spyer and R.J. Miller: 5-Hydroxytryptamine–3 receptors modulate synaptic activity in the rat nucleus tractus solitarius in vitro. Brain Res. 1992; 589: 62–68.

380 W.T. Talman and S.J. Lewis: Altered cardiovascular responses to glutamate and acetylcholine microinjected into the nucleus tractus solitarii of the SHR. Clin. Exp. Hyperten. 1991; 13: 661–668.

381 H.N. Sapru: Cholinergic mechanisms subserving cardiovascular function in the medulla and spinal cord. Prog. Brain Res. 1989; 81: 171–179.

382 K. Tsukamoto, M. Yin and A.F. Sved: Effect of atropine injected into the nucleus tractus solitarius on the regulation of blood pressure. Brain Res. 1994; 648: 915.

383 W.T. Talman and S.C. Robertson: Glycine, like glutamate, microinjected into the nucleus tractus solitarii of rat decreases arterial pressure and heart rate. Brain Res. 1989; 477: 7–13.

384 M.D. Cassell, L. Roberts and W.T. Talman: Glycine-containing terminals in the rat dorsal vagal complex. Neuroscience 1992; 50: 907–920.

385 W.T. Talman, J.M. Colling and S.C. Robertson: Glycine microinjected into nucleus tractus solitarii of rat acts through cholinergic mechanisms. Am. J. Physiol. 1991; 260: H1326–H1331.

386 H. Matsuguchi, F.M. Sharabi, F.J. Gordon, A.K. Johnson and P.G. Schmid: Blood pressure and heart rate responses to microinjection of vasopressin into the nucleus tractus solitarius region of the rat. Neuropharmacol. 1982; 21: 687–693.

387 K.A. King and C.C. Pang: Cardiovascular effects of injections of vasopressin into the nucleus tractus solitarius in conscious rats. Brit. J. Pharmacol. 1987; 90: 531–536.

388 Q.J. Pittman and L.G. Franklin: Vasopressin antagonist in nucleus tractus solitarius/vagal area reduces pressor and tachycardia responses to paraventricular nucleus stimulation in rats. Neurosci. Lett. 1985; 56: 155–160.

389 V.J. Massari, P.J. Hornby, E.K. Friedman, T.A. Milner, R.A. Gills and P.J. Gad: Dis-

tribution of neuropeptide Y-like immunoreactive perikarya and processes in the medulla of the cat. Neurosci. Lett. 1990; *115*: 37–42.

390   V.M. Pickel, J. Chan and V.J. Massari: Neuropeptide Y-like immunoreactivity in neurons of the solitary tract nuclei: vesicular localization and synaptic input from GABAergic terminals. Brain Res. 1989; *476*: 265–278.

391   C.J. Tseng, R. Mosqueda-Garcia, M. Appalsamy and D. Robertson: Cardiovascular effects of neuropeptide Y in rat brainstem nuclei. Circ. Res. 1989; *64*: 55–61.

392   L. Grundemar, C. Wahlestedt and D.J. Reis: Long-lasting inhibition of the cardiovascular responses to glutamate and the baroreceptor reflex elicited by neuropeptide Y injected into the nucleus tractus solitarius of the rat. Neurosci. Lett. 1991; *122*: 135–139.

393   L. Grundemar, C. Wahlestedt and D.J. Reis: Neuropeptide Y acts at an atypical receptor to evoke cardiovascular depression and to inhibit glutamate responsiveness in the brainstem .J. Pharmacol. Exp. Therap. 1991; *258*: 633–638.

394   D.B. Averil, D.I. Diz, K.L. Barnes and C.M. Ferrario: Pressor responses of angiotensin II microinjected into the dorsomedial medulla of the dog. Brain Res. 1987; *414*: 294–300.

395   R. Casto and M.I. Phillips: Neuropeptide action in nucleus tractus solitarius: angiotensin specificity and hypertensive rats. Am. J. Physiol. 1985; *249*: R341–R347.

396   R. Rettig, D.P. Healy and M.P. Printz: Cardiovascular effects of microinjections of angiotensin II into the nucleus tractus solitarii. Brain Res.1986; *364*: 233–240.

397   M.J. Campagnole-Santos, D.I. Diz and C.M. Ferrario: Baroreceptor reflex modulation by angiotensin II at the nucleus tractus solitarii. Hypertension 1988; *11*: 167–171.

398   M.A. Petty and W. de-Jong: Enkephalins induce a centrally mediated rise in blood pressure in rats. Brain Res. 1983; *260*: 322–325.

399   M.A. Petty and W. de-Jong: Cardiovascular effects of β-endorphin after microinjection into the nucleus tractus solitarii of the anaesthetized rat. Europ. J. Pharmacol. 1982; *81*: 449–457.

400   L.Y. Koda, N. Ling, R. Benoit, S.G. Madamba and C. Bakhit: Blood pressure following microinjection of somatostatin related peptides into the rat nucleus tractus solitarii. Europ. J. Pharmacol. 1985; *113*: 425–430.

401   M. Vallejo, S. Lightman and I. Marshall: Central cardiovascular effects of calcitonin gene related peptide: interaction with noradrenaline in the nucleus tractus solitarius of rats. Exp. Brain Res. 1988; *70*: 221–224.

402   F.R. Calaresu and C.P. Yardley: Medullary basal sympathetic tone. In: R.M. Berne (Ed.): Annual reviews of physiology, vol 50. Palo Alto: Annual Reviews Inc., 1988; 511–524.

403   W.W. Blessing and D.J. Reis: Inhibitory cardiovascular function of neurons in the caudal ventrolateral medulla of the rabbit: relationship to the area containing A1 noradrenergic cells. Brain Res. 1982; 253: 161–171.

404   T.A. Day, A. Ro and L.P. Renaud: Depressor area within caudal ventrolateral medulla of the rat does not correspond to the A1 catecholamine cell group. Brain Res. 1983; *279*: 299–302.

405   W.W. Blessing and D.J. Reis: Evidence that GABA- and glycine-like inputs inhibit vasodepressor neurons in the caudal ventrolateral medulla of the rabbit. Neurosci. Lett. 1983; *37*: 57–62.

406   R.N. Willette, A.J. Krieger, P.P. Barcas and H.N. Sapru: Medullary-aminobutyric acid (GABA) receptors and the regulation of blood pressure in the rat. J. Pharmacol. Exp. Therap. 1983; *226*: 893–899.

407 J.S. Schwaber: Neuroanatomical substrates of cardiovascular and emotional-auto-
     nomic regulation. In: A. Magro, W. Osswald, D.J. Reis and P. Vanhoutte (Eds.): Cen-
     tral and peripheral mechanisms of cardiovascular regulation, New York: Plenum
     Press, 1986; 353–384.

408 S.K. Agarwal, A.J. Gelsema and F.R. Calaresu: Inhibition of rostral VLM by baror-
     eceptor activation is relayed through caudal VLM. Am. J. Physiol. 1990; 258: R1271–
     R1278.

409 F.J. Gordon: Aortic baroreceptor reflexes are mediated by NMDA receptors in cau-
     dal ventrolateral medulla. Am. J. Physiol. 1987; 252: R628–R633.

410 Y.-W. Li and W.W. Blessing: Localization of vasodepressor neurons in the caudal
     ventrolateral medulla in the rabbit. Brain Res. 1990; 517: 57–63.

411 Z.J. Gieroba, Y.-W. Li and W.W. Blessing: Characteristics of caudal ventrolateral me-
     dullary neurons antidromically activated from rostral ventrolateral medulla in the
     rabbit. Brain Res. 1992; 582: 196–207.

412 I. Jeske, S.F. Morrison, S.L. Cravo and D.J. Reis: Identification of baroreceptor reflex
     interneurons in the caudal ventrolateral medulla. Am. J. Physiol. 1993; 264: R169–
     R178.

413 N. Terui, N. Masuda, Y. Saeki and M. Kumada: Activity of barosensitive neurons in
     the caudal ventrolateral medulla that send axonal projections to the rostral ventro-
     lateral medulla in rabbits. Neurosci. Lett. 1990; 118: 211–214.

414 S.L. Cravo, S.F. Morrison and D.J. Reis: Differentiation of two cardiovascular regions
     within caudal ventrolateral medulla: Am. J. Physiol. 1991; 261: R985–R994.

415 Y.-W. Li, Z.J. Gieroba, R.M. McAllen and W.W. Blessing: Neurons in rabbit caudal
     ventrolateral medulla inhibit bulbospinal barosensitive neurons in rostral medul-
     la. Am J. Physiol. 1991; 261: R44–R51.

416 Y.-W. Li, S.L. Wesselingh and W.W. Blessing: Projections from rabbit caudal medulla
     to C1 and A5 sympathetic premotor neurons, demonstrated with phaseolus leucoag-
     glutinin and herpes simplex virus. J. Comp. Neurol. 1992; 317: 379–395.

417 Y.-W. Li and R.A. Dampney: Expression of c-fos protein in the medulla oblongata
     of conscious rabbits in response to baroreceptor activation. Neurosci. Lett. 1992;
     144: 70–74.

418 K.A. Yamada, R.M. McAllen and A.D. Loewy: GABA antagonists applied to the
     ventral surface of the medulla oblongata block the baroreceptor reflex. Brain Res.
     1984; 297:175–180.

419 S.J. Humphrey and R.B. McCall: Evidence for τ-aminobutyric acid mediation of the
     sympathetic nerve inhibitory response to vagal afferent stimulation. J. Pharmacol.
     Exp. Therap. 1985; 234: 288–297.

420 W.W. Blessing and J.O. Willoughby: Depressor neurons in rabbit caudal medulla do
     not transmit the baroreceptor-vasomotor reflex. Am. J. Physiol. 1987; 253: H777–H786.

421 S.L. Cravo and S.F. Morrison: The caudal ventrolateral medulla is a source of tonic
     sympathoinhibition. Brain Res. 1993; 621: 133–136.

422 W.W. Blessing and Y.-W. Li: Inhibitory vasomotor neurons in the caudal ventrolat-
     eral region of the medulla oblongata. Prog. Brain Res. 1989; 81: 83–97.

423 A.R. Granata, Y. Numao, M. Kumada and D.J. Reis: A1 noradrenergic neurons ton-
     ically inhibit sympathoexcitatory neurons of C1 area in rat brainstem. Brain Res.
     1986; 377: 127–146.

424 H. Kaba, H. Saito, K. Otsuka, K. Seto and M. Kawakami: Effects of estrogen on the
     excitability of neurons projecting from the noradrenergic A1 region to the preop-
     tic and anterior hypothalamic area. Brain Res. 1983; 274: 156–159.

425   H. Kaba, H. Saito, K. Otsuka and K. Seto: Ventrolateral medullary neurons project-
      ing to the medial preoptic-anterior hypothalamic area through the medial forebrain
      bundle: An electrophysiological study in the rat. Exp. Brain Res. 1986; *63*: 369–374.

426   H. Yamashita, H. Kannan and Y. Ueta: Involvement of caudal ventrolateral medulla
      in mediating visceroreceptive information to the hypothalamic paraventricular
      nucleus. In: J. Ciriello, M.M. Caverson and C. Polosa (Eds.): Central Neural Organ-
      ization of Cardiovascular Control. Progress in Brain Research. Amsterdam: Else-
      vier, 1989: vol 81, 293–302.

427   R.M. McAllen and W.W. Blessing: Neurons (presumably A1 cells) projecting from
      the caudal ventrolateral medulla to the region of the supraoptic nucleus respond
      to baroreceptor inputs in the rabbit. Neurosci. Lett. 1987; *73*: 247–252.

428   D.A. Thrivikraman, D.A. Bereiter and D.S. Gann: Catecholamine activity in para-
      ventricular hypothalamus after hemorrhage in cats. Am. J. Physiol. 1989; *257*: H370–
      H376.

429   L. Quitin, J.-Y. Gillon, M. Ghigone, B. Renaud and J.-F. Pujol: Baroreflex-linked vari-
      ations of catecholamine metabolism in the caudal ventrolateral medulla: An 'in vivo'
      electrochemical study. Brain Res. 1987; *425*: 319–336.

430   M. Elam: On the Physiological Regulation of Brain Norepinephrine Neurons in Rat
      Locus Coeruleus. Kompendietryckeriet, Kallered, Goteberg, Sweden.

431   W.W. Blessing, C.B. Jaeger, D.A. Ruggiero and D.J. Reis: Hypothalamic projections
      of medullary catecholamine neurons in the rabbit: a combined catecholamine flu-
      orescence and HRP transport study. Brain Res.Bull. 1982; *9*: 279–286.

432   P.E. Sawchenko and L.W. Swanson: The organization of noradrenergic pathways from
      the brainstem to the paraventricular and supraoptic nuclei in the rat. Brain Res.
      Rev. 1982; *4*: 275–325.

433   E. Mills and S.C. Wang: Liberation of antidiuretic hormone: location of ascending
      pathways. Am. J. Physiol. 1964; *207*: 1399–1404.

434   W. Feldberg and S.M. Rocha: Vasopressin release produced in anaesthetized cats
      by antagonists of GABA abd glycine. Brit. J. Pharmacol. 1978; *62*: 99–106.

435   W.W. Blessing and J.O. Willoughby: Inhibiting the rabbit caudal ventrolateral medulla
      prevents baroreceptor-initiated secretion of vasopressin. J. Physiol. 1985; *367*: 253–265.

436   Z.J. Gieroba, M.J. Fullerton, J.W. Funder and W.W. Blessing: Medullary pathways
      for adrenocorticotropic hormone and vasopressin secretion in rabbits. Am. J. Phys-
      iol. 1992; *262*: R1047–R1056.

437   W.W. Blessing and J.O. Willoughby: Excitation of neuronal function in rabbit cau-
      dal ventrolateral medulla elevates plasma vasopressin. Neurosci Lett. 1985; *58*: 189–
      194.

438   A. Benetos, I. Gavras and H. Gavras: Norepinephrine applied in the paraventricu-
      lar hypothalamic nucleus stimulates vasopressin release. Brain Res. 1986; *381*: 322–
      326.

439   T.A. Day, A.V. Ferguson and L.P. Renaud: Facilitatory influence of noradrenergic
      afferents on the excitability of rat paraventricular nucleus neurosecretory cells. J.
      Physiol. 1984; *355*: 237–249.

440   T.A. Day and L.P. Renaud: Electrophysiological evidence that noradrenergic affer-
      ents selectively facilitate the activity of supraoptic vasopressin neurons. Brain Res.
      1984; *303*: 233–240.

441   B.J. Davis, M.L. Blain, J.R. Sladek and C.D. Sladek: Effects of lesions of hypotha-
      lamic catecholamines on blood pressure, fluid balance, vasopressin and renin in the
      rat. Brain Res. 1987; *405*: 1–15.

442   J. Tanaka, H. Kaba, H. Saito and K. Seto: Inputs from the A1 noradrenergic region to hypothalamic paraventricular neurons in the rat. Brain Res. 1985; *355*: 368–371.

443   J.C.R. Randle, C.W. Bourque and L.P. Renaud: α-Adrenergic activation of rat hypothalamic supraoptic neurons maintained *in vitro*. Brain Res. 1984; *307*: 374–378.

444   T. Imaizumi, A.R. Granata, E.E. Benarroch, A.F. Sved and D.J. Reis: Contributions of arginine vasopressin and the sympathetic nervous system to fulminating hypertension after destruction of neurons of caudal ventrolateral medulla in the rat. J. Hyperten. 1985; *3*: 491–501.

445   J. Minson, J. Chalmers, V. Kapoor, M. Cain and A. Caon: Relative importance of sympathetic nerves and of circulating adrenaline and vasopressin in mediating hypertension after lesions of the caudal ventrolateral medulla in the rat. J. Hyperten. 1986; *4*: 273–281.

446   J. Ciriello, M.M. Caverson and C. Polosa: Function of the ventrolateral medulla in the control of the circulation. Brain Res. Rev. 1986; *111*: 359–391.

447   Y.I. Kim, C.A. Dudley and R.L. Moss: Inhibitory effect of norepinephrine on the single-unit activity of caudally projecting paraventricular neurons. Synapse 1989; *3*: 213–224.

448   H. Yamashita, R.E.J. Dyball, K. Inenaga and K. Kannan: The effects of noradrenaline on supraoptic and paraventricular cells of mice *in vitro*. In: J. Ciriello, F.R. Calaresu, L.P. Renaud and C. Polosa (Eds.): Organization of the autonomic nervous system: central and peripheral mechanisms. New York: Alan Liss Inc. 1987; 417–423.

449   A.J. Silverman, Y.A. Hou and B.J. Oldfield: Ultrastructural identification of noradrenergic nerve terminals and vasopressin-containing neurons of the paraventricular nucleus in the same thin section. J. Histochem. Cytochem. 1983; *31*: 1151–1156.

450   S.C. Wang and S.W. Ranson: Autonomic responses to electrical stimulation of the lower brain stem. J. Comp. Neurol. 1939; *71*: 437–455.

451   D.M. Farlow, A.K. Goodchild and R.A. Dampney: Evidence that vasomotor neurons in the rostral ventrolateral medulla project to the spinal sympathetic outflow via the dorsomedial pressor area. Brain Res. 1984; *298*: 313–320.

452   M. Kumada, R.A. Dampney and D.J. Reis: Profound hypotension and abolition of the vasomotor component of the cerebral ischemic response produced by restricted lesions of medulla oblongata: relationship to the so-called tonic vasomotor center. Circ. Res. 1979; *45*: 63–70.

453   M.E. Clement and R.B. McCall: Lateral tegmental field involvement in the central sympathoinhibitory action of 8-OH DPAT. Brain Res. 1993; *612*: 78–84.

454   C. Vayssettes-Courchay, F. Bouysset, T.J. Verbeuren, H. Schmitt and M. Laubie: Cardiovascular effects of microinjections of quipazine into nuclei of the medulla-oblongata in anaesthetized cats-comparison with L-glutamate. Eur. J. Pharmacol. 1992; *211*: 243–250.

455   M.E. Clement and R.B. McCall: Evidence that the lateral tegmental field plays an important role in the central sympathoinhibitory action of 8-OH-DPAT. Brain Res. 1992; *587*: 115–122.

456   G.L. Gebber and S.M. Barman.: Lateral tegmental field neurons of cat medulla: a potential source of basal sympathetic discharge. J. Neurophysiol. 1985; *54*: 1498–1512.

457   Y. Hirooka, J.W. Polson and R.A. Dampney: Pressor response from rostral dorsomedial medulla is mediated by excitatory amino acid receptors in rostral VLM. Am. J. Physiol. 1994; *267*: R309–R315.

458   P.L. McGeer and E.G. McGeer: Kainic acid: the neurotoxic breakthrough. CRC Crit. Rev. Toxicol. 1982; *10*: 1–26.

459   C. Vayssettes-Courchay, F. Bouysset, T.J. Verbeuren and M. Laubie: Role of the lat-

eral tegmental field in the central sympatho-inhibitory effect of 8-hydroxy–2-(di-n-propylamino)tetralin in the cat. Europ. J. Pharmacol. 1993; *236*: 121–130.

460   M.E. Clement and R.B. McCall: Lateral tegmental field involvement in the central sympathoinhibitory action of 8-OH DPAT. Brain Res. 1993; *612*: 78–84.

461   C. Vayssettes-Courchay, F. Bouysset, T.J. Verbeuren and M. Laubie: Role of the nucleus tractus solitarii and the rostral depressive area in the sympatholytic effect of 8-hydroxy–2-(di-n-propylamino)tetralin in the cat. Europ. J. Pharmacol. 1993; *242*: 37–45.

462   D. Bieger and D.A. Hopkins: Viscerotopic representation of the upper alimentary tract in the medulla oblongata in the rat: the nucleus ambiguus. J. Comp. Neurol. 1987; *262*: 546–562.

463   D.A. Hopkins and J.A. Armour: Medullary cells of origin of physiologically identified cardiac nerves in the dog. Brain Res. Bull. 1982; *8*: 359–365.

464   P.N. Izzo, J. Deuchars and K.M. Spyer: Localization of cardiac vagal preganglionic motoneurones in the rat-immunocytochemical evidence of synaptic inputs containing 5-hydroxytryptamine. J. Comp. Neurol. 1993; *327*: 572–583.

465   S. Nosaka, T. Yamamoto and K. Yasunaga: Localization of vagal cardioinhibitory preganglionic neurons within rat brainstem. J. Comp. Neurol. 1979; *186*: 79–92.

466   D.M. Plecha, W.C. Randall, G.S. Geis and R.D. Wurster: Localization of vagal preganglionic somata controlling sinoatrial and atrioventricular nodes. Am. J. Physiol. 1988; *255*: R703–R708.

467   S.K. Agarwal and F.R. Calaresu: Electrical stimulation of nucleus tractus solitarius excites vagal preganglionic cardiomotor neurons of the nucleus ambiguus in rats. Brain Res. 1992; *574*: 320–324.

468   A.D. Loewy and H. Burton: Nuclei of the solitary tract: efferent projections to the lower brainstem and spinal cord of the cat. J. Comp. Neurol. 1978; *181*: 421–450.

469   S.L. Stuesse and S.E. Fish: Projections to the cardioinhibitory region of the nucleus ambiguus of rat. J. Comp. Neurol. 1984; *229*: 271–278.

470   M.P. Gilbey, D. Jordan, D.W. Richter and K.M. Spyer: Synaptic mechanisms involved in the inspiratory modulation of the vagal cardioinhibitory neurons in the cat. J. Physiol. 1984; *356*: 65–78.

471   A. Pazos and J.M. Palacios: Quantitative autoradiographic mapping of serotonin receptors in the rat brain. I. Serotonin–1 receptors. Brain Res. 1985; *346*: 205–230

472   S. Manaker and H.M. Verderame: Organization of serotonin 1A and 1B receptors in the nucleus of the solitary tract. J. Comp. Neurol. 1990; *301*: 535–553.

473   M.R. Dashwood, M.P. Gilbey, D. Jordan and A.G. Ramage: Autoradiographic localization of 5-HT1A binding sites in the brain stem of the cat. Br. J. Pharmacol. 1988; *94*: 386P.

474   K. Gradin, A. Pettersson, T. Hedner and B. Persson: Acute administration of 8-hydroxy–2-(di-n-propylamino) tetralin (8-OH-DPAT), a selective 5-HT receptor agonist in Sprague-Dawley rat and the spontaneously hypertensive rat. J. Neural Transm. 1985; *62*: 305–319.

475   A.G. Ramage and J.R. Fozard.: Evidence that the putative 5-HT$_{1A}$ receptor agonists 8-OH DPAT and ipsapirone have a central hypotensive action that differs from that of clonidine in anaesthetized cats. Europ J Pharmacol. 1987; *138*: 179–191.

476   A.G. Ramage, W. Wouters and P. Bevan: Evidence that the novel antihypertensive agent, flesinoxan, causes differential sympathoinhibition and also increases vagal tone by a central action, Europ. J. Pharmacol. 1988; *151*: 373–379.

477   J.H. Coote: The central antihypertensive action of 5-hydroxytryptamine: the location of site of action. In: P.R. Saxena, D.I. Wallis, W. Wouters and P. Bevan (Eds.): Cardiovascular Pharmacology of 5-Hydroxytryptamine. Kluwer Academic Publishers, Dordrecht, 1990, 259–270.

478   P. N. Izzo, D. Jordan and A.G. Ramage: Anatomical and pharmacological evidence supporting the involvement of serotonin in the central control of cardiac vagal motoneurones in the anaesthetized cat. J. Physiol. 1988; 406: 19P.

479   D.W. Dalton, W. Feniuk and P.P.A. Humphrey: An investigation into the mechanisms of the cardiovascular effects of 5-hydroxytryptamine in conscious normotensive and Doca-salt hypertensive rats. J. Auton. Nerv. Syst. 1986; 6: 219–229.

480   S.C.E. Sporton, S.L. Shepheard, D. Jordan and A.G. Ramage: Microinjections of 5-HT_{1A} agonists into the dorsal motor vagal nucleus produce a bradycardia in the atenolol-pretreated anaesthetized rat. Brit. J. Pharmacol. 1991; 104: 466–470.

481   R.B. McCall, N.A. Escandon, L.T. Harris and M.E. Clement: Tolerance development to the vagal-mediated bradycardia produced by 5-HT_{1A} receptor agonists. J. Pharmacol. Exp. Therap. 1994; 271: 776–781.

482   J.M. De Voogd and G. Prager: Early clinical experience with flesinoxan, a new selective 5-HT_{1A} receptor agonist. In: P.R. Saxena, D.I. Wallis, W. Wouters and P. Bevan (Eds.): Cardiovascular Pharmacology of 5-Hydroxytryptamine. Kluwer Academic Publishers, Dordrecht, 1990, 259–270.

483   R.G. Bogle, J.G. Pires and A.G. Ramage: Evidence that central 5-HT_{1A} receptors play a role in the von Bezold-Jarisch reflex in the rat. Br. J. Pharmacol. 1990; 100: 757–760.

484   H.A. Futuro-Neto, J.G. Pires, M.P. Gilbey and A.G. Ramage: Evidence for the ability of central 5-HT_{1A} receptors to modulate the vagal bradycardia induced by stimulating the upper airways of anesthetized rabbits with smoke. Brain Res. 1993; 629: 349–354.

Progress in Drug Research, Vol. 46 (E. Jucker, Ed.)
© 1996 Birkhäuser Verlag, Basel (Switzerland)

Development of novel anti-inflammatory agents: A pharmacologic perspective on leukotrienes and their receptors

By William T. Jackson and Jerome H. Fleisch

Lilly Research Laboratories, Eli Lilly & Company, Indianapolis, Indiana, USA

1   Introduction

Inflammation is the body's response to injury. Participation by a variety of cells and endogenous molecules make it a complex physiologic, and often times pathologic, event. Leukotrienes have been well documented to play a significant role, both as mediators of the acute inflammatory response and as contributors to the chronicity of the disorder. Research has concentrated in 3 main areas, understanding interactions of leukotrienes with complementary cell surface receptors, development of inhibitors of their synthesis, and discovery of receptor antagonists that block their pharmacologic effect. The following represents our view of this area with a bias toward medicinal chemistry, pharmacologic, and clinical studies related to our own research interests.

2   Historical perspective

Fifty-seven years have passed since Feldberg and Kellaway [1] first described a material released by cobra venom from perfused guinea pig, cat, dog, or monkey lung and from perfused dog liver. This pharmacologic principle produced a slow delayed contraction of isolated guinea pig jejunum. Two years later, Kellaway and Trethewie [2] extended this observation. They bioassayed perfusate from antigen-challenged guinea pig lung on jejunum and noted the presence of a "slow-reacting smooth muscle-stimulant substance" or SRS. This differed from what would have been expected if the lung only released histamine, which at the time was the presumed mediator of such a response. They concluded that the samples contained an SRS in addition to histamine.

Interest in this problem was rekindled in the mid 1950s by Brocklehurst [3–5] who tested perfusate from antigen-challenged guinea pig lung on unsensitized guinea pig ileum in the presence of pyrilamine, a newly discovered histamine$_1$ receptor antagonist. With the histamine component blocked, the remaining activity was characterized by a slow sustained contraction of the isolated gut. Fractionating the perfusate and armed with only pharmacologic techniques, Brocklehurst found histamine to be rapidly liberated after antigen challenge whereas release of another substance appeared somewhat later. This agent was named SRS-A or Slow Reacting Substance of Anaphylaxis to differentiate it from other SRS types generated by non-immunologic means, e.g. cobra venom. The importance of SRS-A in the pathobiology of anaphylaxis and as a potential contributing factor in obstructive airway disease became obvious even from those seminal experiments.

Brocklehurst's work stimulated exploration of SRS-A by many laboratories. Two major goals guided this effort. The first was to chemically, biochemically, and pharmacologically characterize SRS-A and the second was to develop drugs that antagonized its action or inhibited its synthesis and subsequent release. The connection between leukotrienes and SRS-A waited until the late 1970s to be uncovered. Historical accounts of this crucial chapter have provided the basis for many reviews and symposia [e.g. 6–8] and are beyond the scope of the present communication. However, one of the most important landmarks in this research actually came about 6 years earlier with the disclosure by Augstein et al. [9] of FPL 55712, which was shown to be a selective antagonist of most of the pharmacologic activity found in crude SRS-A. Furthermore, this agent was used to demonstrate that biologic activity attributed to SRS-A was due to its interaction with a membrane-bound receptor on smooth muscle [10–12] and thereby strongly supporting the suggestion that SRS-A was an endogenous substance or group of substances released by cells in response to either antigen-antibody reactions or to certain chemicals. Following characterization of SRS-A, large quantities of pure cysteinyl leukotrienes became available. As was the case with SRS-A, the pharmacologic effects of leukotriene D_4 (LTD$_4$) and leukotriene E_4 (LTE$_4$) were shown to be antagonized by FPL 55712 [13–15]. Thus, FPL 55712 provided a starting point for development of a new class of therapeutic agents, the leukotriene receptor antagonists [16–19], and once again demonstrated the importance of a selective pharmacologic antagonist, coupled with chemically pure agonists and *in vitro* pharmacologic techniques, for revealing and then exploring the pathophysiologic role of newly discovered endogenous molecules.

3   The leukotrienes

Leukotrienes (Fig. 1) belong to a family of C-20 polyunsaturated fatty acids derived from arachidonic acid after its liberation from membrane phospholipids by phospholipase A_2 (PLA$_2$) and subsequent oxygenation by 5-lipoxygenase (5-LO). Synthesis and release of the leukotrienes takes place *de novo* in response to an injurious stimulus such as physical trauma, immediate type hypersensitivity reactions, and exposure to chemicals. Leukotrienes are synthesized by inflammatory cells such as neutrophils, eosinophils, mast cells, basophils, monocytes, and macrophages [20–22]. These cells are by no means the only ones to produce leukotrienes but are the major types involved in inflammatory responses. Leukotrienes can be divided into 2 major classes. Cysteinyl leukotrienes, leukotriene C_4 (LTC$_4$),

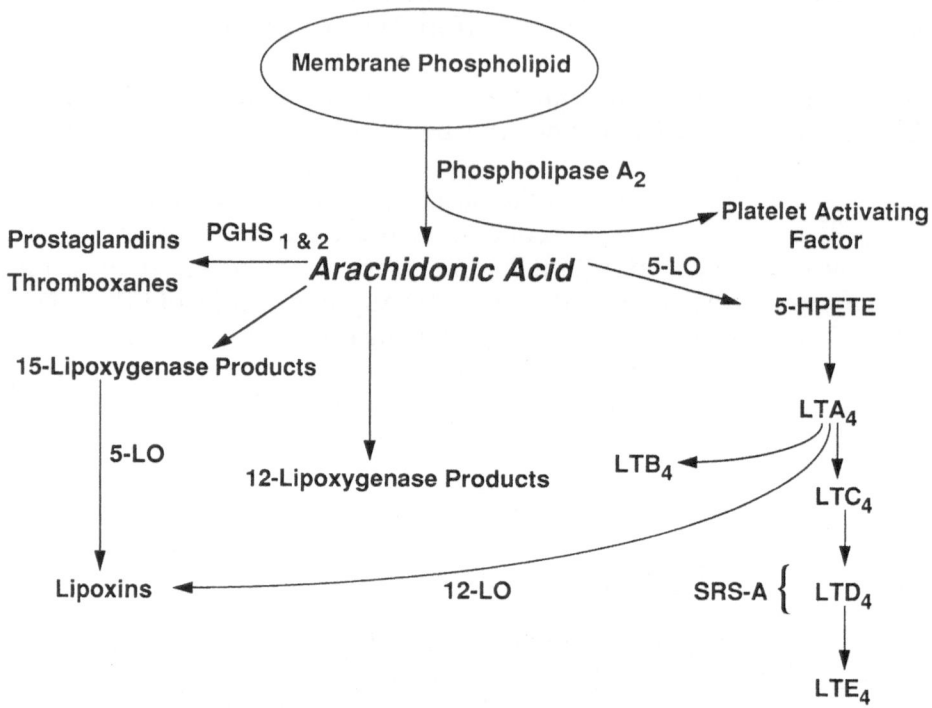

Fig. 1
Formation of arachidonic acid metabolites from cell membranes. Phospholipase A_2 hydrolyzes membrane phospholipids to yield free arachidonic acid which, in turn, is converted to prostaglandins, thromboxanes, leukotrienes, and/or lipoxins.

LTD_4, and LTE_4, the main components of SRS-A [20,21,23], are C-6 substituted eicosatetraenoic acids. LTC_4 and LTD_4 have tri- and dipeptide substitutents at the 6 position from which they get their often cited classification of peptidoleukotrienes or sulfidopeptide leukotrienes. LTE_4 has only a cysteine molecule at C-6. Since cysteine is a common feature of all 3 lipid mediators, the designation of cysteinyl leukotrienes seems more appropriate. LTC_4 is formed by the addition of glutathione to LTA_4, a short-lived intermediate, by the enzyme glutathione S-transferase. Metabolic removal of glutamate from LTC_4 by γ-glutamyltranspeptidase results in the production of LTD_4. Cleavage of glycine from of LTD_4 by an aminopeptidase results in the formation of LTE_4. All 3 mediators have profound pharmacologic effects on the cardiovascular, pulmonary, and gastrointestinal systems and probably work in concert contributing to the pathology of various inflammatory diseases [24]. To different degrees these lipids contract and sometimes relax smooth muscles, decrease myocardial contractility, increase permeability of blood vessels, enhance mucous production, and reduce mucociliary transport [8, 16, 18].

The second group of leukotrienes, initially described by Borgeat and Samuelsson [25–27], are chemically characterized as dihydroeicosatetraenoic acids; LTB_4 has been the most widely studied molecule in this class. Whereas the cysteinyl leukotrienes are generally appreciated for their acute pharmacologic effects, the actions of LTB_4 tend to be a consequence of its ability to direct migration of inflammatory cells (i.e. neutrophils) into a site of injury [28–31]. LTB_4 is not only a potent chemotactic agent but it can also activate these same inflammatory cells to a state from which they release noxious substances into the surrounding milieu [32]. Thus, from a pharmacologic perspective, LTB_4 can be said to function in many situations as both a direct and indirect acting agonist. During a variety of tissue insults, the neutrophil leaves the peripheral circulation and takes up residence in the lung [33]. This margination occurs after the upregulation of CD11b/CD18 adhesion molecules on the surface of the neutrophil followed by attachment of the cell to the complimentary ligand, ICAM-1, on the pulmonary vascular endothelium [34–36]. LTB_4 is a potent stimulant of CD11b/CD18 receptor upregulation. This characteristic formed the basis for an *ex vivo* assay of novel LTB_4 receptor antagonists in human subjects [37]. After these agents were administered, peripheral blood neutrophils were assessed for their ability to upregulate CD11b/CD18 adhesion receptors on their surface in response to LTB_4. The amount of decrease in this process relative to control was considered a measure of receptor antagonist activity.

This review is primarily focused on agonists and antagonists that interact with the leukotriene receptors. Since LTB_4 is a primary interest of our group, special emphasis will be paid to this leukotriene. However, we remind the reader that arachidonic acid release results in the formation of a myriad of substances in addition to the leukotrienes (Fig. 1). These include prostaglandins, thromboxanes, and prostacyclin as examples of cycloxygenase products. Similarly, many lipoxygenase products are produced as a result of arachidonic acid release, an example being the lipoxins [38]. Like the leukotrienes, they are a family of lipoxygenase-derived metabolites formed via the arachidonic acid cascade. These interesting lipid mediators are produced by dual oxygenation of arachidonic acid involving the action of 5-lipoxygenase coupled with either the 12- or 15-lipoxygenase depending on the biochemistry of the involved cells [38, 39].

LXA_4 and LXB_4 which are generated by this process have shown pharmacologic activity on a variety of test systems [38–41].

Our knowledge of the arachidonic acid cascade has expanded dramatically since its initial discovery. Whether all molecules relevant to inflammatory processes have been uncovered is unknown but it appears to have reached a plateau. Leukotriene research has now evolved to the point where greater emphasis is being placed on the clinical development of effective receptor antagonists or synthesis inhibitors rather than on the discovery of new physiologic or pathologic roles for members of this chemical family. We now have sufficient tools at hand to determine whether this group of biologically active substances significantly contributes to human disease.

4   Characterization of leukotriene receptors

Since Paul Erhlich's classic studies over 80 years ago on selectivity of chemotherapeutic agents [42], pharmacologists have been trying to characterize the cell receptors to which natural agonists bind and to understand the mechanism by which those sites are activated. Receptors for histamine, serotonin, acetylcholine and catecholamines serve as examples of entities that have been extensively explored. Leukotriene receptors have not undergone the same scrutiny. Nevertheless, there is now emerging a fair amount of pharmacologic data which makes possible preliminary observations about the properties of these receptors. Final confirmation will have to wait until the receptors are cloned and sequenced.

Receptors for cysteinyl leukotrienes and LTB_4 are different. Each receptor is specific for its own agonist and antagonists. Upon binding to their receptors, LTC_4, LTD_4, and LTE_4 stimulate a different array of biological reactions than those induced by LTB_4. Consequently, in this review we have described the properties of cysteinyl leukotriene receptors separately from those of the LTB_4 receptor.

4.1   Cysteinyl leukotriene receptors

Since the three cysteinyl leukotrienes have a similar lipid backbone but a different amino acid side-chain, one might expect the receptors for these eicosanoids to be heterogenous. Pharmacologic studies carried out on animal tissue with agonists and selective antagonists have supported this concept. Interpretation of these experiments, however, is complicated because in many tissues LTC_4 is rapidly metabolized to LTD_4. This metabolism can be prevented by addition of appropriate inhibitors of γ-glutamyltran-speptidase but these agents need to be used with caution because of possible nonspecific effects on tissues.

Initial indications of the heterogeneity of leukotriene receptors were revealed when pure LTC_4 and LTD_4 became available and their ability to induce contraction of smooth muscle was measured using different tissues. LTD_4 was found by Drazen et al. [13] to be 100-fold more potent at contracting guinea pig lung parenchyma strips than LTC_4. Goldenberg and Subers [43], using rat distal colonic tissue, also found LTD_4 to be a better agonist than LTC_4. Proof of receptor heterogeneity was established with the development of the antagonists FPL 55712 and LY171883 (Fig. 2). Drazen et al. observed that contractions of guinea pig lung parenchymal strips induced by LTD_4 were antagonized by FPL 55712 whereas the compound had no effect on a corresponding LTC_4-induced response [13]. In independent studies, Krell obtained similar results with FPL 55712 [14]. In vitro studies with LY171883 by Fleisch et al. showed this compound to be a specific antagonist of LTD_4 and LTE_4-induced contractions of guinea pig ileum, trachea and lung parenchyma [44a,b]. The small inhibitory effect on LTC_4-stimulated responses (1/50th of the effect on the corresponding LTD_4-activated phenomena) was postulated to be due, in part, to effects on LTD_4, newly formed from metabolism of LTC_4 (Fig. 1).

Subsequently, Snyder and Krell [45] showed that when guinea pig trachea were induced to contract by LTC_4 in the presence of L-serine borate, a γ-glutamyltranspeptidase inhibitor, FPL 55712 no longer antagonized LTC_4-mediated responses. This result clearly showed that LTC_4 bound to a different receptor than LTD_4 in guinea pig trachea. Fleisch et al. [12] found that FPL 55712 competitively antagonized contractions induced with LTD_4 on guinea pig ileum, trachea and parenchyma. The K_B and pA_2 values were similar for trachea and parenchyma tissue but different from those obtained in the ileum, prompting the authors to suggest the existence of different subtypes of the LTD_4 receptor in airway and ileum. Krell et al. [46], conducting experiments in the presence of indomethacin to prevent formation of thromboxane A_2, found that FPL 55712 bound to two distinct LTD_4 receptor subtypes on guinea pig trachea, one with significantly higher affinity for FPL 55712 than the other. In addition, they found that LTE_4 appeared to interact preferentially with the higher affinity receptor for LTD_4. In contrast, contractions of human intralobar airway smooth muscle [47] induced by either LTC_4 or LTD_4 were equally inhibited by FPL 55712, even in the presence of metabolic inhibitors. Similar results were observed with ICI 198,615 (Fig. 3), a more potent selective leuko-

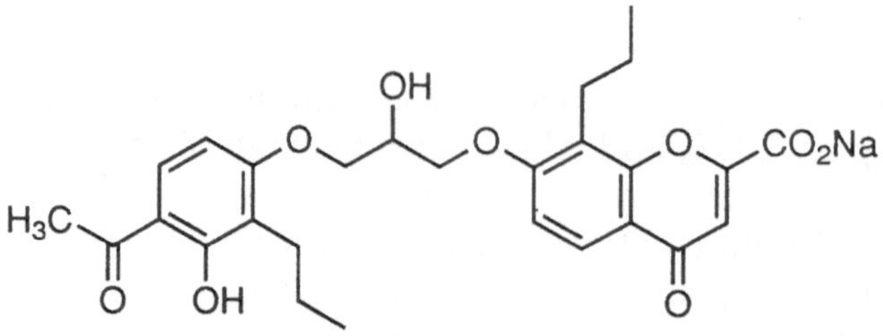

FPL 55712

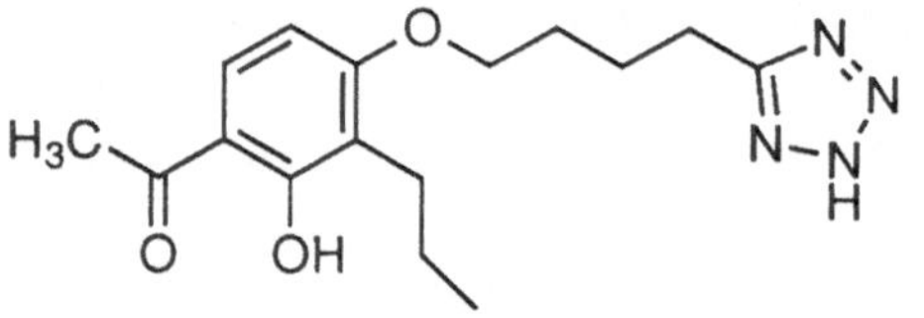

LY171883

Fig. 2
FPL 55712 was the first LTD_4/LTE_4 receptor antagonist to be disclosed. LY171883 established that agents in this chemical class could have oral activity and clinical efficacy in human subjects.

triene receptor antagonist [48]. Additional studies with ICI 204,219 (Fig. 3), an analog of ICI 198,615, indicated that this compound was equally effective at inhibiting contraction of human airway smooth muscle induced by not only LTC_4 and LTD_4 but also by LTE_4 [49]. Interestingly, all three leukotrienes were found to be equipotent in contracting this particular human tissue [49]. When other potent cysteinyl leukotriene receptor antagonists were developed such as ONO-1078, SKF 104353 and MK-571 (Fig. 3), they were also tested for their effects on leukotriene-induced contraction of guinea pig trachea and human bronchus [50–53]. The results were similar. Using guinea pig lung tissue, the compounds were potent antagonists of LTD_4 and LTE_4 but had only marginal or no activity on LTC_4-mediated responses when conversion of LTC_4 to LTD_4 was prevented. However, when experiments were done with human tissue, the compounds were equally active on both LTC_4- and LTD_4-induced contraction. In general, the pK_B values of these antagonists on guinea pig trachea are 0.5–1.0 log higher than on human airways. Some of these same receptor antagonists have also been shown to inhibit leukotriene-induced contraction of guinea pig gall bladder and rat lung strips [54, 55]. However, these compounds are not capable of attenuating leukotriene elicited responses of human pulmonary vein [56], ferret trachea [57], ferret spleen [58] and sheep bronchus [59]. This has led investigators to postulate that there are two receptors for the cysteinyl leukotrienes, one which can be antagonized by the above-mentioned antagonists and a second receptor that is resistant to these agents. Tissues such as human bronchus or human pulmonary vein appear to be homogenous for one or the other leukotriene receptor. Other tissues such as guinea pig trachea and ileum appear to be a mixture of the two receptor types. Recently BAY u9773, a leukotriene analog (Fig. 3), was found to inhibit LTC_4 as well as LTD_4-induced contractions in guinea pig tracheal preparations [60, 61]. Moreover, it was equally effective at inhibiting LTC_4- and LTD_4-induced contractions of human bronchial and venous muscle preparations [56]. Thus, this appears to be the first antagonist developed that binds to the cysteinyl leukotriene receptor which was previously unaffected by the more traditional antagonists. The practice has arisen of referring to the more traditional blocking agents as LTD_4/LTE_4 receptor antagonists because of their selective action on guinea pig responses induced with these two leukotrienes and we will follow this nomenclature throughout this review. However, the receptor nomenclature committee of IUPHAR has recently endorsed an alternate system, using the term $CysLT_1$ for the receptor to which these compounds bind [62].

Results obtained from radioligand binding studies with $[^3H]$-LTD_4 have generally corroborated the findings obtained from isolated smooth muscle experiments. Binding of radioactive LTD_4 to membranes isolated from smooth muscle cells of guinea pig lung [63, 64], guinea pig myocardium [65], human lung [66], sheep trachea [67], the human monocytic leukemia cell, U-937 [68], and the rat basophilic cell line, RBL-1 [69], was found to be stereoselective, specific, and saturable. The antagonists described above were found to competitively inhibit this binding at nanomolar concentrations [70–72]. In addition, the rank order potency of the compounds at inhibiting binding correlated with their pharmacologic effect on smooth muscle responses induced by LTD_4. As observed in smooth muscle contraction studies, the potency of each antagonist at inhibiting binding to human lung receptors was several fold less than that found for guinea pig lung membranes.

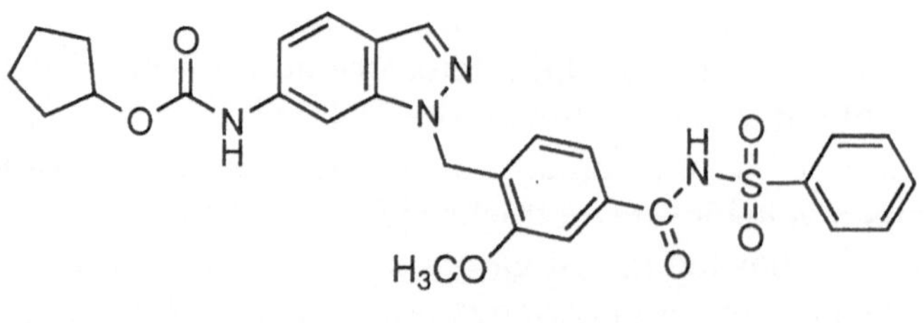

ICI 198,615

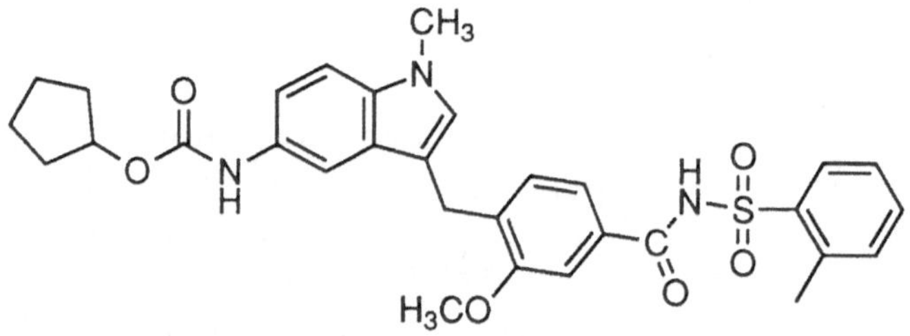

ICI 204,219

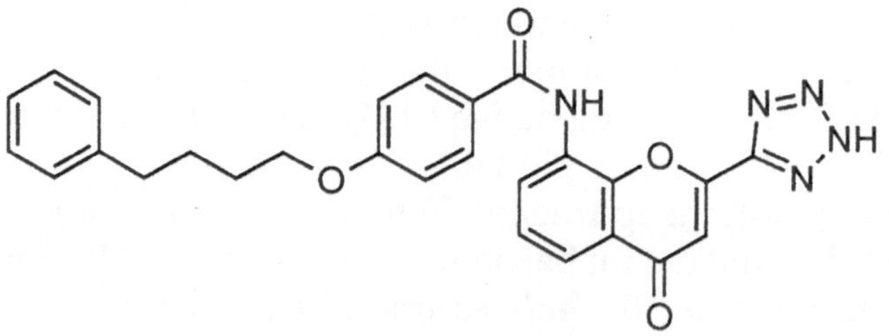

ONO-1078

Fig. 3
Second generation LTD$_4$/LTE$_4$ receptor antagonists. These diverse structures are superior to FPL 55712 and LY171833 in potency.

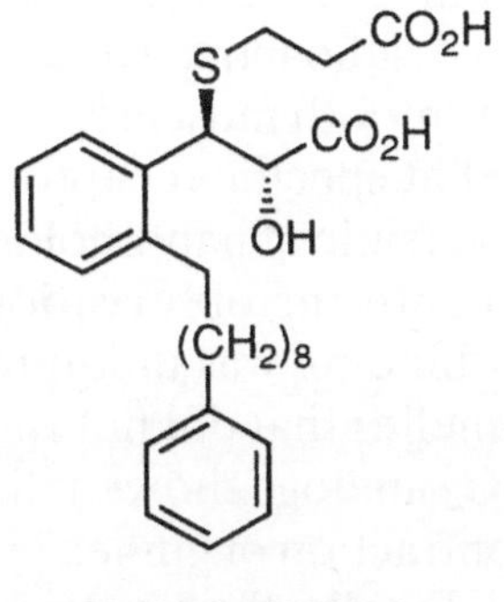

SKF 104353

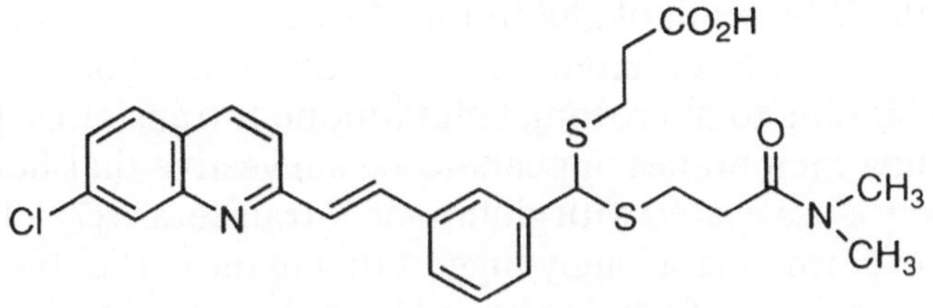

MK-571 (L 660,711)

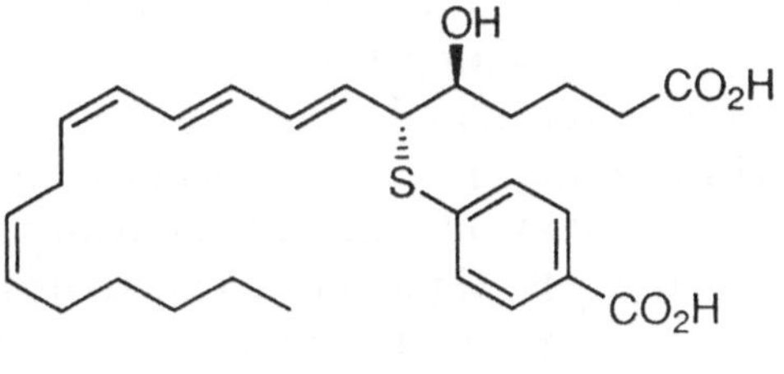

BAY u9773

Fig. 3 (continued)

Studies on [^{3}H] LTC$_4$-binding have not been as illuminating. Initially it was thought that binding of radioactive LTC$_4$ to membranes from guinea pig lung, ileal, and uterine smooth muscle [63, 64, 73, 74], rat lung [75] and human lung [76] occurred at specific receptors because the binding was specific, saturable, and reversible at nanomolar concentrations. However, there were a number of confusing observations. Tissue distribution surveys indicated that LTC$_4$-binding was ubiquitous in nature including tissues and subcellular organelles that did not respond to leukotrienes [77]. Moreover, a series of LTC$_4$ analogs showed divergent results when binding was compared with contraction of guinea pig tracheal and lung smooth muscle preparations [78]. Finally, the binding was not sensitive to regulation by nonhydrolyzable guanine nucleotides or cations. Subsequently, Sun et al. [79a, 79b] showed that substantial amounts of the LTC$_4$-binding that occurred in rat liver cytosol, mitochondrial, and microsomal fractions was to the Ya subunit of glutathione S-transferase. Recently, LTC$_4$-binding activity in differentiated U937 cell membranes has been shown to be due to binding to microsomal glutathione S-transferase [80]. Data with sheep lung membranes appears to be suggestive that here too the binding activity is associated with glutatione S-transferase [72]. Thus, these more recent experiments strongly suggest that in the earlier binding studies significant amounts of labeled ligand bound to transferase and not to an LTC$_4$ receptor.

The signal transduction system for cysteinyl leukotriene receptors has only been partially characterized. Most information collected so far has been on the LTD$_4$ receptor. Binding of this leukotriene to its receptor is specifically regulated by sodium ion, divalent cations calcium and magnesium, and GTP [64, 66, 69, 81–83]. Divalent cations increase the density of ligand binding sites while sodium ions and nonhydrolyzable GTP analogs reduce the affinity of LTD$_4$ for its receptor. These results are consistent with the ternary complex hypothesis originally suggested by Lefkowitz et al. [84]. Thus, it can be envisioned that LTD$_4$, the receptor, along with a G-protein form a coupling unit that subsequently activates additional second messenger systems in the cell. Binding of LTD$_4$ to its receptor in guinea pig membranes promotes the complexing of ligand, receptor, and G-protein. O'Sullivan and Mong [85], using a radiolabeled LTD$_4$ antagonist, [^{3}H]ICI-198,615, suggested that the LTD$_4$ receptor can exist in two affinity states with K$_D$'s of 0.5 and 200 nM. Divalent cations favor formation of the high affinity state. Sodium ion, EDTA, or GTPγS induced a shift to the low affinity state. When all three of these agents were used in combination, the LTD$_4$ receptors were completely converted to the low affinity state. Although a number of G-protein regulated complexes are coupled to adenylate cyclase, support is not strong for intracellular c-AMP as an important second messenger in LTD_4-mediated responses. In fact, Torphy et al. [86] showed that contraction of opossum trachea with LTD_4 caused an increase in tissue levels of cGMP but not cAMP. In addition, LTD_4 did not affect isoproterenol-induced accumulation of cAMP.

There is considerable evidence to suggest that the signal transduction mechanism involves phosphatidylinositol (PI) hydrolysis, followed by calcium mobilization and protein kinase C (PKC) activation. Mong et al. [87] showed that LTD_4 induced a rapid hydrolysis of PI in guinea pig lung with a concomitant formation of inositol phosphates. In addition, binding of LTD_4 to membrane receptors activated phospholipase C, the enzyme that hydrolyzes PI. Pretreatment of guinea pig lung with the specific LTD_4 antagonist, SKF 104353, inhibited LTD_4-induced PI hydrolysis [88]. Studies with the rat basophilic leukemia cell line, RBL-1, yielded similar results. Incubation of these cells with LTD_4 resulted in PI hydrolysis [69] and an increase in PKC activity [89]. Prior treatment of the cells with either SKF 104353 or the PKC inhibitor, staurosporine, inhibited the activation of PKC. Several laboratories have reported elevations in intracellular calcium $[Ca^{++}]i$ upon exposure of cells to LTD_4 [90–94]. The rapid, transient increase in $[Ca^{++}]i$ is derived from both internal stores and extracellular calcium. However, the degree to which either calcium mobilization or influx is involved in LTD_4-induced contractions varies depending on the tissue or cell type. The rise in intracellular calcium upon contraction of guinea pig ileal longitudinal muscle by LTD_4 stems almost exclusively from extracellular calcium since removal of extracellular Ca^{++} by addition of EGTA competely abolished the rise in $[Ca^{++}]i$ [95]. In addition, the time course of $[Ca^{++}]i$ elevation was monophasic and declined very slowly, a pattern expected for calcium influx. This was also true when HL60 cells were stimulated with LTD_4 [90]. However, removal of extracellular calcium did not inhibit or only partially inhibited LTD_4-stimulated $[Ca^{++}]i$ increases in sheep tracheal smooth muscle cells [92], RBL-1 [91], U-937 [93], mesangial cells [94], and contraction of guinea pig lung parenchyma [96, 97]. The implication of these findings is that there are diverse calcium modulatory systems for regulating LTD_4 receptors from different cells and tissues. Subsequent to the activation of PKC, stimulation of cytoplasmic PLA_2 takes place. The nature of how this process occurs has not been extensively studied. A protein that activates a low molecular weight PLA_2 from EL-4 cells but not a high molecular weight enzyme derived from mouse mammary cells has been described [98, 99]. Clark et al. have reported a transient increase in this protein in smooth muscle and endothelial cells following treatment with LTD_4 and inhibition of LTD_4-induced prostanoid synthesis in these cells with antisense oligonucleotides [100]. With the activation of $cPLA_2$, arachidonic acid is released and depending on the cell is metabolized by either the cyclo-oxygenase pathway, the lipoxygenase pathway, or both.

4.2   Leukotriene B_4 receptor

Characterization of the properties and functions of LTB_4 receptors has been ascertained mainly in either intact human neutrophils or isolated neutrophilic membranes. Using high specific activity $[^3H]LTB_4$ and intact purified human neutrophils, Goldman and Goetzl [101] reported that a Scatchard analysis of binding data implied that two classes of LTB_4 receptors existed, a high (K_D, 3.9×10^{-10} M) and a low affinity receptor (K_D, 6.1×10^{-8} M). In addition, studies with stereoisomers of LTB_4 and desensitization experiments by prior exposure to LTB_4 suggested that the high affinity receptor was associated with chemotaxis and adhesion of neutrophils. Similarities between the K_D of the low affinity receptor and the EC_{50} for LTB_4-induced release of lysosomal enzymes or superoxide production, as well as the failure of agonist desensitization to suppress either low affinity binding or enzyme release implied that degranulation and reactive oxygen species production are mediated by the low affinity receptor [101,102]. Subsequent experiments have revealed that the LTB_4 receptor complex consists of a 60 kDa protein [103] that contains the LTB_4 binding site and a 40–41 kDa protein that binds GTP [104]. Affinity of this complex for LTB_4 appears to be modulated by local concentrations of GTP, the higher the concentration of GTP, the lower the affinity for LTB_4 [105]. Further support for the involvement of a G-protein is indicated from studies showing that pertussis toxin, under conditions where it catalyzes ADP-ribosylation of the α subunit of G_i, can completely inhibit chemotaxis and enzyme release induced by LTB_4 [104]. In addition, pertussis toxin treatment reduced the density of high affinity receptors and increased their affinity for LTB_4 threefold. These data suggested a close link between the high affinity receptor subtype and the G-protein. Complexes of receptor protein with a G-protein have been shown for other chemotactic factors and raise the question of whether there is a distinct G-protein for each receptor or whether a common protein is used by all receptor macromolecules. Recent comparative studies on ADP-ribosylation of G-proteins in HL60 membranes by pertussis and cholera toxins led McLeisch and colleagues to conclude that FMLP and LTB_4 receptors are coupled to common G-proteins but the two receptors induce different conformations of the activated α subunit of G_i [106, 107].

Upon activation or inhibition of the formation of second messengers triggered by binding of LTB_4 to its neutrophilic receptor, appropriate regulatory proteins are phosphorylated leading ultimately to activation of cell responses such as chemotaxis, superoxide production, and degranulation. A key enzyme involved in the phosphorylation process is PKC. Stimulation of cells with divalent cationic ionophores, such as ionomycin and A23187, leads to a considerable elevation of intracellular calcium concentrations. This, in turn, causes soluble PKC in the cytosol to translocate to the plasma membrane where it binds diacylglycerol and becomes capable of phosphorylating response-eliciting proteins [108]. However, the mechanism of PKC activation in LTB_4-stimulated cells appears even more complex. O'Flaherty et al. carried out experiments in which they measured binding of phorbol dibutyrate and intracellular calcium concentrations at intervals after LTB_4 stimulation [109]. Their results indicated that LTB_4 induced two sequential mechanisms for translocating PKC. Initially a rapidly reversing response involving calcium transients is involved in movement of PKC to the plasmalemma followed by a second more slowly evolving cytosolic calcium-independent process. In addition, the same investigators found PKC activators to have bidirectional effects on degranulation responses induced by LTB_4 [110]. Low concentrations enhanced, whereas high concentrations inhibited release of lysozyme and β-glucuronidase. The latter effect correlated with a decrease in density of high affinity receptors and elevation of intracellular calcium. These findings appear to indicate that at high amounts of PKC activation, feedback inhibition takes place with the enzyme down-regulating the number of receptors available on the cell surface.

5   Criteria for establishing leukotriene involvement in human disease

To prove that an endogenous substance (mediator) contributes to the pathobiology of a disease, the following criteria need to be satisfied:

1. The body must have the capability to synthesize and release the mediator in response to noxious stimuli or to tissue injury.
2. Elevated levels of the mediators are present in body fluids surrounding involved tissue just prior to or at the peak of the disorder.
3. Exogenous administration of chemically pure mediator produces symptoms or induces lesions similar to that observed during the actual pathologic event.

4. Perhaps most important, inhibition of synthesis, release, or pharmacologic activity of the mediator must produce a positive clinical response in patients suffering from the disorder assuming appropriate pharmacokinetics and bioavailability.

Taking the first three factors into consideration and by the use of novel receptor antagonists and enzyme inhibitors, a wealth of information has resulted implicating the leukotrienes in a diverse group of inflammatory diseases. Since this area has matured sufficiently to warrant its own review, we have selected only a few examples to make key points and have highlighted recent preclinical findings which will ultimately translate into a new understanding of human clinical disorders.

6   Development and clinical use of LTD_4/LTE_4 receptor antagonists for treatment of asthma

Given the initial discovery of the cysteinyl leukotrienes as components of SRS/SRS-A, it is not surprising that these mediators were proposed to have significant involvement in human allergic asthma [7,22,111]. As early as 1963, Herxheimer and Streseman [112] reported preliminary results in 9 asthmatic patients who inhaled crude SRS-A. Vital capacity decreased in these subjects. This effect was not seen in normal subjects probably due to the lack of airway hyperreactivity, a key feature of asthma. More recent studies have found elevated levels of leukotrienes in bronchoalveolar lavage fluid or urine from subjects after antigen inhalation [113, 114], during episodes of aspirin-induced asthma [115], after an incidence of exercise-induced asthma [116], and in patients suffering from naturally occurring asthma [117–119]. Inhalation of cysteinyl leukotrienes by human subjects caused an intense bronchospasm at considerably lower concentrations than a similar response elicited to histamine or methacholine [120-122]. Perhaps more important, Arm et al. demonstrated airway hyperreactivity to histamine following inhalation of LTE_4 but not methacholine in asthmatics [123].

FPL 55712, the first cysteinyl leukotriene receptor antagonist, was discovered during evaluation of a series of potential mast cell stabilizers derived from disodiumchromoglycate. This propylhydroxyacetophenone was never developed into a therapeutic agent due to poor oral absorption and a short biological half-life after intravenous administration (124,125). Several research groups attempted to improve the bioavailability of this class of compounds while retaining pharmacologic activity. The first noteworthy success with this approach was the discovery of LY171883, a tetra-zole-substituted acetophenone [126, 44]. This compound was of similar potency to FPL 55712 but had a much longer biological half-life after oral administration. LY171883 was the first LTD_4/LTE_4 receptor antagonist to be evaluated in the clinic for the treatment of human asthma [44, 126, 127]. Although not especially potent by current standards [16–19], it pro-duced significant beneficial effects in a group of mild to moderate asth-matics [128] including improvement in FEV_1, a pulmonary function test that assesses airway patency. Furthermore, a reduction in bronchodilator usage was associated with administration of compound. LY171883 also produced a slight reduction in the bronchospasm that followed cold air inhalation in asthmatics [129] and seemed to have a positive effect in patients who experienced exercise-induced asthma [130]. Together, these initial studies indicated that pharmacologic interference with the action of cysteinyl leukotrienes might prove valuable in the treatment of obstruc-tive airway disease. Unfortunately, LY171883 was withdrawn from clini-cal trials due to toxicity observed in long-term animal studies [131, 132]. Like LY171883, other compounds with similar pharmacologic profiles from various research laboratories showed the potential for clinical effi-cacy in asthma only to have their development discontinued due to bio-availability, pharmaceutical, or toxicological issues. The importance of these early clinical explorations, however, cannot be understated. They established that a new class of pharmaceuticals, with a novel mechanism of action, could positively impact on human asthma, thereby opening the door to many intensive drug discovery programs. Three second genera-tion antagonists, SKF 104353, ICI 204,219 and MK-571 (Fig. 3) have arisen from such efforts and proceeded to advanced stages in clinical trials.

The approach that led to the synthesis of SKF 104353 began by analyz-ing the activity of structural modifications of LTD_4. Elimination of a meth-ylene group between the C-1 and C-5 carbon of LTD_4 led to a molecule with much less agonist activity and some antagonist potency [133, 134]. Further SAR studies revealed that a saturated lipid tail was necessary for antagonist activity but the glycyl unit was not [135, 136]. The near sym-metry of these antagonists suggested that the two polar chains might be functionally interchangeable when the molecule is bound to the LTD_4 receptor. Subsequently, compounds were synthesized with two identical polar chains and the effects of modifications of the polar and lipid regions on receptor antagonism measured [137, 138]. The key observations in these studies were the finding that the triene moiety could be replaced with a phenyl group and attachment to the aromatic ring of a lipid side chain of 10–12 carbon atoms greatly enhanced activity. Inserting a second phenyl group at the end of the lipid chain improved metabolic stability of the compounds. These observations ultimately led to synthesis of the stereo-isomer SKF 104353. This drug has a high affinity for guinea pig lung membrane receptors and is a competitive antagonist of LTD_4 and LTE_4-induced guinea pig tracheal contraction [139,140]. SKF 104353, which has an absolute stereochemistry identical to LTD_4, is a much stronger antagonist than its enantiomer, indicating a highly stereoselective interaction of the drug with the LTD_4 receptor. *In vivo* experiments [141] in guinea pigs showed that the compound was effective at inhibiting LTD_4-induced bronchoconstriction when given as an aerosol, intravenously, or intraduodenally. Clinical studies have been carried out via the inhalation route. SKF 104353 effectively inhibited LTD_4-induced bronchoconstriction in normal subjects and mild asthmatics but not the corresponding response induced by histamine [142, 143]. The drug also was shown to be capable of preventing allergen-induced bronchoconstriction [144]. Pretreatment of patients sensitive to ragweed or cat dander with 640 μg led to inhibition of the early response in 7 of 10 individuals and to complete suppression of the late-phase response in the only two patients who experienced this effect. Finally, 15 min after administering an 800-μg dose to mild asthmatics, SKF 104353 inhibited the drop in FEV_1 resulting from exercise challenge [145].

MK-571 (L-660,711) evolved from identifying a simple styryl quinoline, 3-[2-(2-quinolinyl)-(E)-ethenyl]pyridine, which moderately inhibited binding of [^{3}H]LTD_4 to guinea pig lung membranes and inhibited antigen-induced dyspnea in hyperreactive rats [146]. The strategy used to develop more potent inhibitors was to synthesize and test compounds that would fit a hypothetical model for the LTD_4 receptor derived by Young from analysis of biological data on various LTD_4 analogs [147, 148]. In this model, the receptor consists of three binding sites, a flat lipophilic binding site where the triene fits, an ionic site where the cysteinyl-glycine unit likely interacts by both hydrogen bonding and ionic actions, and a polar site where the carboxyl group binds through H-bonding. Zamboni et al. [146] proposed that the lead structure bound to the flat lipophilic binding site and therefore by adding further lipophilic and polar components they could improve the potency. Initially increased activity was obtained by replacement of the pyridyl moiety with a phenyl group. Substitution of a chlorine molecule at the 7 position on the quinoline ring and attachment of two acidic groups to the 3-position of the aryl ring via a dithioacetal led to a compound with an IC_{50} of 3 nM. Formation of the mono-N, N-dimethylamide derivative (MK-571) improved the activity another 3-fold. *In vitro* pharmacologic studies showed MK-571 to be a potent competitive and selective inhibitor of LTD_4 binding to guinea pig and human lung membranes [52]. LTD_4 and LTE_4-induced contractions of guinea pig trachea and ileum were strongly antagonized. Contractions induced by LTC_4 in the presence of serine borate buffer were not affected. Likewise, responses induced with mediators such as histamine and acetylcholine were not attenuated with MK-571. Contraction of human trachea induced by LTD_4 could also be inhibited but the pA_2 value was a log lower than that obtained in guinea pig trachea. Antigen-induced contractions of guinea pig trachea in the presence of atropine, mepyramine and indomethacin were only partly inhibited because the reaction is not fully mediated by LTD_4. In contrast, anti-IgE mediated contractions of human trachea were completely blocked by MK-571.

In vivo studies [52] demonstrated that bronchoconstriction induced by any of the cysteinyl leukotrienes in anesthetized guinea pigs could be attenuated by intravenous doses of MK-571. In addition, when given intraduodenally, it inhibited LTD_4-induced bronchoconstriction in this species. Studies with conscious squirrel monkeys showed the compound could block both LTD_4-mediated pulmonary responses and those elicited after challenge with Ascaris antigen. Furthermore, ovalbumin-induced airway constriction was inhibited by MK-571 in rats pretreated with methysergide. Intravenous infusion of the compound reduced the early phase and completely blocked the late phase response in Ascaris challenged sheep [149,150]. The early and late responses in allergen challenged Brown-Norway rats were also reduced by the drug [151].

In initial clinical studies, Depré et al. [152] and Kips et al. [153] reported that MK-571 inhibited LTD_4-induced bronchoconstriction in six healthy volunteers and six asthmatic individuals in a double-blind, placebo-controlled, randomized crossover study without significant adverse effects. Normal subjects were given a total of either 28, 86 or 1500 mg of the drug in a regimen consisting of a bolus followed by a continuous infusion. The mean end-of-infusion plasma concentrations were 0.6, 1.9 and 118 µg/ml, respectively. At all of these plasma concentrations, MK-571 completely inhibited bronchoconstriction induced by inhaling 100 µM LTD_4 and therefore no dose-response measurements could be made. Asthmatic patients were administered 27 and 277 mg of the drug in a regimen similar to that used with control subjects. Mean end-of-fusion levels of the drug were 0.7 and 8.6 µg/ml, respectively. The higher dose of drug caused an 84-fold rightward shift of the LTD_4 dose-response curve. Even at the lower dose, a 44-fold shift in the dose-response curve was observed. When the drug was infused in mildly asthmatic men [154] who were challenged with antigen, MK-571 inhibited both the immediate and the late phase response. In addition, pretreatment of stable asthmatics with the compound attenuated exercise-induced bronchoconstriction [155]. Finally, twelve patients with moderately severe asthma who were given an infusion of the drug had a 20% increase in their mean FEV_1 values when compared to placebo treatment [156].

MK-571 is a racemate, containing a chiral center at the methine carbon of the dithio side chain. Both enantiomers are pharmacologically active but the S-enantiomer is slightly more active than the R-enantiomer as an inhibitor of LTD_4 binding to guinea pig lung membranes and LTD_4-induced guinea pig trachea contraction [157]. However, when the enantiomers were studied for their effects on antigen-induced dyspnea in hyperactive rats, the R-enantiomer was approximately 4-fold more potent. This reversal of potencies when the compounds were dosed *in vivo* appears due to higher blood levels and a longer half-life for the R-enantiomer in rats [158]. Extensive *in vitro* and *in vivo* studies with the R-enantiomer (MK-679, verlukast) showed the compound had a pharmacologic profile similar to that of the racemate [53]. In clinical studies MK-679 has been found to block airway obstruction induced by bronchial provocation with inhaled lysine-aspirin in aspirin-sensitive asthmatics [159]. Treatment of eight such patients with 825 mg oral doses of MK-679 caused a bronchodilation that lasted at least nine hours [160]. The average peak improvement in FEV_1 was 18% above the predrug baseline.

ICI 204,219 (Accolate®) is a second generation selective LTD_4/LTE_4 receptor antagonist with a similar pharmacologic profile to FPL 55712 and LY171883 but with greatly enhanced potency [161–165]. Development of this indole derivative originated with separate SAR studies on both FPL 55712 and the cysteinyl leukotrienes. Modifications of FPL 55712 led to a methoxybenzoic acid series incorporating the hydroxyacetophenone group while the leukotriene series focused on the replacement of the triene backbone with phenyl groups [166, 167]. Each effort resulted in benzoic acid compounds with micromolar potency. At this point, it was decided to gain potency by synthesizing molecules with more conformational constraint. This was done by selecting bicyclic indazoles and indoles as a framework to which benzoic acid groups and lipophilic chains could be attached. Optimization of antagonist activity was achieved by studying modifications of the acyl chain, the central heterocyclic template, and the benzoic acid moiety. This ultimately led to synthesis of the potent orally active indole, ICI 204,219 [168–170]. This compound is a competitive antagonist of both LTD_4 and LTE_4-induced guinea pig airway smooth muscle contraction with pK_B values ranging from 9.0 to 9.6 [161]. On isolated human bronchial smooth muscle, the compound competitively antagonized contractions induced by all 3 cysteinyl leukotrienes [171]. The pK_B values were independent of the particular cysteinyl leukotriene used to elicit contraction but as found with other antagonists 10-fold lower than values observed with guinea pig tissue. Activity of the compound is selective since it does not antagonize contraction of guinea pig ileum induced by other agonists [161]. Whether administered orally, intravenously, or as an aerosol, ICI 204,219 is a potent *in vivo* inhibitor of cysteinyl leukotriene induced responses [161]. The compound rapidly reverses bronchoconstriction when administered intravenously at the peak of a leukotriene-induced response. In addition, antigen-induced bronchoconstriction was prevented by prior intravenous dosing of ICI 204,219 and reversed by intravenous administration at the peak of the response.

ICI 204,219 has now successfully undergone extensive clinical evaluation and the results have erased any doubt of a cysteinyl leukotriene involvement in human asthma. Initial studies in normal subjects indicated that a single oral 40-mg dose could inhibit LTD_4-induced bronchoconstriction [162]. A follow-up investigation indicated that the compound also antagonized LTD_4-induced bronchoconstriction in mild asthmatics [172]. Moreover, there was a direct correlation between the plasma concentration of the drug and its protective effect. Subsequently, Taylor et al. [173] evaluated the efficacy of the compound on allergen-induced pulmonary function changes. Ten mild atopic patients were given a single oral 40-mg dose of ICI 204,219 in a double blind placebo controlled crossover study. Two hours later, they were subjected to a bronchial challenge with aerosolized allergen and airway responses assessed for the following 6 hours. ICI 204,219 profoundly attenuated the early fall in FEV_1 and significantly reduced the bronchial reactivity. In a separate investigation Dahlen et al. [174] carried out bronchial provocation studies on 10 atopic asthmatic men and found a 20-mg dose of drug given two hours before antigen challenge inhibited 60% of the acute response. In a more detailed multicenter, dose-ranging study carried out for 6 weeks, a 20 mg twice daily dose decreased nighttime awakenings by 46%, albuterol use by 30%, daytime symptoms by 26% and increased FEV_1 by 11% [165]. Hui and Barnes, in a double-blind study with ten asthmatic patients administered a single 40 mg oral dose, observed a significantly increased FEV_1 above baseline [175]. This was not seen with the placebo control, suggesting that there is a persistent generation of cysteinyl leukotrienes in asthmatics even when subjects are treated with inhaled corticosteroids. The compound also attenuated bronchoconstriction occurring in exercise-induced asthma [176]. In eight male subjects with stable asthma, a 2 hour pretreatment with an oral 20-mg dose of ICI 204,219 reduced the mean maximum percentage fall in FEV_1 following exercise from $36.0 \pm 6.1\%$ to $21.6 \pm 5.9\%$.

7   Role of LTB$_4$ in inflammatory diseases

Although LTB$_4$ has been suggested to play a proinflammatory role in human pathology, receptor antagonists of this leukotriene have not advanced to the stage where they have been vigorously evaluated as potential therapeutic agents. However, at least 4 newly discovered potent orally active compounds in this class, LY293111 [177, 178], SC-53228 [179], CP-105,696 [180], and CGS 25019C [181], are moving along that development path. The current expectation based on a knowledge of the neutrophil chemotactic and cell-activating properties of LTB$_4$, in addition to other pharmacologic activities, such as stimulating release of thromboxane from cells [28, 30–32], would be for LTB$_4$ receptor antagonists to reduce the intensity of those disorders where neutrophils and possibly eosinophils contribute to an inflammatory response. Inflammatory bowel disease (IBD), psoriasis, arthritis, and asthma would appear to be logical targets.

Sharon and Stenson [182] first proposed an involvement for LTB$_4$ in the two major forms of IBD, Crohn's disease and ulcerative colitis. Colonic mucosa from patients with IBD converted more exogenous arachidonic acid to LTB$_4$ than mucosa from control subjects. This was followed by an examination of tissue lipid extracts to identify the chemotactic substance responsible for infiltration of neutrophils, the primary inflammatory cells in that disorder. LTB$_4$ was found in concentrations capable of inducing chemotaxis [182, 183]. Additional experiments supported the connection between maintenance of IBD and generation of LTB$_4$ [184, 185]. With the use of *in vivo* equilibrium dialysis, elevated levels have been reported in the lumen of patients with active ulcerative colitis [186]. The concentration correlated with disease activity by clinical, endoscopic and histological grading and was reduced when patients responded to topical 5-aminosalicylate and prednisolone therapy. Interestingly, sulfasalazine and 5-aminosalicylic acid, some of the primary therapeutic agents used to treat IBD, have 5-lipoxygenase inhibitory activity at pharmacologically relevant concentrations [187, 188].

Kragballe and Voorhees [189] have summarized evidence that LTB$_4$ and other lipoxygenase products have a pathological role in psoriasis. Numerous studies have documented higher levels of 5-lipoxygenase products in involved but not in uninvolved skin from patients with psoriasis [190–192], and a variety of other dermatoses [193–195]. Besides elevated concentrations of LTB$_4$, extremely high levels of arachidonic acid and 12-R-HETE are also found in psoriatic skin lesions. Cunningham et al. [196] and Evans et al. [197] have shown that 12-R-HETE binds to the LTB$_4$ receptor and stimulates the same cell responses as LTB$_4$. Moreover, LTB$_4$ receptor antagonists block 12-R-HETE induced responses [198]. Application of LTB_4 or racemic 12-HETE to human skin results in formation of intraepidermal microabscesses, one of the earliest morphological events seen in the development of psoriasis [199]. In addition, both LTB_4 and racemic 12-HETE have been shown to stimulate epidermal proliferation [200]. Consequently, the two eicosanoids may contribute to both inflammatory and proliferative changes that occur in psoriasis [201]. Unfortunately, despite epidermal and dermal localization of the lesions, and therefore easy drug accessibility, therapy with an appropriate synthesis inhibitor or pharmacologic antagonist has not been forthcoming. Whether due to lack of drug potency, the high levels of eicosanoids relative to antagonist or synthesis inhibitor in the skin, or perhaps a more prominent role by other inflammatory mediators, is presently unknown.

Evidence has also accumulated suggesting a role for LTB_4 in clinical arthritic disorders. Rae et al. [202] has reported greatly elevated levels of LTB_4 in gouty effusions. They also found evidence of this mediator or its metabolites in synovial fluid of rheumatoid arthritics [203]. Several investigators [204–206] have indicated that neutrophils from rheumatoid arthritic patients can be stimulated to produce more LTB_4 than corresponding cells from individuals without disease. Metabolic activity of cells from patients treated with methotrexate [207–209], tenidap sodium [210], fish oil [211, 212], nonsteroidal anti-inflammatory agents [213] or clotrimazole [213] indicated that treatment with all of these drugs reduced the neutrophils ability to produce excessive amounts of LTB_4. In some cases, this effect correlated with reduction of symptoms.

Less obvious is the role played by LTB_4 in the asthmatic state. Initial studies by Lee et al. [214] demonstrated elevated levels of LTB_4 in plasma following induction of anaphylaxis by intravenous administration of antigen in immunologically sensitized guinea pigs. Documentation that this LTB_4 might have emanated from the lung was obtained by Atkins et al. [215] using sensitized guinea pig lung fragments. Antigen challenge of this preparation resulted in release of sufficient LTB_4 to account for the neutrophil chemotactic activity residing in the supernatant fluid. Silbaugh et al. [216] observed a delayed-onset airway obstruction associated with pulmonary granulocyte infiltration during inhalation of LTB_4 in guinea pigs. In concert with these animal studies, Wardlow et al. [217], Shindo et al. [218], and Sampson et al. [219] detected elevated levels of LTB_4 in blood and bronchoalveolar lavage (BAL) fluid from asthmatics. Similarly, Zocca et al. [220] reported increased concentrations of LTB_4 associated with neutrophil influx and late phase bronchospasm in lungs of patients with occupational asthma caused by toluene diisothionate hypersensitivity. An interesting clinical study by Koh et al. [221] has recently added additional support to the hypothesis that LTB_4 is an important neutrophil chemotactic substance in lung after antigen challenge. Ragweed-allergic volunteers were exposed to antigen through a bronchoscope. Examination of neutrophils removed from the lung by bronchoalveolar lavage revealed that they were selectively desensitized in their chemotactic response to LTB_4 but not to anaphylatoxin C5a or formyl-L-methionyl-L-leucyl-L-phenylalanine (fMLP). This selective desensitization suggested that there had been prior exposure to LTB_4. The assumption was therefore made that the neutrophils had been previously exposed to LTB_4 generated in response to the antigen challenge. A similar study by the same group has provided an initial indication that after antigen challenge BAL eosinophils are also desensitized to LTB_4 [222]. More recent studies have suggested a primary role for interleukin-8 (IL-8), a polypeptide cytokine, as possibly the major neutrophil chemotactic factor in lung [223, 224]. This substance joins platelet activating factor (PAF), various bacterial derived peptides, complement C5a, in addition to LTB_4 as important chemoattractants for human neutrophils. Any or all of these substances might participate in the underlying inflammation characteristic of asthma, and other lung diseases such as adult respiratory distress syndrome, interstitial pulmonary fibrosis, chronic bronchitis, and cystic fibrosis. In fact, studies by Thomsen et al. [225] and McCain et al. [226] have pointed to an interrelationship that exists between LTB_4 and IL-8. Similarly, interleukin 5 (IL-5), another cytokine, known to mediate a variety of activities governing eosinophil function including chemotaxis [227, 228], was demonstrated by Yamaoka and Kolb [229] to be produced by human T-cells in response to LTB_4. Clearly, a variety of endogenous molecules participate in the inflammatory process. Whether this indicates mediator redundancy, which would make treatment with antagonists more difficult because of the need to have a specific blocking agent for each mediator, or whether there is a common signal transduction pathway, interruption of which by a single inhibitor could produce significant medical relief will have to wait the introduction of selective enzyme inhibitors and pharmacologic antagonists into clinical medicine.

8   Development of LTB_4 receptor antagonists

The first antagonists of LTB_4 to be reported were structural analogs (Fig. 4). In 1981, Goetzl and Pickett [230] synthesized diacetyl-LTB_4 and found it to be a competitve inhibitor of LTB_4-induced chemotaxis of human neu-

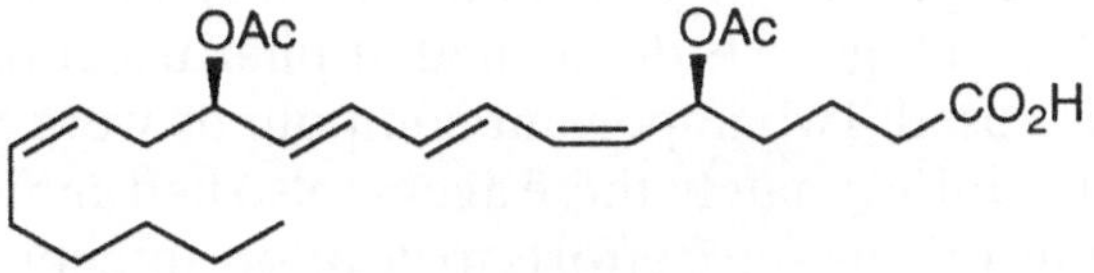

DiAcetyl-LTB$_4$

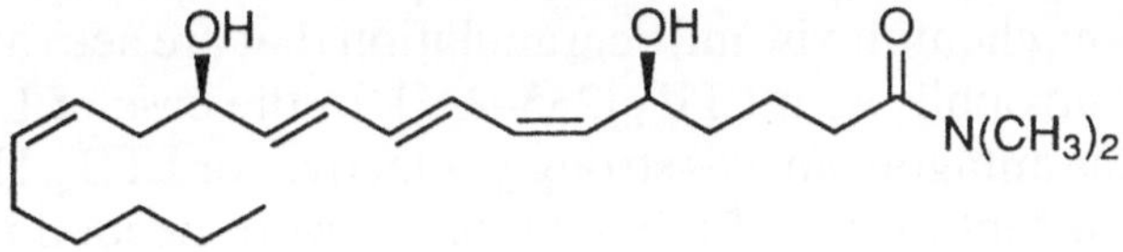

LTB$_4$ Dimethylamide

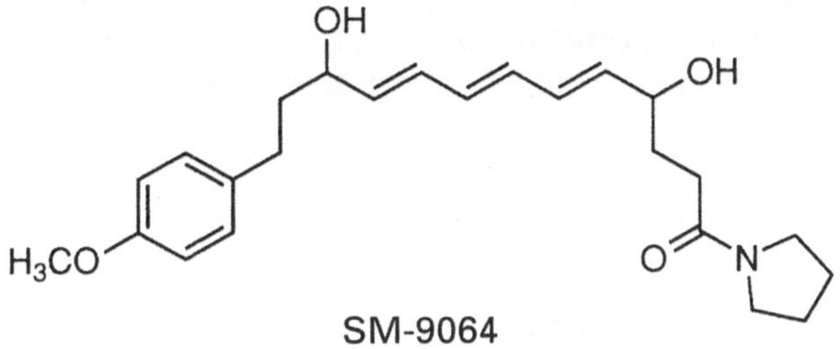

SM-9064

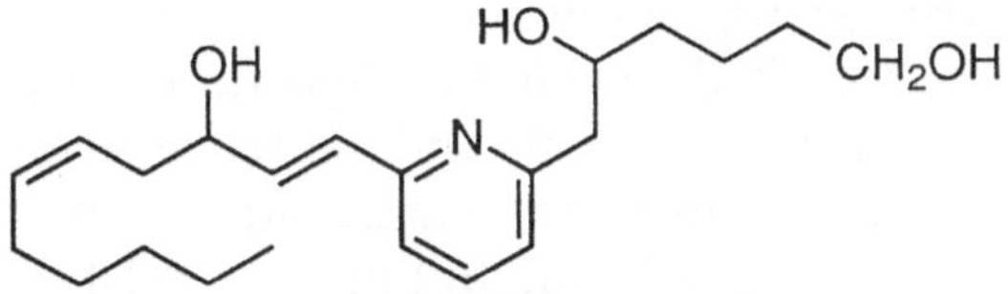

U-75302

Fig. 4
Analogs of LTB$_4$ were the initial LTB$_4$ receptor antagonists to be described.

trophils. The following year, Showell et al. [231] reported that LTB_4 dimethylamide inhibited degranulation of rabbit neutrophils induced by LTB_4. In the mid-1980's antagonists developed at pharmaceutical companies began to be disclosed. Two important compounds were SM-9064 and U-75302 [232–234]. Unfortunately, these agents also had agonist activity. This is not entirely surprising since efforts to develop antagonists from analogs of other biologically active molecules have often yielded partial agonists.

The initial non-LTB_4 analog receptor antagonists were LY255283, LY223982, and SC-41930 (Fig. 5). All of these compounds inhibited not only specific binding of $[^3H]LTB_4$ to the LTB_4 receptor but also cell functions such as aggregation, chemotaxis, and degranulation that are activated upon stimulation of neutrophils with LTB_4 [235–237]. In the case of LY255283 and LY223982, this antagonism was strongly selective for LTB_4. Hundredfold or greater concentrations of the antagonists were needed to inhibit cell activation by other agonists. LY255283 and SC-41930 were developed by modifying acetophenone structures which had previously been found to antagonize LTD_4-mediated responses [237,238]. Efforts to see if benzophenones could substitute for acetophenones led to the discovery of LY223982 [239,240]. The structural changes that convert an acetophenone from an LTD_4 receptor antagonist to an LTB_4 receptor antagonist are quite subtle. In the case of the LY255283 series, it is transposing the short nonpolar chain from the 3- to the 5-position on the phenyl ring. For the SC-41930 series, methoxylating the phenolic hydroxy makes it an LTB_4 receptor antagonist. Although LTD_4 and LTB_4 produce very different responses, the fact that their specific antagonists have structural similarities suggest that the two receptors probably have common features.

Comparisons of the activities of different analogs synthesized during the development of these antagonists give some suggestion as to how they bind to the LTB_4 receptor. In the LY255283 series, maximum activity was achieved when the hydroxyacetophenone contained a short chain alkyl ketone in the 1-position, a free hydroxyl in the 2-position, a hydrogen in the 3-position, a six- or eight-carbon chain linking the oxygen in the 4-position with an acidic function, and a nonpolar substituent in the 5-position [238]. This suggests that LY255283 might bind to the LTB_4 receptor with the acidic group binding where the carboxyl group of LTB_4 attaches, the flat hydroxyalkoxyacetophenone binding where the flat triene unit of LTB_4 binds, and the phenolic hydroxyl group interacting at the site where the C(12)-hydroxyl group fits.

In the evolution of the LY223982 chemical series, two features were found critical for maximizing binding of compound to the LTB_4 receptor on

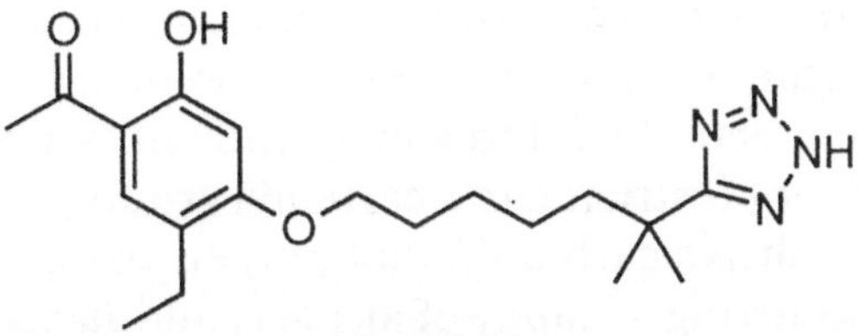

LY255283

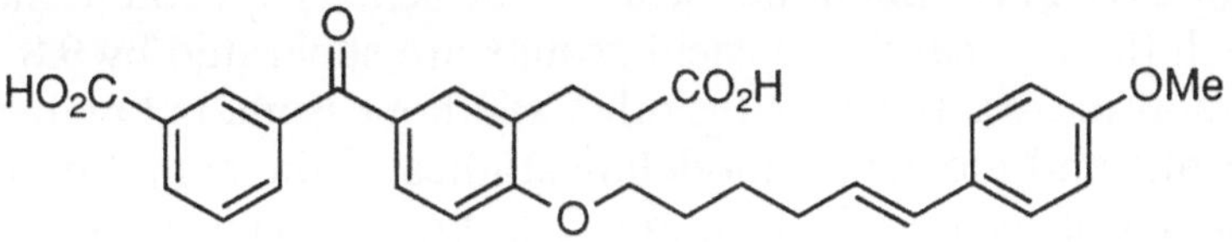

LY223982

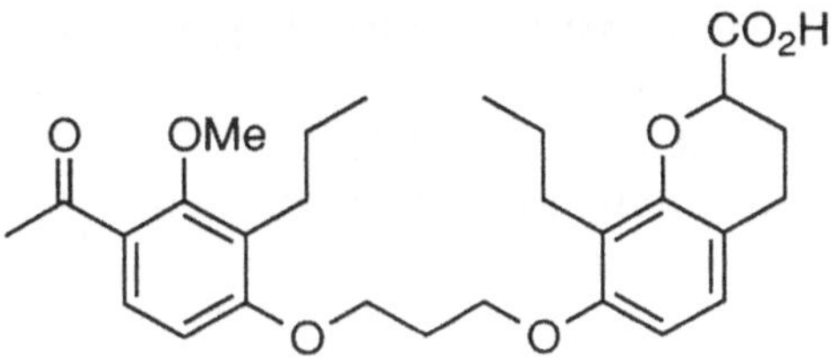

SC-41930

Fig. 5
First compounds not related to LTB$_4$ in structure that were found to selectively inhibit LTB$_4$-mediated events.

human neutrophils. First, it was necessary for the molecule to contain a lipophilic side chain of a particular length [239]. For example, in a series of n-alkoxyl derivatives, optimal activity was observed when the length of the chain was 10 carbons. In addition, terminating the chain with a paramethoxyphenyl moiety greatly enhanced the potency of these structures. The second critical feature of benzophenone antagonists was the presence of acidic groups on each ring [240]. Relative orientation of these groups was important with substitutions in the meta position on each ring yielding maximum activity. Interestingly, the entity linking the two aromatic groups was not restricted to a carbonyl group but could be a variety of other linkers such as a carbinol, ether oxygen, oxime, etc. without much loss of activity occurring. Chaney et al. [241] and Jackson et al. [242] further characterized the spatial arrangement of the two acidic groups by comparing concentration profiles for inhibition of [^{3}H]LTB$_4$ receptor binding of rigid xanthone isomers that mimicked the four major conformational states of benzophenone dicarboxylic acids. They found the isomer in which the two carboxylic acid groups are separated by 9.8 Å to be considerably more active than the other xanthone isomers. On the basis of these results and molecular modeling studies of the compounds, the investigators suggested that the xanthone dicarboxylic acids form a 3-point attachment with the LTB$_4$ receptor in which the aryl acid group, the carbon atoms in one of the rings, and the lipophilic tail bind, respectively, to sites normally occupied by the carboxyl group, the triene carbons, and the hydrophobic tail of LTB$_4$. The other acid group of the antagonists (the propionic moiety of LY223982) binds to a site not available to LTB$_4$. However, the complex of LTB$_4$ with receptor may well be more intricate than this model with the carboxyl group of LTB$_4$ able to oscillate back and forth between the two acid binding sites.

LY223982 lacked oral activity and LY255283, when dosed orally, was only modestly effective at preventing LTB$_4$ produced airway obstruction [243]. To develop a more potent oral drug, structural modifications of LY255283 were made. The strategy used was to divide the parent molecule into three sections, the acetophenone portion, the acid moiety, and a linker piece, and to study the effect of modifications on the activity of each. The effort eventually led to the synthesis of LY293111, a compound with considerably greater oral potency than LY255283. Some of the key compounds made during the project are shown in Fig. 6. Sofia et al. [244, 245] found that substitution of the acetyl group with alkyl or alkoxy moieties led to compounds with enhanced receptor binding and functional antagonistic properties. LY247833, for example, was greater than 10-fold more potent at inhibiting LTB$_4$ receptor binding and LTB$_4$-induced upregulation of CD11b/CD18 than LY255283 [37, 238, 245]. Replacement of the acetyl group with a pyrazole (LY266640) or a p-fluorophenyl moiety (LY306669) also increased *in vitro* activity [246, 247]. However, only the p-fluoro-phenyl-substitution led to enhanced oral activity when tested on LTB$_4$-

induced airway obstruction induced in guinea pigs. Substitution of the tetrazole group with a chroman carboxylic acid (LY247826) did not alter *in vitro* activity on human neutrophils extensively but substantially increased oral activity [248]. Further study of different acid units led to the synthesis of LY285009, a diaryl ether acid, which was found to bind the human neutrophil LTB_4 receptor approximately 1.5-fold more tightly than LY247826 [249]. The presence of the secondary lipophilic propyl group was critical for maximum potency. A major advantage of the diaryl ether acid is its lack of a chiral center and therefore there is no need to resolve enantiomorphs as with chroman carboxylic acids. Coupling of the more active modifications of both the acetophenone and acid portions of the parent molecule resulted in the synthesis of LY293111. This compound binds to the human neutrophil receptor 5-fold more tightly than LY255283 and is 28 times more potent orally.

SC-41930 was the first orally active LTB_4 receptor antagonist to be described [237]. Fretland et al. found the compound able to abrogate neutrophil accumulation at dermal sites where LTB_4 had been injected [250]. Comparison of ED_{50}'s when drug was given intravenously and orally indicated that the compound was readily absorbed. *In vitro* studies showed that SC-41930 inhibited chemotaxis, degranulation, intracellular calcium mobilization, and CD11b/CD18 expression on neutrophils induced by LTB_4 [37, 251]. The ability of the compound to reduce the severity of skin lesions resulting from topical application of either A23187 or PMA and acetic acid-induced colonic inflammation in several species led to clinical trials with SC-41930 for treatment of psoriasis and ulcerative colitis [252–254]. However, this agent proved to have several other activities. Villani-Price et al. showed that SC-41930 could inhibit fMLP, C5a and NaF-stimulated superoxide production and A23187-induced eicosanoid production in human neutrophils and HL60 cells at concentrations only slightly higher than those that inhibited LTB_4-elicited responses [255]. Consequently, some of the anti-inflammatory effects demonstrated with this compound were probably due to other activities in addition to LTB_4 receptor antagonism. SC-41930 has a chiral center and studies with the optical isomers indicated that the (+) enantiomer was 2- to 10-fold more potent as an LTB_4 antagonist than the (–) enantiomer [256].

In 1992, Penning et al. disclosed the discovery of several analogs of SC-41930 with considerably enhanced potency [257]. One of these, SC-50605 (Fig. 7), was 5 to 17-fold more potent than SC-41930 at inhibiting a variety of LTB_4 receptor mediated responses [258]. In addition, it had a longer duration of action than SC-41930 and no activity on lipoxygenases, human

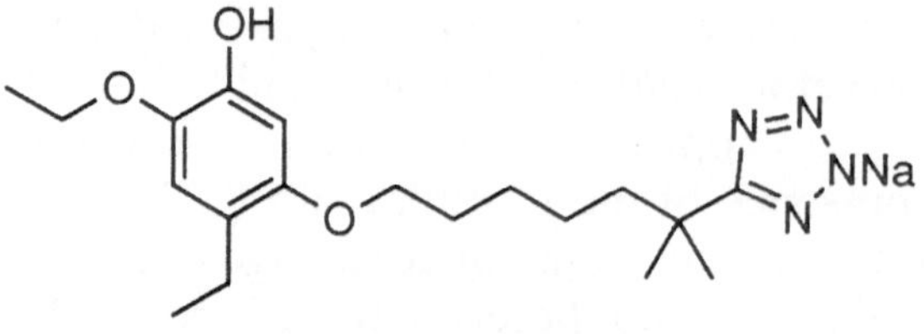

LY247833

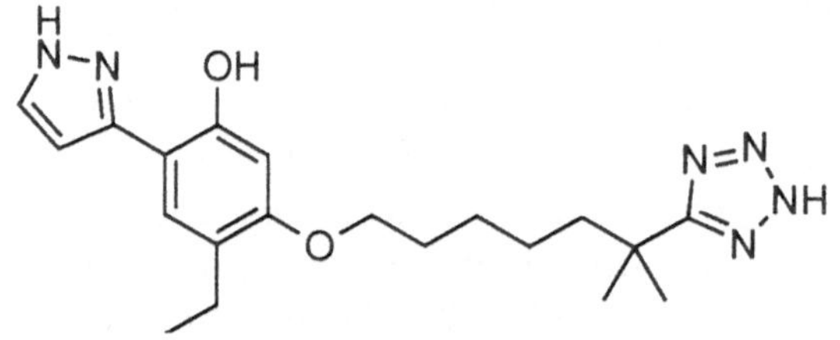

LY266640

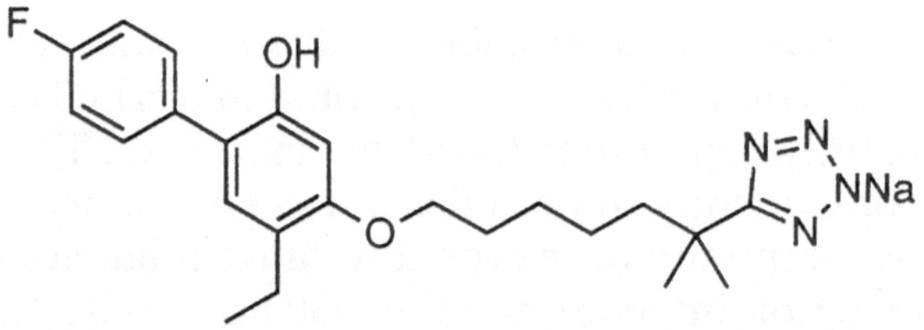

LY306669

Fig. 6
Intermediate structures made during development of LY293111 from LY255283. Replacement of the acetyl and the tetrazole groups on LY255283 with other substituents led to greater potency and improved oral activity.

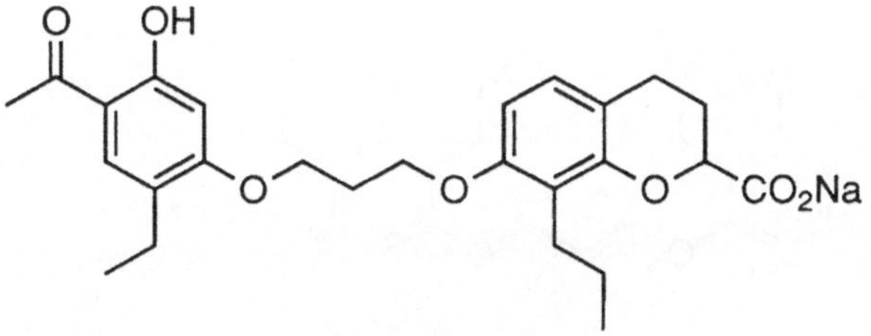

LY247826

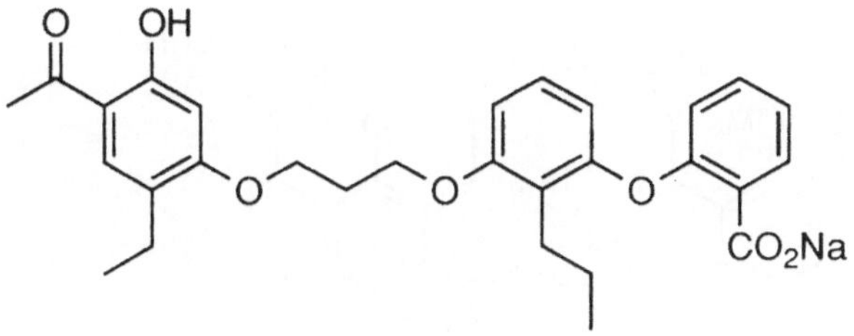

LY285009

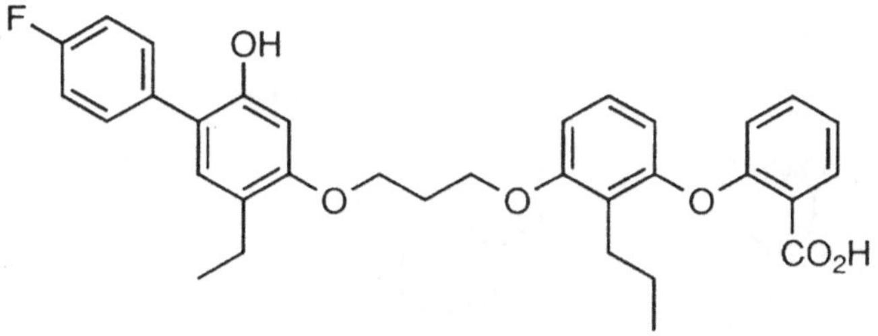

LY293111

Fig. 6 (continued)

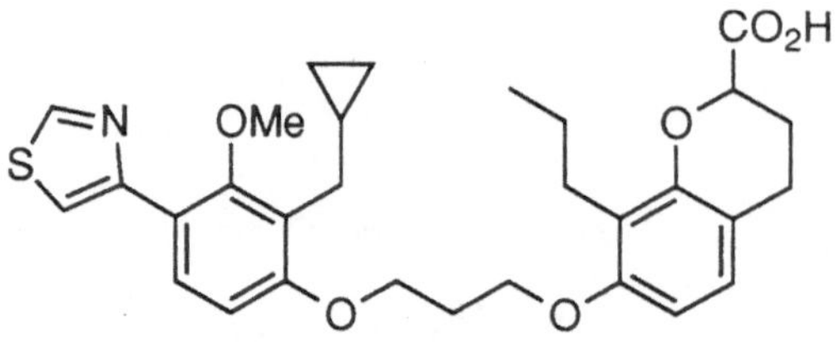

SC-50605

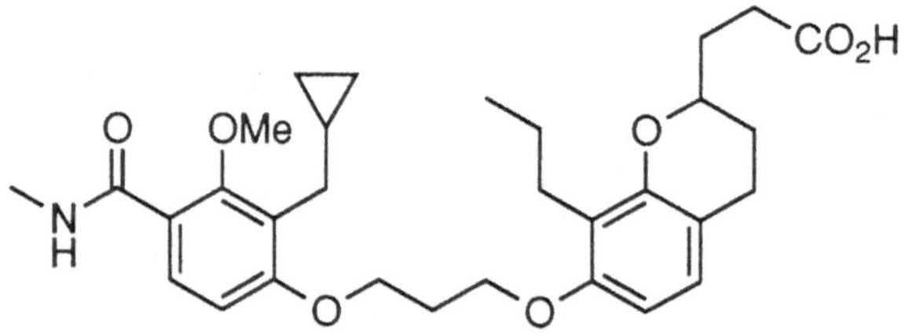

SC-51146

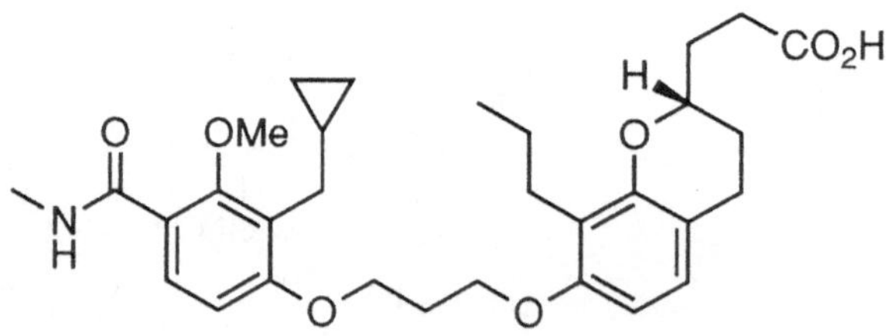

SC-53228

Fig. 7
Analogs of SC-41930 with enhanced potency and greater selectivity.

synovial fluid PLA_2, bovine heart phosphodiesterase, or ram seminal vesicle cyclooxygenase. However, another analog, SC-51146 (Fig. 7), was found to be approximately 2-fold more potent than SC-50605 when applied topically, equipotent when given orally, and 1.4-fold longer in duration of action. As found with SC-41930, the (+) enantiomer SC-53228 (Fig. 7) was more potent than the (−) antipode [259]. At a dose of 20 mg/kg, B.I.D., SC-53228 has been given by gavage to cotton-top tamarins with histologically confirmed acute colitis for a total of 8 weeks [260]. Animals treated in this fashion had improved consistency of the stool and less loss of weight than control tamarins. Neither neutrophils nor abscesses were found in the intestinal crepts of most drug-treated animals. SC-53228 is currently a clinical candidate as therapy for inflammatory bowel disease and psoriasis.

Several other research groups have developed potent LTB_4 receptor antagonists. Some of these are currently in clinical trial. Konno et al. [261] developed a series of β-phenylpropionic acids that eventually led to ONO-4057 (Fig. 8a). At micromolar concentrations, ONO-4057 inhibited neutrophil aggregation and degranulation and antagonized the contraction of lung parenchymal strips induced by LTB_4 but not responses stimulated with LTC_4 and LTD_4 [262]. Intravenous or oral administration of the compound prevented LTB_4-induced neutropenia in guinea pigs and, upon oral dosing of 30 mg/kg, LTB_4-stimulated neutrophil accumulation in the skin was suppressed for more than 6 hours [263].

Kingsbury et al. [264] used a strategy to develop LTB_4 receptor antagonists similar to that used to make U-75302 by building ring-fused analogs of LTB_4 with their restricted conformational freedom from a preferred conformation of LTB_4. SB 201146 and SB 201993 (Fig. 8a) are potent receptor binding compounds without agonist activity that were developed from modifications of LTB_4 in which a pyridine moiety was inserted into the molecule [265, 266]. The latter compound has been reported to be in clinical trial for treatment of psoriasis.

The LTB_4 receptor antagonists developed by Cohen et al. [267, 268] arose from initial observations that the LTD_4 receptor antagonist, Ro23-3544, inhibited LTB_4-induced bronchoconstriction in guinea pigs and LTB_4 binding to isolated human neutrophils [267, 269]. The compound is an o-hydroxyacetophenone tethered to a dihydrochroman acid and hence is structurally similar to SC-41930. By substituting a chromanone group for the o-hydroxyacetophenone and replacing the acidic moiety with an o-substituted phenylpropanoic acid, a 30-fold increase in receptor binding activity was achieved. A further 10-fold improvement in *in vitro* activity was obtained by adding a second alkanoic acid [268]. Recently described Ro-25-4094 (Fig. 8a) exemplifies this series [270].

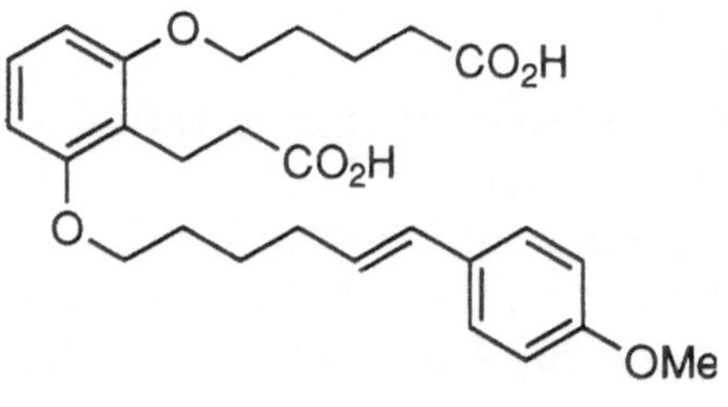

Fig. 8a
Second generation LTB$_4$ receptor antagonists.

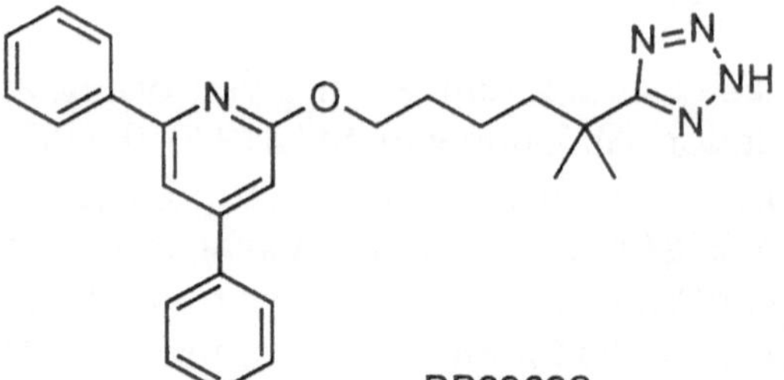

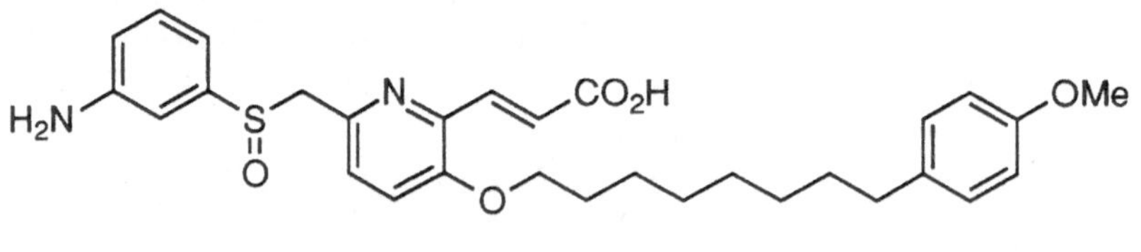

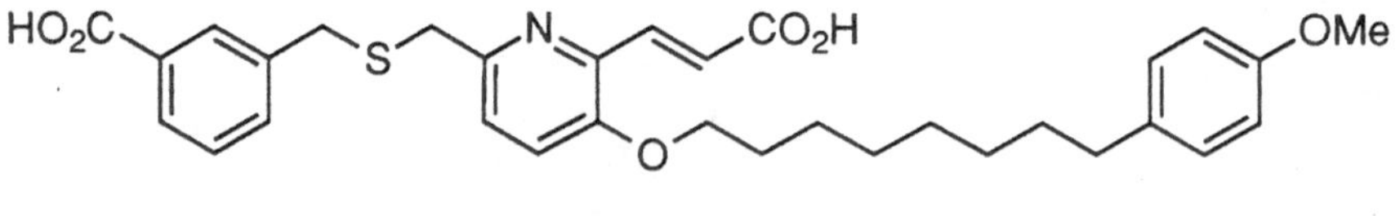

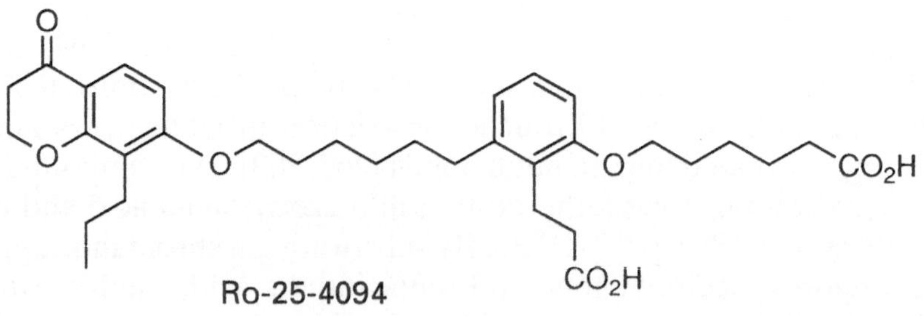

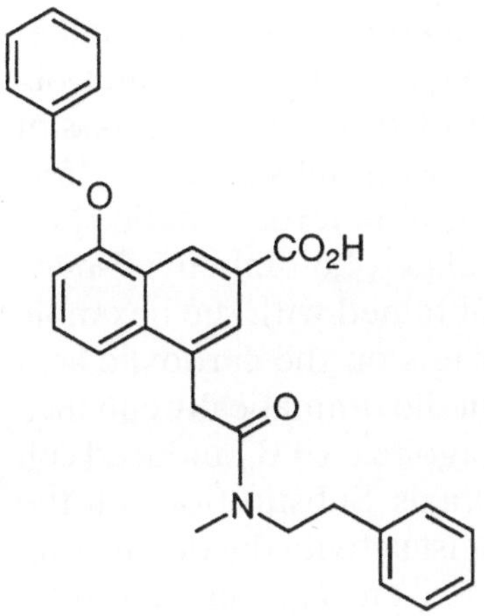

RG 14893

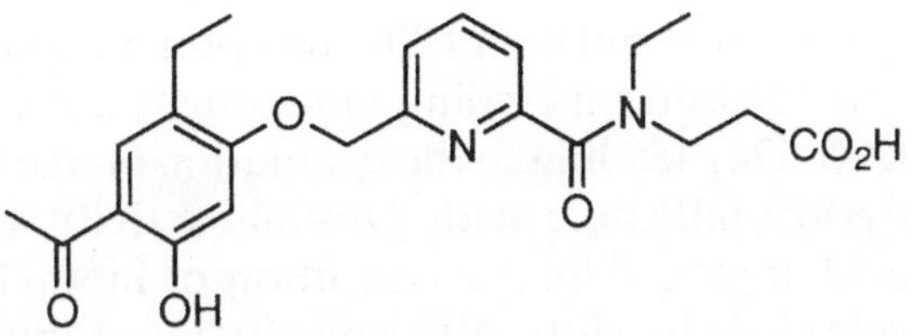

SM-15178

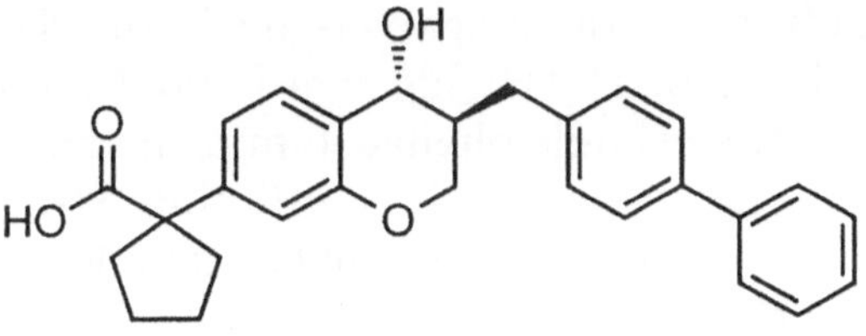

CP-105,696

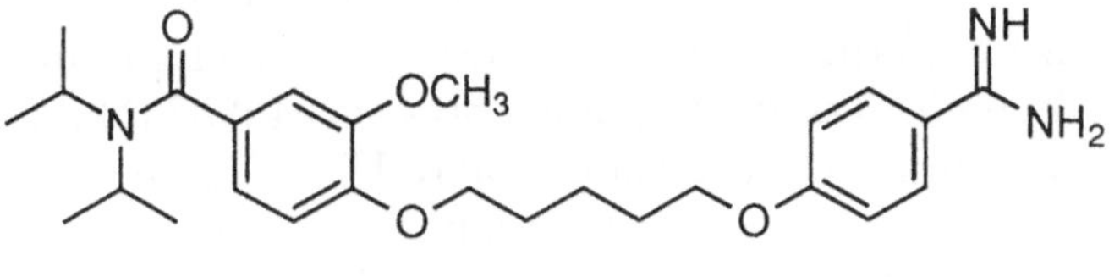

CGS 25019C
(maleate salt)

Fig. 8b
Second generation LTB$_4$ receptor antagonists..

Labaudinière et al. [271] studied a series of ω-[5-(ω-arylalkyl)-2-thienyl] alkanoic acids that were selective and metabolically stable LTA_4 hydrolase inhibitors. During the course of this investigation, some thienylalkanoic acids were found to bind selectively to LTB_4 receptors on guinea pig splenic membranes. This prompted a more detailed study of this class of compounds and their LTB_4 receptor antagonism [272]. Subsequently, effort was focused on finding antagonists containing N-heteroaromatic rings [273, 274], leading to the evaluation of a series of ω-[(4,6-diphenyl-2-pyridyl)oxy]alkanoic acids. Optimal activity was obtained with the hexanoic acid analog. Alpha-substitution of methyl groups on the carboxlic acid side chain had little effect on binding affinity but did dramatically enhance the ability of the compounds to selectively antagonize LTB_4-induced cell functions such as elastase release and chemotaxis. Substitutions on the phenyl rings suggested that for optimal antagonist activity the phenyl ring in the 4-position on the pyridine nucleus must exist in a quasiplanar relationship with the pyridine nucleus. RP69698 (Fig. 8a), which potently inhibited binding to human neutrophils, antagonized LTB_4-induced elastase release, and inhibited LTB_4-induced leukopenia in rabbits was selected for clinical trials.

Recently disclosed LTB_4 receptor antagonists are featured in Fig. 8b. RG 14893 is a compound developed by Huang et al. [275]. Their initial observation was the finding that a simple phenacetamide had moderate binding affinity for LTB_4 receptors on human neutrophils. Structure modifications established that N-methyl-N-phenethylacetamide was a key binding ligand to the LTB_4 receptor. Addition of an acidic function, replacement of a central phenyl ring with other aromatic moieties and optimization of the geometrical relationship of the functional groups led to RG 14983. The compound not only specifically inhibited LTB_4 binding to guinea pig spleen cell membranes and intact human neutrophils but also prevented LTB_4-induced aggregation of guinea pig neutrophils. The antagonist was effective in abrogating *in vivo* LTB_4-induced phenomenon too. When given orally to guinea pigs, RG 14983 inhibited accumulation of neutrophils at dermal sites where LTB_4 had been injected and, when administered intravenously to monkeys at 3 mg/kg, it inhibited LTB_4-induced changes in the circulating neutrophil count.

SM-15178 (Fig. 8b) is a new hydroxyacetophenone derivative that inhibits specific binding of LTB_4 to human neutrophils and modestly antagonizes LTB_4-induced chemotaxis [276, 277]. When administered orally at doses of 40 mg/kg or higher to guinea pigs and mice, the compound inhibited LTB_4-induced bronchoconstriction and arachidonic acid-stimulated neutrophil accumulation.

CP-105,696 (Fig. 8b) was designed using LTB_4 as a structural template and optimizing potency by assuming a three-point attachment of the antagonist to the LTB_4 receptor as had been done for the development of the NK1 receptor antagonist, CP-96,345 [278]. The cyclopentanecarboxylic acid moiety mimicked the ion-pair site. The middle portion provided specificity for the LTB_4 receptor and the biphenyl fit the accessory site originally proposed by Ariens [279] which is a common feature of G protein-coupled receptor antagonists [280]. CP-105,696 is a very potent *in vitro* antagonist [281, 282]. The compound strongly inhibited binding of labeled LTB_4 to both intact human neutrophils and membrane preparations. In addition, it was a potent inhibitor of LTB_4-induced chemotaxis and CD11b/CD18 upregulation. Specificity was shown by its lack of effect on activation of these functions by other chemotactic factors such as C5a, IL-8 and PAF. Interestingly, besides inhibiting LTB_4-induced chemotaxis of neutrophils from mice, monkeys and guinea pigs, CP-105,696 also inhibited LTB_4-stimulated chemotaxis of guinea pig eosinophils and Ca^{++} mobilization in human monocytes. A variety of effects were seen with the compound after *in vivo* administration. CP-105,696, when given 1 hour prior to agonist, inhibited neutrophil and eosinophil infiltration caused by LTB_4 injected into guinea pig dermis [283]. Acute inflammation induced by injecting arachidonic acid intradermally was attenuated in a similar manner by the compound implying that the fatty acid is converted to LTB_4 which, in turn, draws in neutrophils and eosinophils. Like other LTB_4 receptor antagonists, this compound also inhibited neutrophil influx induced by 12-(R)-HETE. As expected for a specific receptor antagonist, neutrophil infiltration in response to C5a was not affected. In contrast, the influx of eosinophils in response to the anaphylatoxin was reduced. This observation is consistent with previous findings that imply C5a induces first an infiltration of neutrophils and then further stimulates these cells to release LTB_4 which, in turn, attracts eosinophils [284]. CP-105,696 has also been shown to have a profound inhibitory effect on development of collagen II-induced arthritis in mice [281, 285, 286]. Administration of daily doses from 0.1 to 10 mg/kg commencing the day prior to immunization with collagen II inhibited the development of clinical symptoms 4 weeks later in a dose-dependent manner. Induction of an accelerated form of the disease by injection of IL-1 into immunized mice was also abrogated by administration of the compound. Effectiveness of the compound was substantiated by histological evaluation of the knee joints of the animals. At 10 mg/kg, the drug completely prevented infiltration of inflammatory cells, pannus formation, and cartilage destruction. Several facts indicate that the efficacy of the drug was due to its antagonism of the LTB_4

receptor on neutrophils and not to some effect on the immunopathology of the disease. Doses of drug that inhibited progression of the disease also inhibited neutrophil infiltration induced by injecting LTB_4 intradermally in mice. The drug was just as efficacious at arresting the accelerated form of the disease when given one day prior to the first injection of IL-1 as when administered daily throughtout the immunization period. Moreover, the compound had no effect on circulating levels of collagen II antibody. Finally, MK-591, a FLAP inhibitor and ZD-2138, a 5-lipoxygenase inhibitor, also attenuated the severity of the IL-1 mediated disease [285]. Taken together, these results imply that neutrophil infiltration into the joints of the arthritic mice and the subsequent tissue destruction is significantly mediated by LTB_4.

CGS 25019C (Fig. 8b) differs from all other LTB_4 receptor antagonists in that the ionic group on the molecule is not acidic but a basic amidine group. Several amidines were initially discovered to have moderate binding affinity to the LTB_4 receptor. Subsequent testing of additional compounds of this type led to the observation that pentamidine could inhibit specific LTB_4 binding at high nanomolar concentrations [287]. Elimination of one of the amidine groups led to a dramatic improvement in receptor affinity. However, replacement of the second amidine by other basic or isosteric groups such as a guanidino moiety resulted in great loss of activity. The tether piece connecting the two aromatic rings is a spacer whose optimal activity length is 7 atoms. In addition to inhibition of binding of LTB_4 to human neutrophils, CGS 25019C also blocked LTB_4-induced neutrophil functions such as calcium release, chemotaxis, and aggregation [270]. Specificity was shown by inability of CG 25019C to inhibit receptor binding of LTD_4 or C5a or functional assays mediated by C5a, PAF, or fMLP. The compound also did not inhibit LTB_4 production by neutrophils or the activity of the two cyclooxygenase enzymes. *In vivo* activity was initially demonstrated by finding that CGS 25019C inhibited LTB_4-induced neutropenia in rats [288]. The compound was also an effective therapeutic agent in two animal models of inflammation. When given orally 0.5 hour before applying arachidonic acid to the ears of mice, the compound inhibited the resultant edema and neutrophil influx into the ear that occurs during the hour following induction of inflammation [288]. In addition, CGS 25019C prevented symptom development in murine collagen-induced arthritis in a dose-dependent manner when given daily by oral administration commencing the day after initiating the insult [270]. CGS 25019C is currently in clinical trial for the treatment of rheumatoid arthritis. As is being done with the clinical trials for LY293111 and CP-105,696, the *ex vivo* analysis of LTB_4-induced CD11b/CD18 expression by blood neutrophils is being used as a marker of the *in vivo* efficacy of the compound [181,289]. CGS 25019C dose-dependently inhibited this response *in vitro* using either human, monkey, or mouse blood. Following oral administration of the compound to mice, blood was collected one hour later and the amount of LTB_4-stimulated CD11b/CD18 upregulation measured. The amidine appeared to be absorbed and circulating in a pharmacologically active form. There was no attenuation of constituative CD11b/CD18 expression. In a Phase I single dose safety study, CGS 25019C was absorbed and circulated at concentrations sufficient to inhibit CD11b/CD18 upregulation induced by LTB_4. Surprisingly, in a 7-day multidose study with CGS 25019C, once-a-day dosing was found to be superior to administering an equal dose B.I.D [181]. Antagonism of LTB_4-induced CD11b/CD18 expression measured at peak and trough time intervals after 1 and 7 days of drug dosing showed no cumulative effect of the compound or development of tolerance. The 300 mg single daily dose provided > 50% inhibition throughout the entire 24-hour period.

9   Treatment of asthma and IBD with a 5-lipoxygenase inhibitor

Inhibition of leukotriene biosynthesis with a 5-lipoxygenase inhibitor in patients has provided important evidence supporting a role for leukotrienes in asthma. Zileuton [290–292] was the first 5-lipoxygenase inhibitor to be extensively evaluated in a clinical setting. Israel et al. [293] found this agent able to increase tolerance of asthmatics to hyperventilation of cold dry air by 47%. Using an *ex vivo* blood assay, they found synthesis of LTB_4 reduced by 74%. These results indicated that leukotriene release occurs during cold dry air inhalation and suggested that greater enzyme inhibition might translate into a more marked reduction in bronchospasm following challenge. Recently, this same group found that symptoms improved in aspirin-sensitive asthmatics following administration of Zileuton [294]. One of the most clinically important studies with Zileuton was a randomized, double-blind, placebo controlled evaluation in mild to moderate asthmatics [295]. The major element of this study lies in the fact that patients suffered from spontaneously occurring disease and not an acute bronchospasm accompanied by inflammatory cells which was induced by a laboratory procedure. Urinary LTE_4 was reduced in these individuals by 39% after 4 weeks of treatment with 600 mg Zileuton four times a day. Despite this modest reduction in urinary LTE_4, pulmonary function was improved, symptoms were decreased, and β-receptor agonist usage decreased by 24%. Clearly, this study highlighted lipoxygenase products as one factor contributing to the chronicity of asthma.

Initial studies in IBD patients with Zileuton demonstrated that 5-lipoxygenase inhibition can substantially lower levels of LTB_4 in rectal dialysates [296]. Subsequently, an early phase II, 28-day clinical trial found Zileuton, 800-mg single daily dose, to have an overall positive effect in a group of patients with mild to moderately active ulcerative colitis [297]. However, histological improvement was not noted. A second phase II study employed 800 mg Zileuton, twice a day. LTB_4 levels in rectal dialysates fell 72% [298]. Symptomatic relief was noted, but there was certainly not a major improvement with respect to all measured parameters. Whether this indicates that greater 5-lipoxygenase inhibition is required or that leukotrienes only mediate to a modest extent the pathology of this disease is presently unknown.

10   Role of leukotrienes in other diseases

Adult respiratory distress syndrome (ARDS), an acute noncardiogenic pulmonary edema [299], like the chronic inflammatory lung diseases, has been associated with the generation of leukotrienes . Early evidence of a link between leukotrienes and ARDS was provided by Matthay et al. [300]. They contrasted levels of eicosanoids in pulmonary edema fluid from patients with ARDS with those from individuals suffering with a cardiac-derived pulmonary edema. Their results showed elevated levels of LTD_4 in lung fluid from the former group. More recent clinical studies have presented evidence in support of their findings [301, 302]. Interestingly, Fauler et al. [303] showed enhanced levels of urinary LTE_4 in patients suffering from multiple trauma not associated with ARDS. However, in those individuals who eventually developed ARDS, the levels were considerably higher. Other pulmonary diseases in which leukotrienes have been implicated include bronchitis [304, 305] and cystic fibrosis [303, 306]. In addition, clinical studies have implicated, or at least provided evidence for the involvement of leukotrienes in other human disorders including cold urticaria [307], multiple sclerosis [308], subarachnoid hemorrhage [309], uveitis [310], and hepatorenal syndrome [311, 312] as well as other liver diseases [313]. At the very least, leukotrienes probably contribute to some of the overt symptomatology characteristics of these abnormalities. However, the possibility exists that leukotrienes are the key mediators of the pathobiology and hence interference with their synthesis or blockade of their pharmacologic receptors may have profound ameliorating effects on the course of a disease.

11 Conclusion

After nearly 6 decades of exploring the pharmacology, physiology, bio-chemistry, molecular biology, and pathology of slow reacting substances/leukotrienes and their receptors, modern medicine is on the threshold of receiving new therapies for the treatment of inflammatory diseases. Drugs with the ability to inhibit the synthesis or action of cysteinyl leukotrienes and dihydroxyleukotrienes are on the horizon. Their importance cannot be understated given the wealth of evidence linking lipid mediators with the process of inflammation. Proven clinical success on a large scale will lead to development of even newer chemical entities that will uniquely alter this arm of the arachidonic acid cascade.

12 Addendum

Since completion of this review, several significant advances have been reported. Ono Pharmaceutical Company became the first to commercialize an LTD_4/LTE_4 receptor antagonist having recently received approval to market ONO-1078 (pranlukast) for asthma in Japan [314]. Regulatory submissions for ICI 204,219 (zafirlukast) have been filed in the UK, the United States and other countries [315]. Recent data presented at the European Congress of Allergology and Clinical Immunology in Madrid (June 25–30, 1995) indicated that in large patient studies, zafirlukast reduced asthma symptoms by twice as much as placebo [315]. Another potent LTD_4/LTE_4 receptor antagonist, montelukast sodium, also known as MK-0476, (1-((((1(R)-(3-(2-(7-chloro-2-quinolinyl)-(E)-ethenyl)phenyl)(3-2-(1-hydroxy-1-methylethyl)phenyl)propyl)thio)methyl)cyclopropane)acetic acid sodium salt, has been described. This agent is a second generation styryl quinoline thioether with a pharmacologic profile superior to that of MK-571 and MK-679. Like its predecessors it binds potently to the $CysLT_1$ subtype of LTD_4/LTE_4 receptors but its binding is less affected by the presence of plasma proteins such as human serum albumin. Bioavailability and clearance studies in animals revealed that montelukast is absorbed when given orally and has a much longer $T_{1/2}$ than the other styryl quinolines. A single oral 4-hour pretreatment dose of the compound inhibited both the early and late phase bronchoconstriction occurring in squirrel monkeys challenged with an ascaris antigen aerosol [316]. An additional advantage of this compound is that it does not induce peroxisomal enzymes or cause liver weight increases in mice [317]. Initial clinical studies have indicated that when given orally to mild asthmatics montelukast was a potent and long-lasting inhibitor of LTD_4-induced bronchoconstriction and improved baseline FEV_1 values [318, 319]. The compound is presently in phase III trials. The 5-lipoxygenase inhibitor, Zileuton, was recommended for approval by the U.S. FDA's pulmonary-allergy drugs advisory committee for treatment of asthmatics whose disease is at a stage where daily inhaled beta receptor agonists are needed to control bronchospasm symptoms [320]. The development of CP-105,696 has been suspended due to the long half-life of 420 hours in human subjects [321]. In a small study involving 12 atopic male asthmatics dosed orally with LY293111 prior to being challenged with antigen, this LTB_4 receptor antagonist significantly reduced influx of neutrophils into the bronchoalveolar space, a finding which further substantiates that LTB_4 is involved in the inflammatory phase of asthma [322].

References

1   W. Feldberg and C.H. Kellaway: J. Physiol. 94, 187 (1938).
2   C.H. Kellaway and E.R. Trethewie: Q. J. Exp. Physiol. 30, 121 (1940).
3   W.E. Brocklehurst, in : Ciba Foundation Symposium on Histamine (Ed. G.E.W. Wolstenholme and C.M. O'Connor; Churchill, London 1956), p. 175.
4   W.E. Brocklehurst: J. Physiol. 151, 416 (1960).
5   W.E. Brocklehurst, in: SRS-A and Leukotrienes (Ed. P.J. Piper; John Wiley & Sons, Chichester, U. K. 1981), p. 7.
6   H.R. Morris, G.W. Taylor, C.M. Jones, P.J. Piper, J.R. Tippins and M.N. Samhoun, in: SRS-A and Leukotrienes (Ed. P.J. Piper; John Wiley & Sons, Chichester, U. K. 1981) p. 19.
7   B. Samuelsson, in: SRS-A and Leukotrienes (Ed. P.J. Piper; John Wiley & Sons, Chichester, U. K. 1981) p. 45.
8   B. Samuelsson: Adv. Prostaglandin, Thromboxane, Leukotriene Res. 15,1 (1985).
9   J. Augstein, J.B. Farmer, T.B. Lee, P. Sheard and M.L. Tattersall: Nature (London) New Biol. 245, 215 (1973).
10   J.M. Drazen, R.A. Lewis, S.I. Wasserman, R.P. Orange and K.F. Austen: J. Clin. Invest. 63, 1 (1979).
11   J.H. Fleisch, K.D. Haisch and S.M. Spaethe: J. Pharmacol. Exp. Ther. 221, 146 (1982).
12   J.H. Fleisch, L.E. Rinkema and S.R. Baker: Life Sci. 31, 577 (1982).
13   J.M. Drazen, K.F. Austen, R.A. Lewis, D.A. Clark, G. Goto, A. Marfat and E.J. Corey: Proc. Natl. Acad. Sci. USA 77, 4354 (1980).
14   R.D. Krell, R. Osborn, L. Vickery, K. Falcone, M. O'Donnell, J. Gleason, C. Kinzig and D. Bryan: Prostaglandins 22, 387 (1981).
15   J.H. Fleisch, L.E. Rinkema and W.S. Marshall: Biochem. Pharmacol. 33, 3919 (1984).
16   D.W. Snyder and J.H. Fleisch: Annu. Rev. Pharmacol. Toxicol. 29, 123 (1989).
17   J.A. Salmon and L.G. Garland: Prog. Drug Res. 37, 9 (1991).
18   C.D. Perchonock, T.J. Torphy and S. Mong: Drugs Fut. 12, 871 (1987).
19   J.S. Sawyer and D.L. Saussy, Jr.: Drug News Perspect. 6, 139 (1993).

20   R.A. Lewis, J.M. Drazen, E.J. Corey and K.F. Austen, in: SRS-A and Leukotrienes (Ed. P.J. Piper; John Wiley & Sons, Chichester, U. K. 1981) p. 101.

21   R.A. Lewis and K.F. Austen: J. Clin. Invest. 73, 889 (1984).

22   J.M. Drazen, B. Pichurko, W. Maguire and E. Israel, in: Asthma: Its Pathology and Treatment (Ed. M. A. Kaliner, P. J. Barnes and C. G. A. Persson; Marcel Dekker, New York 1991). p. 301.

23   D. Keppler: Rev. Physiol. Biochem. Pharmacol. 121, 92 (1992).

24   W.R. Henderson, Jr.: Ann. Intern. Med. 121, 684 (1994).

25   P. Borgeat and B. Samuelsson: Proc. Natl. Acad. Sci. USA 76, 2148 (1979).

26   P. Borgeat and B. Samuelsson: J. Biol. Chem. 254, 2643 (1979).

27   P. Borgeat and B. Samuelsson: Proc. Natl. Acad. Sci. USA 76, 3213 (1979).

28   R.M. McMillan and S.J. Foster: Agents Actions 24, 114 (1988).

29   A.W. Ford-Hutchinson, M.A. Bray, M.V. Doig, M.E. Shipley and M.J.H. Smith: Nature (London) 286, 264 (1980).

30   A.W. Ford-Hutchinson: Crit. Rev. Immunol. 10, 1 (1990).

31   P. Borgeat and P.H. Naccache: Clin. Biochem. 23, 459 (1990).

32   D.W. Goldman, L.A. Gifford, T. Marotti, C.H. Koo and E.J. Goetzl: Fed. Proc. 46, 200 (1987).

33   W. König, W. Schönfeld, M. Raulf, M. Köller, J. Knöller, J. Scheffer and J. Brom: Eicosanoids 3, 1 (1990).

34   T.M. Carlos and J.M. Harlan: Immunol. Rev. 114, 5 (1990).

35   R.M. Strieter, N.W. Lukacs, T.J. Standiford and S.L. Kunkel: Thorax 48, 765 (1993).

36   J.M. Pilewski and S.M. Albelda: Am. Rev. Respir. Dis. 148, S31 (1993).

37   P. Marder, R.M. Schultz, S.M. Spaethe, M.J. Sofia and D.K. Herron: Prostaglandins, Leukotrienes Essent. Fatty Acids 46, 265 (1992).

38   C.N. Serhan: J. Bioenerg. Biomembr. 23, 105 (1991).

39   C.N. Serhan: Biochim. Biophys. Acta 1212, 1 (1994).

40   J. Rokach and B. Fitzsimmons: Transplant. Proc. 38, Suppl. 4, 7 (1986).

41   S.-E. Dahlén, L. Franzén, J. Raud, C.N. Serhan, P. Westlund, E. Wikström, T. Björck, H. Matsuda, S.E. Webber, C.A. Veale, T. Puustinen, J. Haeggstrom, K.C. Nicolaou and B. Samuelsson, in: Lipoxins (Ed. P.Y.-K. Wong and C.N. Serhan; Plenum Publishing Corporation, New York 1988) p. 107.

42   P. Erhlich: Lancet 2, 445 (1913).

43   M.M. Goldenberg and E.M. Subers: Eur. J. Pharmacol. 78, 463 (1982).

44   (a) J.H. Fleisch, L.E. Rinkema, K.D. Haisch, D. Swanson-Bean, T. Goodson, P.P.K. Ho and W.S. Marshall: J. Pharmacol. Exp. Ther. 233, 148 (1985). (b) J.H. Fleisch, L.E. Rinkema, C.A. Whitesitt and W.S. Marshall: Adv. Inflammation Res. 12, 173 (1988).

45   D.W. Snyder and R.D. Krell: J. Pharmacol. Exp. Ther. 231, 616 (1984).

46   R.D. Krell, B.S. Tsai, A. Berdoulay, M. Barone and R.E. Giles: Prostaglandins 25, 171 (1983).

47   C.K. Buckner, R.D. Krell, R.B. Laravuso, D.B. Coursin, P.R. Bernstein and J.A. Will: J. Pharmacol. Exp. Ther. 237, 558 (1986).

48   D.W. Snyder, R.E. Giles, R.A. Keith, Y.K. Yee and R.D. Krell: J. Pharmacol. Exp. Ther. 243, 548 (1987).

49   R.D. Krell, D. Aharony, C.K. Buckner and E.J. Kusner: Adv. Prostaglandins, Thromboxane, Leukotriene Res. 20, 119 (1990).

50   T. Obata, Y. Okada, M. Motoishi, N. Nakagawa, T. Terawaki and H. Aishita: Jpn. J. Pharmacol. 60, 227 (1992).

51   D.W.P. Hay, R.M. Muccitelli, S.S. Tucker, L.M. Vickery-Clark, K.A. Wilson, J.G. Glea-

son, R.F. Hall, M.A. Wasserman and T.J. Torphy: J. Pharmacol. Exp. Ther. *243*, 474 (1987).

52   T.R. Jones, R. Zamboni, M. Belley, E. Champion, L. Charette, A.W. Ford-Hutchinson, R. Frenette, J.-Y. Gauthier, S. Leger, P. Masson, C.S. McFarlane, H. Piechuta, J. Rokach, H. Williams, and R.N. Young: Can. J. Physiol. Pharmacol. *67*, 17 (1989).

53   T.R. Jones, R. Zamboni, M. Belley, E. Champion, L. Charette, A.W. Ford-Hutchinson, J.-Y. Gauthier, S. Leger, A. Lord, P. Masson, C. S. McFarlane, K. M. Metters, C. Pickett, H. Piechuta and R.N. Young: Can. J. Physiol. Pharmacol. *69*, 1847 (1991).

54   R.C. Falcone and R.D. Krell: J. Pharmacol. Exp. Ther. *262*, 1095 (1992).

55   P. Norman, T.S. Abram, N.J. Cuthbert, S.R. Tudhope and P.J. Gardiner: Eur. J. Pharmacol. *271*, 73 (1994).

56   C. Labat, J.L. Ortiz, X. Norel, I. Gorenne, J. Verley, T.S. Abram, N.J. Cuthbert, S.R. Tudhope, P. Norman, P. Gardiner and C. Brink: J. Pharmacol. Exp. Ther. *263*, 800 (1992).

57   D.W. Snyder and R.D. Krell: Prostaglandins *32*, 189 (1986).

58   P.J. Gardiner, P. Norman, N.J. Cuthbert, S.R. Tudhope and T.S. Abram: Eur. J. Pharmacol. *238*, 19 (1993).

59   N.J. Cuthbert, T.S. Abram and P.J. Gardiner: Ann. N. Y. Acad. Sci. *629*, 405 (1991).

60   N.J. Cuthbert, S.R. Tudhope, P.J. Gardiner, T.S. Abram, P. Norman, A.M. Thompson, R.J. Maxey and M.A. Jennings: Ann. N. Y. Acad. Sci. *629*, 402 (1991).

61   S.R. Tudhope, N.J. Cuthbert, T.S. Abram, M.A. Jennings, R.J. Maxey, A.M. Thompson, P. Norman and P.J. Gardiner: Eur. J. Pharmacol. *264*, 317 (1994).

62   Robert A. Coleman R.M. Eglen, R.L. Jones, S. Narumiya, T. Shimizu, W.L. Smith, S.-E. Dahlén, J.M. Drazen, P.L. Gardiner, W.T. Jackson, T.R. Jones, R.D. Krell and S. Nicosia: Adv. Prostaglandin, Thromboxane and Leukotriene Res. *23*, 283 (1995).

63   G.K. Hogaboom, S. Mong, H.-L. Wu, and S.T. Crooke: Biochem. Biophys. Res. Commun. *116*, 1136 (1983).

64   R.F. Bruns, W.J. Thomsen and T.A. Pugsley: Life Sci. *33*, 645 (1983).

65   G.K. Hogaboom, S. Mong, J.M. Stadel and S.T. Crooke: J. Pharmacol. Exp. Ther. *233*, 686 (1985).

66   M.A. Lewis, S. Mong, R.L. Vessella and S.T. Crooke: Biochem. Pharmacol. *34*, 4311 (1985).

67   S. Mong, G. Chi-Rosso, D.W. Hay and S.T. Crooke: Mol. Pharmacol. *34*, 590 (1988).

68   H.M. Sarau and S. Mong: Adv. Prostaglandins, Thromboxane, Leukotriene Res. *19*, 180 (1989).

69   H.M. Sarau, S. Mong, J.J. Foley, H.-L. Wu and S.T. Crooke: J. Biol. Chem. *262*, 4034 (1987).

70   D. Aharony and R.D. Krell: Ann. N. Y. Acad. Sci. *629*, 125 (1991).

71   E.A. Frey, D.W. Nicholson and K.M. Metters: Eur. J. Pharmacol. *244*, 239 (1993).

72   K.M. Metters, Y. Gareau, A. Lord, C. Rochette and N. Sawyer: J. Pharmacol. Exp. Ther. *270*, 399 (1994).

73   S.L. Levinson: Pharmacologist *25*, 201 (1983).

74   A.F. Welton, S. Nicosia, H.J. Crowley and D. Oliva: Fed. Proc. *42*, 2091 (1983).

75   S.-S. Pong, R.N. DeHaven, F.A. Kuehl, Jr., and R.W. Egan: J. Biol. Chem. *258*, 9616 (1983).

76   G.E. Rovati, D. Oliva, L. Sautebin, G.C. Folco, A.F. Welton and S. Nicosia: Biochem. Pharmacol. *34*, 2831 (1985).

77   S. Krilis, R.A. Lewis, E.J. Corey and K.F. Austen: Proc. Natl. Acad. Sci. USA *81*, 4529 (1984).

78　S. Mong, H.-L. Wu, M.O. Scott, M.A. Lewis, M.A. Clark, B.M. Weichman, C.M. Kinzig, J.G. Gleason and S.T. Crooke: J. Pharmacol. Exp. Ther. *234*, 316 (1985).

79a　F.F. Sun, L.-Y. Chau, B. Spur, E.J. Corey, R.A. Lewis and K.F. Austen: J. Biol. Chem. *261*, 8540 (1986).

79b　F.F. Sun, L.-Y. Chau and K.F. Austen: Fed. Proc. *46*, 204 (1987).

80　K.M. Metters, N. Sawyer and D.W. Nicholson: J. Biol. Chem. *269*, 12816 (1994).

81　S.-S. Pong and R.N. DeHaven: Proc. Natl. Acad. Sci. USA *80*, 7415 (1983).

82　S. Mong, H.-L. Wu, G.K. Hogaboom, M.A. Clark and S.T. Crooke: Eur. J. Pharmacol. *102*, 1 (1984).

83　S. Mong, H.-L. Wu, G.K. Hogaboom, M.A. Clark, J.M. Stadel and S.T. Crooke: Eur. J. Pharmacol. *106*, 241 (1985).

84　R.J. Lefkowitz, J.M. Stadel and M.G. Caron: Annu. Rev. Biochem. *52*, 159 (1983).

85　B.P. O'Sullivan and S. Mong: Mol. Pharmacol. *35*, 795 (1989).

86　T.J. Torphy, M. Burman, L.W. Schwartz and M.A. Wasserman: J. Pharmacol. Exp. Ther. *237*, 332 (1986).

87　S. Mong, K. Hoffman, H.-L. Wu and S.T. Crooke: Mol. Pharmacol. *31*, 35 (1987).

88　S. Mong, H.-L. Wu, J. Miller, R.F. Hall, J.G. Gleason and S.T. Crooke: Mol. Pharmacol. *32*, 223 (1987).

89　R.V.K. Vegesna, S. Mong and S.T. Crooke: Eur. J. Pharmacol. *147*, 387 (1988).

90　L. Baud, E.J. Goetzl and C.H. Koo: J. Clin. Invest. *80*, 983 (1987).

91　S. Mong, H.-L. Wu, A. Wong, H.M. Sarau and S.T. Crooke: J. Pharmacol. Exp. Ther. *247*, 803 (1988).

92　S. Mong, J. Miller, H.-L. Wu, and S.T. Crooke: J. Pharmacol. Exp. Ther. *244*, 508 (1988).

93　D.L. Saussy, Jr., H.M. Sarau, J.J. Foley, S. Mong and S.T. Crooke: J. Biol. Chem. *264*, 19845 (1989).

94　M.S. Simonson, P. Mené, G.R. Dubyak and M.J. Dunn: Am. J. Physiol. *255*, C771 (1988).

95　D. Oliva, M.R. Accomazzo, S. Giovanazzi and S. Nicosia: J. Pharmacol. Exp. Ther. *268*, 159 (1994).

96　B.M. Weichman, R.M. Muccitelli, S.S. Tucker and M.A. Wasserman: J. Pharmacol. Exp. Ther. *225*, 310 (1983).

97　P. Sirois, M. Lauzière and P. Braquet: Prostaglandins *31*, 1117 (1986).

98　M.A. Clark, T.M. Conway, R.G.L. Shorr and S.T. Crooke: J. Biol. Chem. *262*, 4402 (1987).

99　M.R. Steiner, J.S. Bomalaski and M.A. Clark: Biochim. Biophys. Acta *1166*, 124 (1993).

100　M.A. Clark, L.E. Özgür, T.M. Conway, J. Dispoto, S.T. Crooke and J.S. Bomalaski: Proc. Natl. Acad. Sci. USA *88*, 5418 (1991).

101　D.W. Goldman and E.J. Goetzl: J. Exp. Med. *159*, 1027 (1984).

102　H. Sumimoto, K. Takeshige and S. Minakami: Biochim. Biophys. Acta *803*, 271 (1984).

103　D.W. Goldman, L.A. Gifford, R.N. Young, T. Marotti, M.K.L. Cheung and E.J. Goetzl: J. Immunol. *146*, 2671 (1991).

104　D.W. Goldman, F.-H. Chang, L.A. Gifford, E.J. Goetzl and H.R. Bourne: J. Exp. Med. *162*, 145 (1985).

105　J.W. Sherman, E.J. Goetzl and C.H. Koo: J. Immunol. *140*, 3900 (1988).

106　K.R. McLeish, P. Gierschik, T. Schepers, D. Sidiropoulos and K.H. Jakobs: Biochem. J. *260*, 427 (1989).

107　T.M. Schepers and K.R. McLeish: Biochem. J. *289*, 469 (1993).

108　A.S. Kraft and W.B. Anderson: Nature (London) *301*, 621 (1983).

109　J.T. O'Flaherty, D.P. Jacobson, J.F. Redman and A.G. Rossi: J. Biol. Chem. *265*, 9146 (1990).

110 J.T. O'Flaherty, J.F. Redman and D.P. Jacobson: J. Immunol. *144*, 1909 (1990).

111 J.P. Arm and T.H. Lee: Clin. Sci. *84*, 501 (1993).

112 H. Herxheimer and E. Stresemann: J. Physiol. *165*, 78P (1963).

113 S.E. Wenzel, G.L. Larsen, K. Johnston, N.F. Voelkel and J.Y. Westcott: Am. Rev. Respir. Dis. *142*, 112 (1990).

114 C.M. Smith, P.E. Christie, R.J. Hawksworth, F. Thien and T.H. Lee: Am. Rev. Respir. Dis. *144*, 1411 (1991).

115 P.E. Christie, P. Tagari, A.W. Ford-Hutchinson, S. Charlesson, P. Chee, J.P. Arm and T.H. Lee: Am. Rev. Respir. Dis. *143*, 1025 (1991).

116 Y. Kikawa, T. Miyanomae, Y. Inoue, M. Saito, A. Nakai, Y. Shigematsu, S. Hosoi and M. Sudo: J. Allergy Clin. Immunol. *89*, 1111 (1992).

117 A.J. Wardlaw, H. Hay, O. Cromwell, J.V. Collins and A.B. Kay: J. Allergy Clin. Immunol. *84*, 19 (1989).

118 K. Shindo, Y. Matsumoto, Y. Hirai, M. Sumitomo, T. Amano, K. Miyakawa, M. Matsumura and T. Mizuno: J. Intern. Med. *228*, 91 (1990).

119 A.P. Sampson, C.P. Green, D.A. Spencer, P.J. Piper and J.F. Price: Ann. N. Y. Acad. Sci. *692*, 437 (1991).

120 L.J. Smith, P.A. Greenberger, R. Patterson, R.D. Krell and P.R. Bernstein: Am. Rev. Respir. Dis. *131*, 368 (1985).

121 E. Adelroth, M.M. Morris, F.E. Hargreave and P.M. O'Byrne: N. Engl. J. Med. *315*, 480 (1986).

122 J.M. Drazen: Chest *89*, 414 (1986).

123 J.P. Arm, B.W. Spur and T.H. Lee: J. Allergy Clin. Immunol. *82*, 654 (1988).

124 P. Sheard, T.B. Lee and M.L. Tattersall: Monogr. Allergy *12*, 245 (1977).

125 B. Mead, L.H. Patterson and D.A. Smith: J. Pharm. Pharmacol. *33*, 682 (1981).

126 W.S. Marshall, T. Goodson, G.J. Cullinan, D. Swanson-Bean, K.D. Haisch, L.E. Rinkema and J.H. Fleisch: J. Med. Chem. *30*, 682 (1987).

127 G.D. Phillips, P. Rafferty, C. Robinson and S.T. Holgate: J. Pharmacol. Exp. Ther. *246*, 732 (1988).

128 M.L. Cloud, G.C. Enas, J. Kemp, T. Platts-Mills, L.C. Altman, R. Townley, D. Tinkelman, T. King, Jr., E. Middleton, A.L. Sheffer, E.R. McFadden, Jr., and D.S. Farlow: Am. Rev. Respir. Dis. *140*, 1336 (1989).

129 E. Israel, E.F. Juniper, J.T. Callaghan, P.N. Mathur, M.M. Morris, A.R. Dowell, G.G. Enas, F.E. Hargreave and J.M. Drazen: Am. Rev. Respir. Dis. *140*, 1348 (1989).

130 G. Shaker, M.M. Glovsky, D. Kebo, S. Glovsky and A. Dowell: J. Allergy Clin. Immunol. *81*, 315 (1988).

131 D.M. Hoover, A.M. Bendele, W.P. Hoffman, P.S. Foxworthy and P.I. Eacho: Fundam. Appl. Toxicol. *14*, 123 (1990).

132 A.M. Bendele, D.M. Hoover, R.B. van Lier, P.S. Foxworthy and P.I. Eacho: Fundam. Appl. Toxicol. *15*, 676 (1990).

133 J.G. Gleason, T.W. Ku, M.E. McCarthy, B.M. Weichman, D. Holden, R.R. Osborn, B. Zabko-Potapovich, B. Berkowitz and M.A. Wasserman: Biochem. Biophys. Res. Commun. *117*, 732 (1983).

134 B.M. Weichman, M.A. Wasserman, D.A. Holden, R.R. Osborn, D.F. Woodward, T.W. Ku and J.G. Gleason: J. Pharmacol. Exp. Ther. *227*, 700 (1983).

135 C.D. Perchonock, I. Uzinskas, T.W. Ku, M.E. McCarthy, W.E. Bondinell, B.W. Volpe and J.G. Gleason: Prostaglandins *29*, 75 (1985).

136 T.W. Ku, M.E. McCarthy, B.M. Weichman and J.G. Gleason: J. Med. Chem. *28*, 1847 (1985).

137 C.D. Perchonock, M.E. McCarthy, K.F. Erhard, J.G. Gleason, M.A. Wasserman, R.M. Muccitelli, J.F. DeVan, S.S. Tucker, L.M. Vickery, T. Kirchner, B.M. Weichman, S. Mong, S.T. Crooke, J.F. Newton: J. Med. Chem. *28*, 1145 (1985).

138 C.D. Perchonock, I. Uzinskas, M.E. McCarthy, K.F. Erhard, J.G. Gleason, M.A. Wasserman, R.M. Muccitelli, J.F. DeVan, S.S. Tucker, L.M. Vickery, T. Kirchner, B.M. Weichman, S. Mong, M.O. Scott, G. Chi-Rosso, H.-L. Wu, S.T. Crooke and J.F. Newton: J. Med. Chem. *29*, 1442 (1986).

139 J.G. Gleason, R.F. Hall, C.D. Perchonock, K.F. Erhard, J.S. Frazee, T.W. Ku, K. Kondrad, M.E. McCarthy, S. Mong, S.T. Crooke, G. Chi-Rosso, M.A. Wasserman, T.J. Torphy, R.M. Muccitelli, D.W. Hay, S.S. Tucker, L. Vickery-Clark: J. Med. Chem. *30*, 959 (1987).

140 D.W.P. Hay, R.M. Muccitelli, S.S. Tucker, L.M. Vickery-Clark, A. Wilson, J.G. Gleason, R.F. Hall, M.A. Wasserman and T.J. Torphy: J. Pharmacol. Exp. Ther. *243*, 474 (1987).

141 T.J. Torphy, J.F. Newton, M.A. Wasserman, L. Vickery-Clark, R.R. Osborn, L.S. Bailey, L.P. Yodis, D.C. Underwood and D.W.P. Hay: J. Pharmacol. Exp. Ther. *249*, 430 (1989).

142 J.M. Evans, N.C. Barnes, J.T. Zakrzewski, H.P. Glenny, P.J. Piper and J.F. Costello: Br. J. Clin. Pharmacol. *26*, 677P (1988).

143 G.F. Joos, J.C. Kips, M. Puttemans, R.A. Pauwels and M.E. Van Der Straeten: J. Allergy Clin. Immunol. *83*, 187 (1989).

144 P.S. Creticos, S. Bodenheimer, A. Albright, L.M. Lichtenstein and P.S. Norman: J. Allergy Clin. Immunol. *83*, 187 (1989).

145 M. Robuschi, E. Riva, L.M. Fuccella, E. Vida, R. Barnabe, M. Rossi, G. Gambaro, S. Spagnotto and S. Bianco: Am. Rev. Respir. Dis. *145*, 1285 (1992).

146 R. Zamboni, M. Belley, E. Champion, L. Charette, R. DeHaven, R. Frenette, J.Y. Gauthier, T.R. Jones, S. Leger, P. Masson, C.S. McFarlane, K. Metters, S.S. Pong, H. Piechuta, J. Rokach, M. Thérien, H.W.R. Williams and R.N. Young: J. Med. Chem. *35*, 3832 (1992).

147 R.N. Young: Adv. Prostaglandins, Thromboxane, Leukotriene Res. *19*, 643 (1989).

148 R.N. Young: Drugs Fut. *13*, 745 (1989).

149 W.M. Abraham and J.S. Stevenson: FASEB J. *2*, A1057 (1988).

150 W.M. Abraham: Adv. Prostaglandin, Thromboxane, Leukotriene Res. *20*, 201 (1990).

151 S. Sapienza, D.H. Eidelman, P.M. Renzi and J.G. Martin: Am. Rev. Respir. Dis. *142*, 353 (1990).

152 M. Depré, D.J. Margolskee, J.Y.K. Hsieh, A. Van Hecken, A. Buntinx, I. De Lepeleire, J.D. Rogers and P.J. De Schepper: Eur. J. Clin. Pharmacol. *43*, 427 (1992).

153 J.C. Kips, G.F. Joos, I. De Lepeleire, D.J. Margolskee, A. Buntinx, R.A. Pauwels and M.E. Van Der Straeten: Am. Rev. Respir. Dis. *144*, 617 (1991).

154 J.B. Rasmussen, L.-O. Eriksson, D.J. Margolskee, P. Tagari, V.C. Williams and K.-E. Andersson: J. Allergy Clin. Immunol. *90*, 193 (1992).

155 P.J. Manning, R.M. Watson, D.J. Margolskee, V.C. Williams, J.I. Schwartz and P.M. O'Byrne: N. Engl. J. Med. *323*, 1736 (1990).

156 J. Gaddy, R.K. Bush, D. Margolskee, V.C. Williams and W. Busse: J. Allergy Clin. Immunol. *85*, 197 (1990).

157 J.Y. Gauthier, T. Jones, E. Champion, L. Charette, R. Dehaven, A.W. Ford-Hutchinson, K. Hoogsteen, A. Lord, P. Masson, H. Piechuta, S.S. Pong, J.P. Springer, M. Thérien, R. Zamboni and R.N. Young: J. Med. Chem. *33*, 2841 (1990).

158 D.J. Tocco, F.A. deLuna, A.E.W. Duncan, J.H. Hsieh and J.H. Lin: Drug Metab. Dispos. *18*, 388 (1990).

159   B. Dahlén, M. Kumlin, D.J. Margolskee, C. Larsson, H. Blomqvist, V.C. Williams, O. Zetterström and S.-E. Dahlén: Eur. Respir. J. *6*, 1018 (1993).

160   B. Dahlén, D.J. Margolskee, O. Zetterström and S.-E. Dahlén: Thorax *48*, 1205 (1993).

161   R.D. Krell, D. Aharony, C.K. Buckner, R.A. Keith, E.J. Kusner, D.W. Snyder, P.R. Bernstein, V.G. Matassa, Y.K. Yee, F.J. Brown, B. Hesp and R.E. Giles: Am. Rev. Respir. Dis. *141*, 978 (1990).

162   L.J. Smith, S. Geller, L. Ebright, M. Glass and P.T. Thyrum: Am. Rev. Respir. Dis. *141*, 988 (1990).

163   S.R. Findlay, J.M. Barden, C.B. Easley and M. Glass: J. Allergy Clin. Immunol. *89*, 1040 (1992).

164   K.M. O'Shaughnessy, I.K. Taylor, B. O'Connor, F. O'Connell, H. Thomson and C.T. Dollery: Am. Rev. Respir. Dis. *147*, 1431 (1993).

165   S.L. Spector, L.J. Smith, M. Glass and the ACCOLATE™ Asthma Trialists Group: Am. J. Respir. Crit. Care Med. *150*, 618 (1994).

166   F.J. Brown, P.R. Bernstein, L.A. Cronk, D.L. Dosset, K.C. Hebbel, T.P. Maduskuie, Jr., H.S. Shapiro, E.P. Vacek, Y.K. Yee, A.K. Willard, R.D. Krell and D.W. Snyder: J. Med. Chem. *32*, 807 (1989).

167   P.R. Bernstein, D.W. Snyder, E.J. Adams, R.D. Krell, E.P Vacek and A.K. Willard: J. Med. Chem. *29*, 2477 (1986).

168   F.J. Brown, Y.K. Yee, L.A. Cronk, K.C. Hebbel, R.D. Krell and D.W. Snyder: J. Med. Chem. *33*, 1771 (1990).

169   V.G. Matassa, T.P. Maduskuie, Jr., H.S. Shapiro, B. Hesp, D.W. Snyder, D. Aharony, R.D. Krell and R.A. Keith: J. Med. Chem. *33*, 1781 (1990).

170   Y.K. Yee, P.R. Bernstein, E.J. Adams, F.J. Brown, L.A. Cronk, K.C. Hebbel, E.P. Vacek, R.D. Krell and D.W. Snyder: J. Med. Chem. *33*, 2437 (1990).

171   C.K. Buckner, J.S. Fedyna, J.L. Robertson, J.A. Will, D.M. England, R.D. Krell and R. Saban: J. Pharmacol. Exp. Ther. *252*, 77 (1990).

172   L.J. Smith, M. Glass and M.C. Minkwitz: Clin. Pharmacol. Ther. *54*, 430 (1993).

173   I.K. Taylor, K.M. O'Shaughnessy, R.W. Fuller and C.T. Dollery: Lancet *337*, 690 (1991).

174   S.-E. Dahlén, B. Dahlén, E. Eliasson, H. Johansson, T. Björck, M. Kumlin, K. Boo, J. Whitney, S. Binks, B. King, R. Stark and O. Zetterström: Adv. Prostaglandin, Thromboxane, Leukotriene Res. *21*, 461 (1990).

175   K.P. Hui and N.C. Barnes: Lancet *337*, 1062 (1991).

176   J.P. Finnerty, R. Wood-Baker, H. Thompson and S.T. Holgate: Am. Rev. Respir. Dis. *145*, 746 (1992).

177   W.T. Jackson, R.J. Boyd, L.L. Froelich, R.M. Schultz, D.L. Saussy, Jr., C.R. Roman, J.H. Fleisch, M.J. Sofia and J.S. Sawyer: World Congress Inflammation '93. Vienna, October (1993), Abst. P75.

178   S.A. Silbaugh, P.W. Stengel, S.L. Cockerham, L.L. Froelich, A.M. Bendele, M.J. Sofia, J.S. Sawyer and W.T. Jackson: World Congress Inflammation '93. Vienna, October (1993), Abst. P76.

179   D.J. Fretland, C.P. Anglin, D.L. Widomski, D. Baron, R.D. Gokhale, L.K. Mathur, S.K. Paulson, J.C. Stolzenbach, S. Docter, S.W. Djuric, T.D. Penning and S. Yu: 7th International Conference Inflammation Research Association, White Haven, PA, Sept. (1994), Abst. W5.

180   K. Koch, L.S. Melvin, Jr., L.A. Reiter, M.S. Biggers, H.J. Showell, R.J. Griffiths, E.R. Pettipher, B. Hackman, J.B. Cheng, A.J. Milici, R. Breslow, M.J. Conklyn, C.A. Farrell, M.A. Smith, E. Salter, N.S. Doherty and K. Cooper: 7th International

Conference Inflammation Research Association, White Haven, PA, Sept. (1994), Abst. W6.

181 S. Uziel-Fusi, R. Stevens, J. Morgan, L. Martin, B. Mandell, A. Raychaudhuri, B. Kotyuk, B. Seligmann, C. Healy, M. Morrissey, P. Simon and P. Marshall: 7th International Conference Inflammation Research Association, White Haven, PA, Sept. (1994), Abst. W24.

182 P. Sharon and W.F. Stenson: Gastroenterology 86, 453 (1984).

183 E.A. Lobos, P. Sharon and W.F. Stenson: Dig. Dis. Sci. 32, 1380 (1987).

184 W.F. Stenson: Scand. J. Gastroenterol. 25 (Suppl. 172), 13 (1990).

185 D.J. Fretland, S.W. Djuric and T.S. Gaginella: Prostaglandins, Leukotrienes Essent. Fatty Acids 41, 215 (1990).

186 K. Lauritsen, L.S. Laursen, K. Bukhave and J. Rask-Madsen: Gastroenterology 91, 837 (1986).

187 O.H. Nielsen, K. Bukhave, J. Elmgreen and I. Ahnfelt-Rønne: Dig. Dis. Sci. 32, 577 (1987).

188 S.T. Nielsen, L. Beninati and C.B. Buonato: Scand. J. Gastroenterol. 23, 272 (1988).

189 K. Kragballe and J.J. Voorhees: Acta Derm. Venereol. Suppl. (Stockh) 120, 12 (1985).

190 S.D. Brain, R.D.R. Camp, F.M. Cunningham, P.M. Dowd, M.W. Greaves and A. Kobza Black: Br. J. Pharmacol. 83, 313 (1984).

191 K. Fogh, T. Herlin and K. Kragballe: J. Invest. Dermatol. 92, 837 (1989).

192 T. Ruzicka: Eicosanoids 1, 59 (1988).

193 S.F. Talbot, P.C. Atkins, E.J. Goetzl and B. Zweiman: J. Clin. Invest. 76, 650 (1985).

194 K. Fogh, T. Herlin and K. Kragballe: J. Allergy Clin. Immunol. 83, 450 (1989).

195 M.W. Greaves and R.D.R. Camp: Arch. Dermatol. Res. 280 [Suppl], S33 (1988).

196 F.M. Cunningham, M.W. Greaves and P.M. Woollard: Br. J. Pharmacol. 87, 107P (1986).

197 J.F. Evans, Y. Leblanc, B.J. Fitzsimmons, S. Charleson, D. Nathaniel and C. Léveillé: Biochim. Biophys. Acta 917, 406 (1987).

198 D.J. Fretland, D.L. Widomski, R.L. Shone, T.D. Penning, J.M. Miyashiro and S.W. - Djuric: Prostaglandins, Leukotrienes Essent. Fatty Acids 38, 169 (1989).

199 P.M. Dowd, A. Kobza Black, P.M. Woollard and M.W. Greaves: J. Invest. Dermatol. 84, 349 (1985).

200 C.-C. Chan, L. Duhamel and A. Ford-Hutchinson: J. Invest. Dermatol. 85, 333 (1985).

201 R.D.R. Camp, A.I. Mallet, F.M. Cunningham, E. Wong, P.M. Woollard, P. Dowd, A. Kobza Black and M.W. Greaves: Br. J. Dermatol. 113, Suppl. 28, 98 (1985).

202 S.A. Rae, E.M. Davidson and M.J.H. Smith: Lancet 2, 1122 (1982).

203 E.M. Davidson, S.A. Rae and M.J.H. Smith: Ann. Rheum. Dis. 42, 677 (1983).

204 J. Elmgreen, O.H. Nielsen and I. Ahnfelt-Rønne: Ann. Rheum. Dis. 46, 501 (1987).

205 J.J. Belch, A. O'Dowd, D. Ansell and R.D. Sturrock: Scand. J. Rheumatol. 18, 213 (1989).

206 D.M. Smith, J.A. Johnson and R.A. Turner: Clin. Exp. Rheumatol. 7, 471 (1989).

207 R.I. Sperling, J.S. Coblyn, J.K. Larkin, A.I. Benincaso, K.F. Austen and M.E. Weinblatt: Arthritis Rheum. 33, 1149 (1990).

208 R.I. Sperling, A.I. Benincaso, R.J. Anderson, J.S. Coblyn, K.F. Austen and M.E. Weinblatt: Arthritis Rheum. 35, 376 (1992).

209 J.L. Leroux, M. Damon, C. Chavis, A. Crastes de Paulet and F. Blotman: J. Rheumatol. 19, 863 (1992).

210 W.D. Blackburn, Jr., L.W. Heck, L.D. Loose, J.D. Eskra and T.J. Carty: Arthritis Rheum. 34, 204 (1991).

211   J.M. Kremer, W. Jubiz, A. Michalek, R.I. Rynes, L.E. Bartholomew, J. Bigaouette, M. Timchalk, D. Beeler and L. Lininger: Ann. Intern. Med. *106*, 497 (1987).

212   L.G. Cleland, J.K. French, W.H. Betts, G.A. Murphy and M.J. Elliott: J. Rheumatol. *15*, 1471 (1988).

213   D.M. Smith, Jr., H. Gonzales, J.A. Johnson, R.C. Franson and R.A. Turner: Int. J. Immunopharmacol. *11*, 45 (1989).

214   T.H. Lee, E. Israel, J. Drazen, A.G. Leitch, J. Ravalese, E.J. Corey, D.R. Robinson, R.A. Lewis and K.F. Austen: J. Immunol. *136*, 2575 (1986).

215   P.C. Atkins, M. Valenzano, E.J. Goetzl, W.D. Ratnoff, F.M. Graziano and B. Zweiman: J. Allergy Clin. Immunol. *83*, 136 (1989).

216   S.A. Silbaugh, P.W. Stengel, S.L. Cockerham, L.L. Froelich, A.M. Bendele, S.R. Baker and W.T. Jackson: Am. Rev. Resp. Dis. *145*, A284 (1992).

217   A.J. Wardlaw, H. Hay, O. Cromwell, J.V. Collins and A.B. Kay: J. Allergy Clin. Immunol. *84*, 19 (1989).

218   K. Shindo, Y. Matsumoto, Y. Hirai, M. Sumitomo, T. Amano, K. Miyakawa, M. Matsumura and T. Mizuno: J. Intern. Med. *228*, 91 (1990).

219   A.P. Sampson, C.P. Green, D.A. Spencer, P.J. Piper and J.F. Price: Ann. N. Y. Acad. Sci. *629*, 437 (1991).

220   E. Zocca, L.M. Fabbri, P. Boschetto, M. Plebani, M. Masiero, G.F. Milani, F. Pivirotto and C.E. Mapp: J. Appl. Physiol. *68*, 1576 (1990).

221   Y.Y. Koh, R. Dupuis, M. Pollice, K.H. Albertine, J.E. Fish and S.P. Peters: Am. J. Respir. Cell Mol. Biol. *8*, 493 (1993).

222   C.J. Kim, G.C. Kane, J.G. Zangrilli, S.K. Cho, Y.Y. Koh and S.P. Peters: Prostaglandins *47*, 393 (1994).

223   A.R. Huber, S.L. Kunkel, R.F. Todd, III, and S.J. Weiss: Science *254*, 99 (1991).

224   S.L. Kunkel, T. Standiford, K. Kasahara and R.M. Strieter: Exp. Lung Res. *17*, 17 (1991).

225   M.K. Thomsen, C.G. Larsen, H.K. Thomsen, D. Kirstein, T. Skak-Nielsen, I. Ahnfelt-Rønne and K. Thestrup-Pedersen: J. Invest. Dermatol. *96*, 260, 1991.

226   R.W. McCain, E.P. Holden, T.R. Blackwell and J.W. Christman: Am. J. Respir. Cell Mol. Biol. *10*, 651 (1994).

227   J.M. Wang, A. Rambaldi, A. Biondi, Z.G. Chen, C.J. Sanderson and A. Mantovani: Eur. J. Immunol. *19*, 701 (1989).

228   T. Ohnishi, H. Kita, D. Weiler, S. Sur, J.B. Sedgwick, W.J. Calhoun, W.W. Busse, J.S. Abrams and G.J. Gleich: Am. Rev. Respir. Dis. *147*, 901 (1993).

229   K.A. Yamaoka and J.-P. Kolb: Eur. J. Immunol. *23*, 2392 (1993).

230   E.J. Goetzl and W.C. Pickett: J. Exp. Med. *153*, 482 (1981).

231   H.J. Showell, I.G. Otterness, A. Marfat and E.J. Corey: Biochem. Biophys. Res. Comm. *106*, 741 (1982).

232   M. Namiki, Y. Igarashi, K. Sakamoto, T. Nakamura and Y. Koga: Biochem. Biophys. Res. Commun. *138*, 540 (1986).

233   C.F. Lawson, D.G. Wishka, J. Morris and F.A. Fitzpatrick: J. Lipid Mediators *1*, 3 (1989).

234   B.M. Taylor, N.J. Crittenden, M.N. Bruden, D.G. Wishka, J. Morris, I.M. Richards and F.F. Sun: Prostaglandins *42*, 211 (1991).

235   W.T. Jackson, R.J. Boyd, L.L. Froelich, T. Goodson, N.G. Bollinger, D.K. Herron, B.E. Mallett and D.M. Gapinski: FASEB J. *2*, A1110, 1988.

236   W.T. Jackson, R.J. Boyd, L.L. Froelich, B.E. Mallett and D.M. Gapinski: J. Pharmacol. Exp. Ther. *263*, 1009 (1992).

237   S.W. Djuric, P.W. Collins, P.H. Jones, R.L. Shone, B.S. Tsai, D.J. Fretland, G.M. Butchko,

D. Villani-Price, R.H. Keith, J.M. Zemaitis, L. Metcalf, R.F. Bauer: J. Med. Chem. *32*, 1145 (1989).

238   D.K. Herron, T. Goodson, N.G. Bollinger, D. Swanson-Bean, I.G. Wright, G.S. Staten, A.R. Thompson, L.L. Froelich and W.T. Jackson: J. Med. Chem. *35*, 1818 (1992).

239   D.M. Gapinski, B.E. Mallett, L.L. Froelich and W.T. Jackson: J. Med. Chem. *33*, 2807 (1990).

240   D.M. Gapinski. B.E. Mallett, L.L. Froelich and W.T. Jackson: J. Med. Chem. *33*, 2798 (1990).

241   M.O. Chaney, L.L. Froelich, D.M. Gapinski, B.E. Mallett and W.T. Jackson: Receptor *2*, 169 (1992).

242   W.T. Jackson, R.J. Boyd, L.L. Froelich, D.M. Gapinski, B.E. Mallett and J.S. Sawyer: J. Med. Chem. *36*, 1726 (1993).

243   S.A. Silbaugh, P.W. Stengel, S.L Cockerham, C.R. Roman, D.L. Saussy, Jr., S.M. Spaethe, T. Goodson, Jr., D.K. Herron and J.H. Fleisch: Eur. J. Pharmacol. *223*, 57 (1992).

244   M.J. Sofia, W.T. Jackson, D.L. Saussy, Jr., S.A. Silbaugh, L.L. Froelich, S.L. Cockerham and P.W. Stengel: BioMed. Chem. Lett. *2*, 1669 (1992).

245   M.J. Sofia, D.L. Saussy, Jr., W.T. Jackson, P. Marder, S.A. Silbaugh, L.L. Froelich, S.L. Cockerham and P.W. Stengel: BioMed. Chem. Lett. *2*, 1675 (1992).

246   R.W. Harper, W.T. Jackson, L.L. Froelich, R.J. Boyd, T.E. Aldridge and D.K. Herron: J. Med. Chem. *37*, 2411 (1994).

247   M.J. Sofia, P. Floreancig, N.J. Bach, S.R. Baker, S.L Cockerham, J.H. Fleisch, L.L. Froelich, W.T. Jackson, P. Marder, C.R. Roman, D.L. Saussy, Jr., S.M. Spaethe, P.W. Stengel and S.A. Silbaugh:J. Med. Chem. *36*, 3978 (1993).

248   M.J. Sofia, P. Floreancig, W.T. Jackson, P. Marder, D.L. Saussy, Jr., S.A. Silbaugh, S.L. Cockerham, L.L. Froelich, C.R. Roman, P.W. Stengel and J.H. Fleisch: BioMed. Chem. Lett. *3*, 1147 (1993).

249   J.S. Sawyer, R.F. Baldwin, D.L. Saussy, Jr., L.L. Froelich and W.T. Jackson: BioMed. Chem. Lett. *3*, 1985 (1993).

250   D.J. Fretland, D.L. Widomski, J.M. Zemaitis, S.W. Djuric and R.L. Shone: Inflammation *13*, 601 (1989).

251   B.S. Tsai, D. Villani-Price, R.H. Keith, J.M. Zemaitis, R.F. Bauer, R. Leonard, S.W. - Djuric, and R.L. Shone: Prostaglandins *38*, 655 (1989).

252   D.J. Fretland, D.L. Widomski, J.M. Zemaitis, R.E. Walsh, S. Levin, S.W. Djuric, R.L. Shone, B.S. Tsai and T.S. Gaginella: Inflammation *14*, 727 (1990).

253   D.J. Fretland, S. Levin, B.S. Tsai, S.W. Djuric, D.L. Widomski, J.M. Zemaitis, R.L. Shone and R.F. Bauer: Agents Actions *27*, 395 (1989).

254   D.J. Fretland, D. Widomski, B.S. Tsai, J.M. Zemaitis, S. Levin, S.W. Djuric, R.L. Shone and T.S. Gaginella: J. Pharm. Exp. Ther. *255*, 572 (1990).

255   D. Villani-Price, D.C. Yang, R.E. Walsh, D.J. Fretland, R.H. Keith, G. Kocan, J.F. - Kachur, T.S. Gaginella and B.S. Tsai: J. Pharmacol. Exp. Ther. *260*, 187 (1992).

256   D.J. Fretland, D.L. Widomski, C.P. Anglin, S.Yu and S.W. Djuric: Chirality *4*, 353 (1992).

257   T.D. Penning, S.W. Djuric, S.H. Docter, S.S. Yu, D. Spangler, C.P. Anglin, D.J. Fretland, J.F. Kachur, R.H. Keith, B.S. Tsai, D. Villani-Price and D.L. Widomski: 6th International Conference Inflammation Research Association, White Haven, PA, Sept (1992) Abst. P108.

258   D.J. Fretland, D.L. Widomski, C.P. Anglin, T.D. Penning, S. Yu and S.W. Djuric: Inflammation *17*, 353 (1993).

259   S.W. Djuric, S.H. Docter, S.S. Yu, D. Spangler, B.S. Tsai, C.P. Anglin, T.S. Gaginella, J.F. Kachur, R.H. Keith, T.J. Maziasz, D. Villani-Price, T.S. Rao, R.E. Walsh, D.L. Widomski and D.J. Fretland: BioMed. Chem. Lett 4, 811 (1994).

260   N. Clapp, J. Tanner, R. Carson, J. Fuhr, L. Adams, C. Anglin, S. Paulson, T. Sanderson, D. Widomski and D. Fretland: 7th International Conference Inflammation Research Association, White Haven, PA, Sept. (1994), Abst. W18.

261   M. Konno, S. Sakuyama, T. Nakae, N. Hamanaka, T. Miyamoto and A. Kawasaki: Adv. Prostaglandin, Thromboxane, Leukotriene Res. 21, 411 (1990).

262   K. Kishikawa, N. Matsunaga, T. Maruyama, R. Seo, M. Toda, T. Miyamoto and A. Kawasaki: Adv. Prostaglandin, Thromboxane, Leukotriene Res. 21, 407 (1990).

263   K. Kishikawa, N. Tateishi, T. Maruyama, R. Seo, M. Toda and T. Miyamoto: Prostaglandins 44, 261 (1992).

264   W.D. Kingsbury, I. Pendrak, J.D. Leber, J.C. Boehm, B. Mallet, H.M. Sarau, J.J. Foley, D.B. Schmidt and R.A. Daines: J. Med. Chem. 36, 3308 (1993).

265   R.A. Daines, P.A. Chambers, I. Pendrak, D.R. Jakas, H.M. Sarau, J.J. Foley, D.B. - Schmidt and W.D. Kingsbury: J. Med. Chem. 36, 3321 (1993).

266   R.A. Daines, P.A. Chambers, I. Pendrak, D.R. Jakas, H.M. Sarau, J.J. Foley, D.B. - Schmidt, D.E. Griswold, L.D. Martin and W.D. Kingsbury: J. Med. Chem. 36, 2703 (1993).

267   N. Cohen and K.A. Yagaloff: Curr. Opin. Invest. Drugs 3, 13 (1994).

268   N. Cohen, F.T. Bizzarro, W.F. May, K. Toth, F.K. Lee, P.J. Heslin, K.A. Yagaloff, L.S. - Franco, W.M. Selig and M.P. Weitz: 205th American Chemical Society Meeting, Denver, Book of Abstracts, Part 1, MEDI: 137 (1993).

269   N. Cohen, G. Weber, B.L. Banner, R.J. Lopresti, B. Schaer, A. Focella, G.B. Zenchoff, A.-M. Chiu, L. Todaro, M. O'Donnell, A.F. Welton, D. Brown, R. Garippa, H. Crowley and D.W. Morgan: J. Med. Chem. 32, 1842 (1989).

270   D. Roland: Inflammation Res. Assoc. Newsletter 3 (2), 3 (1994).

271   R. Labaudinière, G. Hilboll, A. Leon-Lomeli, H.-H. Lautenschläger, M. Parnham, P. Kuhl and N. Dereu: J. Med. Chem. 35, 3156 (1992).

272   R. Labaudinière, G. Hilboll, A. Leon-Lomeli, B. Terlain, F. Cavy, M. Parnham, P. Kuhl and N. Dereu: J. Med. Chem. 35, 3170 (1992).

273   R. Labaudinière, W. Hendel, B. Terlain, F. Cavy, O. Marquis and N. Dereu: J. Med. Chem. 35, 4306 (1992).

274   R. Labaudinière, N. Dereu, F. Cavy, M.-C. Guillet, O. Marquis and B. Terlain: J. Med. Chem. 35, 4315 (1992).

275   F.-C. Huang, W.-K. Chan, J.D. Warus, M.M. Morrissette, K.J. Moriarty, M.N. Chang, J.J. Travis, L.S. Mitchell, G.W. Nuss and C.A. Sutherland: J. Med. Chem. 35, 4253 (1992).

276   H. Kawakami, N. Ohmi and H. Nagata: BioMed. Chem Lett. 4, 1461 (1994).

277   N. Ohmi, C. Tani, K. Yamada and M. Fukui: Inflammation 18, 129 (1994).

278   J.A. Lowe, III, S.E. Drozda, R.M. Snider, K.P. Longo, S.H. Zorn, J. Morrone, E.R. Jackson, S. McLean, D.K. Bryce, J. Bordner, A. Nagahisa, Y. Kanai, O. Suga and M. Tsuchiya: J. Med. Chem. 35, 2591 (1992).

279   E.J. Ariens, A.J. Beld, J.F. Rodrigues de Miranda and A.M. Simonis: in The Receptors: A Comprehensive Treatise, (Ed. R. D. O'Brien; Plenum, New York, 1979) 1, p. 33.

280   B.E. Evans, K.E. Rittle, M.G. Bock, R.M. DiPardo, R.M. Freidinger, W.L. Whitter, G.F. Lundell, D.F. Veber, P.S. Anderson, R.S.L. Chang, V.J. Lotti, D.J. Cerino, T.B. Chen, P.J. Kling, K.A. Kunkel, J.P. Springer and J. Hirshfield: J. Med. Chem. 31, 2235 (1988).

281   K. Koch, L.S. Melvin, Jr., L.A. Reiter, M.S. Biggers, H.J. Showell, R.J. Griffiths, E.R. Pettipher, J.B. Cheng, A.J. Milici, R. Breslow, M.J. Conklyn, M.A. Smith,

B.C. Hackman, N.S. Doherty, E. Salter, C.A. Farrell and G. Schulte: J. Med. Chem. *37*, 3197 (1994).

282   H.J. Showell, R. Breslow, M.J. Conklyn, C.A. Farrell, J.S. Pillar, G.P. Hingorani, E.R. Pettipher, R.J. Griffiths, J.B. Cheng, N.S. Doherty, L.S. Melvin, Jr., L.A. Reiter, M.S. Biggers, and K. Koch: 7th International Conference Inflammation Research Association, White Haven, PA, Sept. (1994), Abst. P22.

283   E.R. Pettipher, E.D. Salter, R.J. Griffiths, K. Koch, N.S. Doherty and H.J. Showell: 7th International Conference Inflammation Research Association, White Haven, PA, Sept. (1994), Abst. P26.

284   E.R. Pettipher, E.D. Salter and H.J. Showell: Br. J. Pharmacol. *113*, 117 (1994).

285   R.J. Griffiths, E.R. Pettipher, K. Koch, M.A. Smith, N.S. Doherty, A.J. Milici, D.N. Scampoli and H.J. Showell: 7th International Conference Inflammation Research Association, White Haven, PA, Sept. (1994), Abst. P100.

286   R.J. Griffiths, E.R. Pettipher, K. Koch, C.A. Farrell, R. Breslow, M.J. Conklyn, M.A. Smith, B.C. Hackman, D.J. Wimberly, A.J. Milici, D.N. Scampoli, J.B. Cheng, J.S. Pillar, C.J. Pazoles, N.S. Doherty, L.S. Melvin, L.A. Reiter, M.S. Biggars, F.C. Falkner, D.Y. Mitchell, T.E. Liston, and H.J. Showell: Proc. Natl. Acad. Sci. USA *92*, 517 (1995).

287   R.J. Fujimoto, A.J. Main, L.I. Barsky, M. Morrissey, R. Cadilla, C. Boehm, Y. Zhang, H. Suh, J.B. Boxer, D.B. Powers, R.A. Doti, C.T. Healy, B.E. Seligmann, S. Uziel-Fusi, M.F. Jarvis, M.A. Sills, R.H. Jackson, K.E. Lipson, M.H. Chin, T.C. Pellas, G. Pastor, L.R. Fryer, A.A. Raychaudhuri and B.L. Kotyuk: 7th International Conference Inflammation Research Association, White Haven, PA, Sept. (1994), Abst. P29.

288   A. Raychaudhuri, B. Kotyuk, T.C. Pellas, G. Pastor, L.R. Fryer, S. Uziel-Fusi, M. Morrissey and A. Main: 7th International Conference Inflammation Research Association, White Haven, PA, Sept. (1994), Abst. P34.

289   J. Morgan, R. Stevens, S. Uziel-Fusi, B. Seligmann, W. Haston, H. Lau, M. Hayes, W.L. Hirschhorn, S. Saris and A. Piraino: Clin. Pharmacol. Ther. *55*, 199 (1994).

290   G.W. Carter, P.R. Young, D.H. Albert, J. Bouska, R. Dyer, R.L. Bell, J.B. Summers and D.W. Brooks: J. Pharmacol. Exp. Therap. *256*, 929 (1991).

291   R.L. Bell, P.R. Young, D. Albert, C. Lanni, J.B. Summers, D.W. Brooks, P. Rubin and G.W. Carter: Int. J. Immunopharmacol. *14*, 505 (1992).

292   L.G. Garland and J.A. Salmon: Drugs Fut. *16*, 547 (1991).

293   E. Israel, R. Dermarkarian, M. Rosenberg, R. Sperling, G. Taylor, P. Rubin and J.M. Drazen: N. Engl. J. Med. *323*, 1740 (1990).

294   E. Israel, A.R. Fischer, M.A. Rosenberg, C.M. Lilly, J.C. Callery, J. Shapiro, J. Cohn, P. Rubin and J.M. Drazen: Am. Rev. Respir. Dis. *148*, 1447 (1993).

295   E. Israel, P. Rubin, J.P. Kemp, J. Grossman, W. Pierson, S.C. Siegel, D. Tinkelman, J.J. Murray, W. Busse, A.T. Segal, J. Fish, H.B. Kaiser, D. Ledford, S. Wenzel, R. Rosenthal, J. Cohn, C. Lanni, H. Pearlman, P. Karahalios and J.M. Drazen: Ann. Intern. Med. *119*, 1059 (1993).

296   L.S. Laursen, J. Naesdal, K. Bukhave, K. Lauritsen and J. Rask-Madsen: Lancet *335*, 683 (1990).

297   C. Collawn, P. Rubin, N. Perez, J. Bobadilla, G. Cabrera, E. Reyes, J. Borovoy and D. Kershenobich: Am. J. Gastroenterol. *87*, 342 (1992).

298   L.S. Laursen, K. Lauritsen, K. Bukhave, J. Rask-Madsen, O. Jacobsen, J. Naesdal, H. Goebell, B. Peskar, P.D. Rubin, L.J. Swanson, J.W. Kesterson, A. Keshavarzian, R. Kozarek, S. Hanauer, D. Cort and W.F. Stenson: Eur. J. Gastroenterol. Hepatol. *6*, 209 (1994).

299 T.M. Hyers, in: Adult Respiratory Distress Syndrome (Ed. W.M. Zapol and F. - Lemaire; Marcel Dekker, Inc., New York, 1991) p. 23.

300 M.A. Matthay, W.L. Eschenbacher and E.J. Goetzl: J. Clin. Immunol. 4, 479 (1984).

301 A.H. Stephenson, A.J. Lonigro, T.M. Hyers, R.O. Webster and A.A. Fowler: Am. Rev. Respir. Dis. 138, 714 (1988).

302 G.R. Bernard, V. Korley, P. Chee, B. Swindell, A.W. Ford-Hutchinson and P. Tagari: Am. Rev. Respir. Dis. 144, 263 (1991).

303 J. Fauler, D. Tsikas, M. Holch, A. Seekamp, M.L. Nerlich, J. Sturm and J.C. Frölich: Clin. Sci. 80, 497 (1991).

304 B.R.C. O'Driscoll, O. Cromwell and A.B. Kay: Clin. Exp. Immunol. 55, 397 (1984).

305 W. Luck, T. Simmet, E.W. Schmidt and B.A. Peskar, in: Prostaglandins In Clinical Research: Cardiovascular System (Alan R. Liss, Inc., New York, 1989) p. 259.

306 P. Greally, A.J. Cook, A.P. Sampson, R. Coleman, S. Chambers, P.J. Piper and J.F. Price: J. Allergy Clin. Immunol. 93, 100 (1994).

307 N.H. Maltby, P.W. Ind, R.C. Causon, R.W. Fuller and G.W. Taylor: Clin. Exp. Allergy 19, 33 (1989).

308 I. Neu, J. Mallinger, A. Wildfeuer and L. Mehlber: Acta Neurol. Scand. 86, 586 (1992).

309 P. Paoletti, P. Gaetani, G. Grignani, L. Pacchiarini, V. Silvani and R. Rodriguez y Baena: J. Neurosurg. 69, 488 (1988).

310 J.A. Parker, E.J. Goetzl and M.H. Friedlaender: Arch. Ophthalmol. 104, 722 (1986).

311 M. Huber, S. Kastner, J. Scholmerich, W. Gerok and D. Keppler: Eur. J. Clin. Invest. 19, 53 (1989).

312 K.P. Moore, G.W. Taylor, N.H. Maltby, D. Siegers, R.W. Fuller, C.T. Dollery and R. Williams: J. Hepatol. 11, 263 (1990).

313 M. Uemura, U. Buchholz, H. Kojima, A. Keppler, P. Hafkemeyer, H. Fukui, T. Tsujii and D. Keppler: Hepatology 20, 804 (1994).

314 Scrip World Pharm. News 2011, 21 (1995).

315 Scrip World Pharm. News 2039, 22 (1995); 2050, 6 (1995).

316 T.R. Jones, M. Labelle, M. Belley, E. Champion, L. Charette, J. Evans, A.W. Ford-Hutchinson, J.-Y. Gauthier, A. Lord, P. Masson, M. McAuliffe, C.S. McFarlane, K.M. Metters, C. Pickett, H. Piechuta, C. Rochette, I.W. Rodger, N. Sawyer, R.N. Young, R. Zamboni and W.M. Abraham: Can. J. Physiol. Pharmacol. 73, 191 (1995).

317 M. Labelle, M. Belley, Y. Gareau, J.Y. Gauthier, D. Guay, R. Gordon, S.G. Grossman, T.R. Jones, Y. Leblanc, M. McAuliffe, C. McFarlane, P. Masson, K.M. Metters, N. Ouimet, D.H. Patrick, H. Piechuta, C. Rochette, N. Sawyer, Y.B. Xiang, C.B. Pickett, A.W. Ford-Hutchinson, R.J. Zamboni and R.N. Young: BioMed. Chem. Lett. 5, 283 (1995).

318 A. Botto, I. DeLepeleire, F. Rochette, T.F. Reiss, J. Zhang, S. Kundu, and M. Decramer: Am. J. Respir. Crit Care Med. 149, A465 (1994).

319 C.A. Sorkness, T.F. Reiss, J. Zhang, S. Kundu, H. Cheng, R. Amin, W. Stricker and W.W. Busse: Am. J. Respir. Crit. Care Med. 149, A216 (1994).

320 Scrip World Pharm. News 2017/18, 29 (1995).

321 R.J. Griffiths: Second World Conference on Inflammation, Brighton, UK, 1995.

322 D.J. Evans, L.J. Coulby, S.M. Spaethe, E. Van Alstyne, P. Pechous, P.J. Barnes and B.J. O'Connor: Amer. J. Respi. Crit Care Med. 151, A680 (1995).

Progress in Drug Research, Vol. 46 (E. Jucker, Ed.)
© 1996 Birkhäuser Verlag, Basel (Switzerland)

Drugs affecting plasma fibrinogen levels. Implications for new antithrombotic strategies

M. Margaglione, E. Grandone, F.P. Mancini and G. Di Minno

I.R.C.C.S. "Casa Sollievo della Sofferenza", S. Giovanni Rotondo (FG) and Clinical Medica, Istituto di Medicina Interna e Malattie Dismetaboliche, Nuovo Policlinico, Napoli, Italy

1   Summary

Current evidence indicates that plasma fibrinogen is synthesized by the liver; that genetic and environmental factors regulate plasma fibrinogen levels; that interleukin-6 (IL-6) affects the synthesis of plasma fibrinogen by mechanisms involving protein kinase C, and that during the acute-phase response, monocytes generate a variety of monokines including IL-6. Certain drugs and nutrients have been reported to lower plasma fibrinogen levels. The mechanism(s) involved in this effect is poorly understood. However, since most of these substances quantitatively and/or qualitatively affect monocytes, the possibility that these drugs affect plasma fibrinogen levels via these cells should be considered.
In addition to fibrinogen, IL-6 also regulates the synthesis of other acute-phase proteins. Especially when combined, major risk factors for atherosclerosis cause vascular injury that triggers inflammatory events. This raises the issue of whether high plasma fibrinogen levels are just the epiphenomenon of as yet unknown events in thrombosis and atherosclerosis. Thus, the issue to be addressed is whether high plasma fibrinogen concentrations should be lowered or should they serve to suggest strong interventions on established risk factors. As for other risk factors, fibrinogen measurements in population-based studies, in parallel with measurements of established risk factors will help define appropriate directions to be followed to gain insight into the issue and define new antithrombotic strategies.

2   Introduction

In 1980, Meade et al. [1] first reported an association between hemostatic variables and cardiovascular death. In their prospective study, these authors reported that persons who died from coronary heart disease (CHD) had had, at recruitment, fibrinogen levels significantly higher than survivors or persons dying from other causes. In addition, they found that the association of fibrinogen with CHD was independent of established risk factors and stronger than the association with serum cholesterol. This issue was confirmed in the Goteborg [2] and in the Framingham [3] studies. Like other epidemiological studies devoted to this issue [4–8], both these studies extended the predictive value of high plasma fibrinogen levels with respect to stroke, and established the independent nature of high plasma fibrinogen level with respect to other well known risk factors such as cigarette smoking, hematocrit, high plasma glucose, and high plasma lipoproteins.

Several lines of evidence have documented that fibrinogen is involved in major mechanisms thought to be crucial in thrombosis and atherosclerosis such as platelet aggregation [9], blood rheology [10, 11], endothelial cell injury [12], and cell proliferation [13]. On the other hand, over the last fifteen years, the hypothesis that hemostatic components are involved in atherosclerosis and in its thrombotic complications has been confirmed and extended [14–16]. Cigarette smoking [17] and high plasma lipid levels have been shown to affect the hemostatic system [9], and gelatinous and fibrous plaques have been documented to be very rich in fibrin(ogen) degradation products [18–20]. Thus, it has been postulated that high plasma fibrinogen levels might have a pathogenetic significance in the thrombotic complications of atherosclerosis [14]. This has fostered the search for drugs able to lower the plasma levels of this protein.

3   Regulation of plasma fibrinogen levels

Current knowledge of the mechanisms regulating the expression of the fibrinogen genes may be helpful for a better understanding of the mechanisms of the action of drugs affecting plasma fibrinogen levels and for identifying new potential strategies of intervention against thrombotic complications of atherosclerosis.

The fibrinogen molecule consists of two subunits each composed of three chains ($A\alpha$, $B\beta$, and γ) held together by disulfide bridges [21, 22]. The genes for the three chains are closely located, in the long arm of chromosome 4 (4q28) [23, 24]. The expression of the gene for the $B\beta$ chain has been shown to be the rate-limiting step in the assembly of plasma fibrinogen [25, 26]. However, more recently the stimulation of any one of the fibrinogen genes has been reported to raise the transcription genes of the other two [27], and the translation as well as the production of the respective polypeptide products. Genetic heritability is currently thought to largely account for the total interindividual variability of plasma fibrinogen concentrations [28–30]. The clinical relevance of this concept has been emphasized by a report by Humphries et al. [31]. These authors used three enzymes to identify different restriction fragment lenght polymorphisms of the fibrinogen genes. One of the polymorphisms, located within the promoter region of the $B\beta$–chain gene, was found to be associated with higher plasma levels of fibrinogen. The authors estimated that these genotypic variations accounted for 4–9% of the variance of plasma fibrinogen concentrations. When the data obtained with these enzymes were combined, these polymorphins accounted for up to 15% of the interindividual variability of plasma levels of fibrinogen. The extent to what genetic variations play a quantitative role in the regulation of fibrinogen synthesis has been disputed by others (reviewed in ref. [32]). However, all the authors agree that genetic components regulate, to some extent, the expression of the fibrinogen genes [32–34].

The possibility of gene-environment interaction in the regulation of plasma fibrinogen levels was raised almost fifteen years ago by Fuller et al. [35, 36]. They showed that the synthesis of fibrinogen was controlled by an indirect feedback mechanism in which fibrinogen/fibrin degradation products induced the release from monocytes of a monokine, the so-called hepatocyte-stimulating factor (HSF). This factor stimulates the synthesis of fibrinogen mRNA. Also cigarette smoking has been suggested [17] to induce the production on the gene of the hepatocyte-stimulating factor by monocytes. This may help explain the strong relationship between plasma fibrinogen levels and cigarette smoking. An effect comparable to that of fibrinopeptides can be achieved by stimulation of monocytes with *E. Coli* lipopolysaccharide. Following stimulation with this lipopolysaccharide, monocytes release interleukin-1 (IL-1) and tumor necrosis factor (TNF) [37]. Some studies were carried out to define whether these two monokines could act as a HSF [38]. This did not appear to be the case: increasing concentrations of TNF and/or IL-1 did not induce fibrinogen mRNA. In contrast, the effect of the HSF was mimicked by TPA [39], a phorbol ester and a tumor promoter, whose cellular effects are known to be mediated by the activation of protein kinase C. In the late '80s, a 26 kDa molecule appeared to mimic the HSF effect [40]. Using a recombinant protein, it was found that IL-6, which modulates the plasma levels of the majority of the acute-phase proteins, was indistinguishable from HSF [41, 42]. Within the regulatory region of the Bβ-fibrinogen an IL-6 response sequence has been identified and a polymorphism modulating the effects of IL-6 on the plasma regulation of IL-6 has been demonstrated [32]. It was also documented that the effect of IL-6 on the expression of fibrinogen genes is modulated by IL-1, TNF [43–45] and transforming growth factor β (TGF-β) [46]. IL-1 and TNF stimulate fibroblasts, endothelial cells and keratinocytes to synthesize IL-6 [43, 44], thus amplifying the process. However, IL-1 also downregulates the mRNA for the IL-6 receptor [45], thus reducing the stimulation of fibrinogen synthesis, due to increased IL-6 levels [46]. On the other hand, IL-6 suppresses IL-1 and TNF mRNA transcription [44]. Binding of IL-6 to its receptor involves the activation of protein kinase C and of a liver-specific nuclear protein [47, 48].

4   Drugs affecting plasma fibrinogen levels

4.1   n-3 fatty acids

Dietary changes in fat and fish intake have been reported to lower the risk of reccurrence of myocardial infarction [49]. A prolonged administration of n-3 fatty acids is associated with the impairment of several monocyte functions such as the synthesis of TNF, IL-1, PAF and of proinflammatory substances such as leukotrienes [50–52]. Dietary supplementation with n-3 fatty acids (fish oils) [53–56], or with olive oil [57], lowers plasma fibrinogen levels. TNF and IL-1 stimulate a variety of cells to synthesize IL-6. This raises the possibility that the fibrinogen lowering effects of n-3 fatty acids involves to some extent the effects of these substances on the monocyte synthesis of IL-6 as well as on that of leukotrienes. On the other hand, monocyte and neutrophil chemotaxis are also lowered by n-3 fatty acids administration [58]. Such effects imply a general downregulation of the immune system by n-3 fatty acids. Several mediators of the inflammatory process are involved in the regulation of the acute-phase response and may explain the effects of n-3 fatty acids on plasma fibrinogen levels. In addition, the impaired production of these potent mitogens could affect certain proliferative response within the vessel wall [59]. In Table 1 some recognized factors known to effect plasma fibrinogen levels are reported.

Table 1
Factors that affect plasma fibrinogen levels

Enhance	Reduce
Cigarette smoking	Physical exercise
Oral contraceptive drugs	n-3 fatty acids
Positive energy balance	Ticlopidine
Diabetes mellitus	Fibrates
Pregnancy	Alcohol
High dietary fat intake	Pentoxifilline
Increasing age	Dipiridamole
Menopause	
Inflammation, thrombin, endotoxin	
Prostaglandins, hormones	
Vascular damage	

4.2   Ticlopidine

Almost ten years ago, a study [60] showed that the administration of ticlopidine was associated with the lowering of plasma levels of fibrinogen. This has been confirmed by other authors [61]. Reports from several major clinical trials [62–64], in which ticlopidine has been shown to prevent thrombotic complications of atherosclerosis, suggest a direction to be followed to elucidate this finding. In about 2% of the subjects studied, the administration of ticlopidine was associated with a marked reduction of the number of circulating white cells. In larger numbers of these patients, ticlopidine caused measurable effects on certain hepatocyte functions [65]. In addition, we have found that this drug affects major functions of the monocyte membrane such as the sodium/hydrogen countertransport (Margaglione et al., unpublished observations).

4.3   Phosphodiesterase inhibitors

Several data show that the administration of phosphodiesterase inhibitors, such as pentoxiphilline and dipyramidole lowers plasma fibrinogen levels [66–70]. On the other hand, Zakarski et al. [71, 72] showed that an analog of dipyramidole reduced plasma levels of fibrinogen and increased the life expectancy of patients with lung cancer. There is no direct explanation for the mechanism of these drugs. However, protein kinase C is involved in the regulation of plasma fibrinogen levels [39]. In several cell systems, high levels of cAMP regulate the effects of protein kinase C [73, 74]. Phosphodiesterase inhibitors increase intracellular levels of cAMP [75].

4.4   Lipid-modifying agents

These drugs are known to affect plasma levels of lipoproteins, and, by interacting with endothelial cells, help release factors that affect major functions of monocytes such as chemotaxis. Drugs affecting lipids and lipoproteins may thus lower plasma fibrinogen by an indirect mechanism.
Fibric acid derivatives (fibrates), are reported to play a role in the regulation of plasma fibrinogen levels [76]. They have an aromatic fatty acid structure different from that of saturated or unsaturated fatty acids [77]. Fibrates interact with a nuclear receptor that belongs to the steroid receptor superfamily of ligand-activated transcription factors [78].
Other members of the superfamily are the receptors for vitamins A and D and for thyroid hormones. Some reports [79, 80] show that the administration of certain fibrates lowers plasma fibrinogen levels. The data on

gemfibrozil have been challenged recently [81]. Differences exist between different fibrates with respect to their ability to affect plasma fibrinogen levels. Bezafibrate seems to be the most effective agent, in this respect, individuals with highest plasma fibrinogen levels being the most sensitive to the lowering effect [80]. Few isolated reports pointed to a lowering effect of probucol on plasma fibrinogen concentrations [82]. This drug has, among other properties, the ability to activate the cholesteryl ester transport protein system [83] and to prevent the oxidation of a series of variables [84, 85].

4.5   Ethanol

It is well known that chronic alcoholics have lower than normal levels of fibrinogen [17, 29, 86]. Several data indicate that ethanol exerts a direct injurious effect on hepatocytes [87]. However, clinical practice also indicates that chronic alcoholics are at high risk for developing infections. In keeping with this, some data indicate that alcohol affects major functions of monocytes [88]. Therefore, it is conceivable that, in addition to an effect on hepatocytes, alcohol may also affect some monocyte functions involved in the regulation of plasma fibrinogen levels.

5   Conclusions

It has been stressed that IL-6 is the major regulator of the expression of fibrinogen genes. Parallel with studies on the effects of IL-6 on the regulation of plasma fibrinogen, other studies document that this interleukin

Table 2
Regulation by IL-6 of acute-phase plasma proteins

Increase	Decrease
Fibrinogen	Prealbumin
Haptoglobulin	Albumin
C3 of complement	Inter a1-Antitripsin
Serum amyloid	a1-Lipoprotein
Ceruloplasmin	Transferrin
C-Reactive protein	
a2-Antiplasmin	
a1-Proteinase inhibitor	
a1-Antitrypsin	
a1-Antichimotrypsin	

is an important factor in the regulation of the immune as well as the hematopoietic system (Table 2). Monocytes, stimulated by different agonists, synthesize and secrete IL-1, IL-6, and TNF. In addition to fibrinogen, this complex network regulates the synthesis of other acute-phase proteins as well. None of the drugs discussed above has a documented direct effect on the regulation of plasma fibrinogen concentrations. In contrast, most of them play a role in the modulation of the immune response. Since an hematological stress syndrome has been described in atherosclerosis [89], this raises the issue whether high plasma fibrinogen is just the index of as yet unknown phenomena in atherosclerosis and in its thrombotic complications. A possible answer to this question could be provided by simultaneous measurements of fibrinogen and other acute-phase proteins such as prothrombin and haptoglobin. However these data are not available.

6   Perspectives

The perspectives on this issue have to take into consideration the concept of fibrinogen as an acute-phase reactant. If raised plasma fibrinogen is the response to the severity of the vascular damage taking place, a strategy to be followed to lower plasma fibrinogen should involve strong interventions on risk factors that may cause (or enhance) vascular damage. In addition to its pathophysiological significance, information from such studies would be essential to develop new directions to understand, prevent and cure thrombotic complications of atherosclerosis. As of now, the extent to which raised levels of fibrinogen in subjects at risk for developing stroke and myocardial infarction reflect a vascular injury and/or the effect of molecular variations is unclear. However, high levels of fibrinogen may greatly amplify an inflammatory response. Inflammation facilitates vascular permeability, the latter allowing fibrinogen to penetrate the intima and be transformed into fibrin by procoagulant activities of perturbed monocytes and endothelial cells [14]. Moreover, in spite of the unsolved issues in the field, the epidemiological data so far available are strong enough to indicate that high plasma fibrinogen levels should be checked to predict stroke and myocardial infarction. In view of this, we believe that studies in cohorts of healthy young people will help answer the unsolved issues in the field and provide a major direction to be followed to extrapolate from molecular markers to pharmacology.

References

1   Meade T.W., Chakrabarti R., Haines A.P. et al.: Haemostatic function and cardio-vascular death: early results of a prospective study. Lancet *1*, 1050–1054 (1980).

2   Wilhelmsen K., Svardsudd K., Korsan-Bengsten K., Larson B., Welin L., Tibblin G.: Fibrinogen as a risk factor for stroke and myocardial infarction. N Engl J Med *311*, 501–505 (1984).

3   Kannel W.B., Wolf P.A., Castelli W.P., D'Agostino R.B.: Fibrinogen and risk of car-diovascular disease. The Framingham Study. JAMA *258*: 1183–1186 (1987).

4   Balleisen L., Bailey J., Epping P.H., Shulte H., van de Loo J.: Epidemiological study on factor VII, factor VIII and fibrinogen in an industrial population. I. Baseline data on the relation to age, gender, body weight, smoking, alcohol, pill using and meno-pause. Thromb Haemost *54,* 475–479 (1985).

5   Stone M.C., Thorpe J.M.: Plasma fibrinogen as a major coronary risk factor. J R Coll Gen Pract *35*, 565–569 (1985).

6   Meade T.W., Brozovic M., Chakrabarti R.R. et al.: Haemostatic function and ischemic heart disease: Principal results of the Northwick Park Heart Study. Lancet *2*, 533–537 (1986).

7   Welin L., Svardsudd K., Wilhelmsen L., Larsson B., Tibblin G.: Analysis of risk fac-tors of stroke in a cohort of men born in 1913. N Engl J Med *317*, 521–526 (1987).

8   Lee A.J., Smith W.C.S., Lowe G.D.O., Tunstall-Pedoe H.: Plasma fibrinogen and cor-onary risk factors: the scottish heart health study. J Clin Epidem *43*, 913–919 (1990).

9   Packham M.A., Mustard J.F.: The role of platelets in the development and compli-cations of atherosclerosis. Semin Haematol *23*, 8–26 (1986).

10   Lowe G.D.O.: Blood rheology in arterial disease. Clin Sci *71*, 137–146 (1986).

11   Leonard E.F.: Rheology in thrombosis, in: Colman R.W., Hirsh J., Marder V.J., Salz-man E.W. (Eds.): Hemostasis and thrombosis: basic principles and clinical practice. 2nd ed. Philadelphia: Lippincot 1987, 1111–1122.

12   Smith E.B., Staples E.M., Dietz H.S., Smith R.H.: Role of endothelium in seques-tration of lipoprotein and fibrinogen in aortic lesions, thrombi and graft pseudo-intimas. Lancet *2*, 812–816 (1979).

13   Levesque J.P., Hatzfeld A., Hatzfeld J.: Fibrinogen mitogenic effect on hemopoietic cell lines: control via receptor modulation. Proc. Natl. Acad. Sci. USA *83*, 6494–7 (1986).

14   Di Minno G., Mancini M.: Measuring plasma fibrinogen to predict stroke and myo-cardial infarction. Arteriosclerosis *10*, 1–7 (1990).

15   York J.L., Benjamin W.: Quantitative studies on the relationship of fibrinogen and "fibrin" in intima and atherosclerotic plaque. Throm Res *18*, 717–724 (1980).

16   Smith E.B.: Fibrinogen, fibrin and fibrin degradation products in relation to athero-sclerosis. Clin Haematol *15*, 355–370 (1986).

17   Meade T.W., Imeson J., Stirling Y.: Effects of changes in smoking and other charac-teristics on clotting factors and the risk of ischaemic heart disease. Lancet *ii*, 986–989 (1987).

18   Haust M.D., Wyllie J.C., Moke R.H.: Electron microscopy of fibrin in human athe-rosclerotic lesions. Exp Mol Pathol *4*, 205–216 (1965).

19   Kao V.C.Y., Wissler R.W.: A study of the immuochemical localization of serum lipop-roteins and other plasma proteins in human atherosclerotic lesions. Exp Mol Pathol *4*, 465–479 (1965).

20   Francis C.W., Markham R.E. Jr., Marder V.J.: Demonstration of *in situ* fibrin degra-dation in pathologic thrombi. Blood *63*, 1216–1224 (1984).

21   Henschen A., McDonagh J.: Fibrinogen, fibrin and factor XIII. In: Blood Coagulation. Zwaal RFA, Hemker HC (eds.). Elsevier, Amsterdam 1986, pp.171–241.

22   Hoeprich P.D., Doolittle R.F.: Dimeric half-momlecules of human fibrinogen are joinedthrough disulphide bonds in an antiparallel orientation. Biochemstry 22,2049 55 (1983).

23   Marino M.W., Fuller G.M., Elder F.F.B.: Chromosomal localisation of human and rat alpha, beta and gamma fibrinogen genes by in situ hybridation. Cytogenet Cell Genet. 42, 36–41 (1986).

24   Buetow K.H., Shiang R., Nakamura Y. et al.: A multipoint genetic map and new RFPLsfor human chromosome 4. Cytogenet. Cell Genet. 51, 973 (1989).

25   Yu S., Sher B., Kudryk B., Redman C.M.: Intracellular assembly of human fibrinogen. J Biol Chem 258, 13407–13410 (1983).

26   Yu S., Sher B., Kudryk B., Redman C.M.: Intracellular assembly of human fibrinogen. J Biol Chem 259, 10574–10581 (1984).

27   Roy S., Mukhopadhyay G., Redman C.: Regulation of fibrinogen assembly. J. Biol. Chem 265, 6389–6393 (1990).

28   Roy S., Overton O., Redman C.: Overexpression of any fibrinogen chain by Hep G2 cells specifically elevates the expression of the other two chains. J. Biol. Chem. 269, 691–695 (1994).

29   Hamsten A., Iselius L., De Faire U., Blomback M.: Genetic and cultural inheritance of plasma fibrinogen concentration. Lancet i, 988– 990 (1987).

30   Berg K., Kierulf P.: DNA polymorphisms at fibrinogen loci and plasma fibrinogen concentrations. Clin. Genet. 36, 229–235 (1989).

31   Humphries S.E., Cook M., Dubowitz M., Stirling Y., Meade T.W.: Role of genetic variation at the fibrinogen locus in determination of plasma fibrinogen concentrations. Lancet i, 1452–1455 (1987).

32   Margaglione M., Grandone E., Di Minno G.: Genetic modulation of plasma fibrinogen concentrations. Implications for thrombotic complication of atherosclerosis. J. Thrombos. Thrombolys. 1995 (in press).

33   Meade T.W., Chakrabarti, Haines A.P., North W.R.S., Stirling Y.: Characteristics affecting fibrinolytic activity and plasma fibrinogen concentrations. Lancet i, 153–156 (1979).

34   Balleisen L., Bailey J., Epping P.H. et al.: Epidemiology study on Factor VII, Factor VIII and Fibrinogen in an industrial population. I. Baseline data on the relation to age, gender, body weight, smoking, alchool, pill using and menopause. Thromb. Haemstas. 54, 475–479 (1985).

35   Ritchie D.G., Levy B.A., Adams M.A., Fuller G.M.: Regulation of fibrinogen synthesis by plasmin-derived fragments of fibrinogen and fibrin: An indirect feedback pathway. Proc Natl Acad Sci 79, 1530–1534 (1982).

36   Ritchie D.G., Fuller G.M.: Hepatocyte-stimulating factor: a monocyte derived acutephase regulatory protein. Ann New York Acad Sci, 490–500 (1983).

37   Hermann F., Martelsmann R.: Polypeptides controlling hematopoietic cell development andactivation. Blut 58, 117 (1989).

38   Baumann H., Richards C., Gauldie J.: Interaction among hepatocyte-stimulating factors, interleukin 1 and glucocorticoids for regulation of acute phase plasma proteins in human hepatoma (Hep G2) cells. J. Immunol. 139, 4122–8 (1987).

39   Evans E., Courtois G.M., Kilian P., Fuller G.M., Crabtree G.R.: Induction of fibrinogen and a subset of acute phase response genes involves a novel monokine which is mimicked by phorbol esters. J Biol Chem 262, 10850–854 (1987).

40   Poupart P. et al.: B cell growth modulating and differentiating activity of recombinant human 26-kd protein (BSF-2, HuINF-β_2, HPGF). EMBO J. 6, 1219 (1987).

41   Le J., Vilcek J.: Interleukin-6: a multifunctional cytokine regulating immune reactions and the acute phase protein response. Lab Invest 61, 588–602 (1989).

42   Heinrich P.C., Castell J.V., Andus T.: Interleukin 6 and the acute phase response. Biochem J 265, 621–636 (1990).

43   Ramadori G., Van Damme J., Reter H., Meyer-Zum-Buschenfelte H.M.: Interleukin 6, the third mediator of acute phase reaction, modulates hepatic protein synthesis in human and mouse. Comparison with interleukin lβ and tumor necrosis factor. Eur. J. Immunol. 18, 1259–64 (1988).

44   Schindler R., Mancilla J., Enders S. et al.: Correlations and interactions in the production of inteleukin 6 (IL-6), IL-1 and tumor necrosis factor (TNF) in human blood mononuclear cells: IL-6 supresses IL-1 and TNF. Blood 75, 40 (1990).

45   Dinarello C.A.: Interleukin-1 and interleukin-1 antagonism. Blood 77, 1627–1652 (1991).

46   Hassan J., Chelucci C., Peschle C., Sorrentino V.: Transforming growth factor β (TGF-β) inhibits expression of fibrinogen and factor VII in a hepatoma cell line. Thromb. Haemostas. 67, 478–483 (1992).

47   Poli V., Cortese R.: Interleukin 6 induces a liver-specific nuclear protein that binds to the promoter of acute-phase genes. Proc Natl Acad Sci 86, 8202–8206 (1989).

48   Poli V., Mancini F.P., Cortese R.: IL-6DBP, a nuclear protein involved in interleukin-6 signal transduction, defines a new family of leucine zipper proteins related to C/EBO. Cell 63, 643–653 (1990).

49   Burr M.L., Fehiky A.M., Gilbert J.F., Rogers S., Holliday R.M., Sweetnam P.M., Elwood P.C., Deadman N.M.: Effects of changes in fat, fish and fibreintakes on death and myocardial infarction: diet and reinfarction trial (DART). Lancet 2, 757-761 (1989).

50   Endres S., Ghorbani R., Kelley V.E., Georgilis K., Lonnemann G., van der Meer J., Cannon J.G., Rogers T.S., Klempner, Weber P., Schaefer E.J., Wolff S.M., Dinarello C.A.: The effect of dietary supplementation with n-3 polyunsaturated fatty acids on the synthesis of interleukin-1 and tumor necrosis factor by mononuclear cells. New Engl J Med 320, 265–271 (1989).

51   Sperling R.J., Robin J.L., Kylander K.A., Lee T.K., Lewis R.A., Austen K.F.: The effects of n-3 polyunsaturated fatty acids on the generation of platelet activating factor-acether by human monocytes. J Immunol 139, 4186–4191 (1987).

52   Takayashi R., Manku M.S., Horrobin D.F.: Impaired platelet aggregation and thromboxane generation in essential fatty-acid deficient rats. J Nutr 117, 1520–1526 (1987).

53   Hostmark A.T., Bjerkedal T., Kierulf P., Flaten H., Ulshagen K.: Fish oil and plasma fibrinogen. Br Med J 297, 180– 181 (1988).

54   Radack K., Deck C., Huster G.: Dietary supplementation with low-dose fish oils lowers fibrinogen levels: a randomized, double-blind controlled study. Ann Intern Med 111, 757–758 (1989).

55   Schmidt E.B., Varming K., Ernst E., Dyerberg J.: Dose-response studies on the effect of n-3 polyunsaturated fatty acids on lipids and haemostasis. Thromb Haemost 63, 1–5 (1990).

56   Venter C.S., Vorster H.H., van der Nest D.G.: Comparison between physiological effects of konjac-glucomannan and propionate in baboons fed "western" diets. J Nutr 120, 1046–1053 (1990).

180   M. Margaglione, E. Grandone, F.P. Mancini and G. Di Minno

57   Oosthuizen W., Vorster H.H., Jerling J.C. et al.: Both fish and olive oil lowered plasma
       fibrinogen in women with high baseline fibrinogen levels. Thrombos. Haemostas.
       72, 557–62 (1994).
58   Schmidt E.B., Pedersen J.O., Varming K. et al.: n-3 fatty acids and leukocyte chem-
       iotaxis. Effects in hyperlipidemia and dòse-response studies in health men. Arteri-
       oscleros. Thrombos. 11, 429–435 (1991).
59   Goodnight S.H.: Fish oil: effects on atherogenesis and thrombosis. Curr Op Lipidol
       1, 334–340 (1990).
60   Aukland A., Hurlow R.A., George A.J., Stuart J.: Platelet inhibition with ticlopidine
       in atherosclerotic intermittent claudication. J. Clin. Pathol. 35, 740–743 (1982).
61   Palareti G., Poggi M., Teoricelli P. et al.: Longterm effect of ticlopidine on fibrino-
       gen and hemorheology in patients with peripheral arterial disease. Thromb. Res. 52,
       621–629 (1988).
62   Balsano F., Coccheri S., Libretti A., Nenci G.G., Catalano M.M., Fortunato G., Grass-
       elli S., Violi F., Hellemans H., Vanhove P.H.: Ticlopidine in the treatment of inter-
       mittent claudication: a 21 month double-blind trial. J Lab Clin Med 114, 84–91 (1989).
63   Balsano F., Rizzon P., Violi F. and the STAI group: Antiplatelet treatment with ticlo-
       pidine in unstable angina: a controlled multicentre clinical trial. Circulation 82, 17–26
       (1990).
64   Janzon L., Bergqvist D., Boberg J., Boberg M., Eriksson J., Lindgarde F., Persson G.:
       Prevention of myocardial infarction and stroke in patients with intermittent claud-
       ication; effects of ticlopidine: Results from STIMS, the Swedish Ticlopidine Multi-
       centre Study. J Int Med 227, 301–308 (1990).
65   McTavish D., Faulds D., Goa K.: Ticlopidine: an updated review of its pharmacol-
       ogy, and therapeutic use in platelet-dependent disorders. Drugs 40, 238–259 (1990).
66   Jarret P.E.M., Moreland M., Browse N.L.: The effect of oxpentifylline on fibrino-
       lytic activity and plasma fibrinogen levels. Curr Med Res Opinion 4, 1492–1495
       (1977).
67   Takamatsu S., Sato K., Takamatsu M., Sakuts S., Mizuno S.: A two year follow up
       study on blood constituents in aged arteriosclerotic patients trteated with pentoxi-
       fylline. Proceedings of the 28th Int Congress of Physiological Sciences, Tübingen,
       West Germany, 1980.
68   Muggeo M., Calabro A., Businaro V., Patussi L., Volpe A., Signorini G.P., Crepaldi G.:
       Blood clotting, fibrinolytic and haemorheological parameters in ischaemic vascu-
       lar disease: the effects of pentoxifylline in the treatment of acute vascular disease.
       Pharmacotherapeutica 3 (suppl 1), 74–90 (1983).
69   Di Perri T., Carandente O., Vittorio O., Guerrini N., Messa G.L.: Studies on the clin-
       ical pharmacology and therapeutic efficacy of pentoxifylline in peripheral obstruc-
       tive arterial disease. Angiology 35, 427–435 (1984).
70   Ott E., Fazekas F., Lechner H.: Haemorheological effects of pentoxifylline in dis-
       turbed blood flow behaviour in patients with cerebrovascular disease. Neurology
       22 (suppl 1), 105–107 (1983).
71   Zacharski L.R., Henderson W.G., Rickles F.R. et al.: Rationale and experimental
       design for the VA Cooperative Study of RA 233 in the treatment of cancer. Am. J.
       Clin. Oncol. 5, 593–609 (1982).
72   Zacharski L.R., Moritz T.E., Baczek L.A. et al.: Effect of RA-233 (Mopidamole) on
       survival in carcinoma of the lung and colon. Final report of the VA Cooperative
       Study 188. J. Natl. Cancer Inst. 80, 90–97 (1988).
73   Watson S.P., McConnel R.T., Lapetina E.G.: The formation of inositol phosphates

in human platelets by thrombin is inhibited by prostacyclin. J. Biol. Chem. *259*, 13199–13203 (1984).

74   Rittenhouse-Simmons S.: Production of diglyceride from phosphatidylinositol in activated human platelets. J Clin Invest *63*, 580–587 (1979).

75˙   Rall T.W.: Evolution of the mechanisms of action of methylxanthines: from calcium mobilizers to antagonists of adenosine receptors. Pharmacologist. *24*, 277–287 (1982).

76   Sirtori C.R., Colli S.: Influences of lipid-modifying agents on hemostasis. Cardiovasc. Drug Ther. *7*, 817–823 (1993).

77   Hertz R., Bar-Tana J., Sujatta M. et al.: The induction of liver peroxisomal proliferation by β,β'-methyl-substituted hexadecanedioic acid (MEDICA 16). Biochem. Pharmacol. *37*, 3571–77 (1988).

78   Issemann I., Green S.: Activation of a member of the steroid hormone receptor superfamily by peroxisome proliferators. Nature *347*, 645–649 (1990).

79   Ciuffetti G., Orecchini G., Siepi D. et al.: Hemorheological activity of gemfibrozil in primary hyperlipidemias. In: Paoletti R. et al. (eds.): Drugs affecting lipid metabolism. Berlin: Springer-Verlag, 1987, 372–375.

80   Niort G., Bukgarelli A., Cassader M., Pagano G.: Effect of short term treatment with bezafibrate on plasma fibrinogen, fibrinopeptide A, platelet activation and blood filterability in atherosclerotic hyperfibrinogenemic patients. Atherosclerosis *71*, 113–119 (1988).

81   Andersen P., Smith P., Seljeflot I., Brataker S., Arnesen H.: Effects of gemfibrozil on lipids and haemostasis after myocardial infarction. Thromb Haemost *63*, 174–177 (1990).

82   Mori J., Wada H., Nagano Y. et al.: Hypercoagulable state in the Watanabe heritable hyperlipidemic rabbit, an animal model for the progression of atherosclerosis. Effect of probucol on coagulation. Thromb. Haemostas. *61*, 140–143 (1989).

83   Franceschini G., Chiesa G., Sirtori C.R.: Probucol increases cholesteryl ester transfer protein activity in hypercholesterolaemic patients. Eur. J. Clin. Invest. *21*, 384–388 (1991).

84   Parthasarathy S., Young S.G., Witzum J.L. et al.: Probucol inhibits oxidative modification of low density lipoprotein. J. Clin. Invest. *77*, 641–644 (1986).

85   Di Minno G., Davi G., Margaglione M. et al.: Abnormally high thromboxane byosinthesis in homozygous homocystinuria. Evidence for platelet involvement and probucol-sensitive mechanism. J. Clin. Invest. *92*, 1400–1406 (1993).

86   Stampfer M.J., Colditz G.A., Willet W.C., Speizer F.E., Hennekens C.: A prospective study of moderate alcohol consuption and the risk of coronary disease and stroke in women. N Engl J Med *319*, 267–273 (1988).

87   Di Minno G., Ames P.R.J.: Developing relationships. Intracerebral bleeding, cardiovascular protection and haemostaic variables in moderate alcohol consumers. Thromb. Haemorrh. Disorders *5*, 1–4 (1992).

88   Bagasra O., Howeedy A., Kajdacsy-Balla A.: Macrophage function in chronic experimental alcoholism. Modulation of surface receptors and phagocytosis. Immunology *65*, 405–409 (1988).

89   Stuart J., George A.J., Davies A.J. et al.: Haematological stress syndrome in atherosclerosis. J. Clin. Pathol. *34*, 464–467 (1981).

Progress in Drug Research, Vol. 46 (E. Jucker, Ed.)
© 1996 Birkhäuser Verlag, Basel (Switzerland)

Aminoglycosides and polyamines: Targets and effects in the mammalian organism of two important groups of natural aliphatic polycations

N. Seiler[1,2], A. Hardy and J.P. Moulinoux

Groupe de Recherche en Thérapeutique Anticancereuse URA CNRS 1529
DRED 1266, Faculté de Médecine, Université de Rennes,
2 avenue du Professeur Léon Bernard, F-35043 Rennes Cedex (France)

---

1   Author for correspondence.
2   Herrn Prof. Dr. Dres. h.c. H. OELSCHLÄGER, meinem langjährigen Freund und selbstlosen Förderer, zum 75. Geburtstag gewidmet.

Introduction

Among the antibiotics isolated in the course of the last 50 years many have several amino groups and even complete polyamine moieties incorporated into their usually rather complex structures. Some of these polyamine- or aminoglycoside-containing antibiotics have antitumoral properties, mostly based on their ability to intercalate into double-stranded DNA and to produce strand breaks. There is a growing interest in these structures since there is hope of finding new therapeutically useful compounds for the treatment of cancer diseases. In the present review we confine ourselves to the "classical" aminoglycoside antibiotics, because they resemble the polyamines – putrescine, spermidine and spermine (Fig. 1) – most closely. The comparison of all aminoglycoside and polyamine-antibiotics with the polyamines would by far exceed the frame of a short review.

The "classical" aminoglycoside antibiotics – gentamicin, tobramycin, amikacin, netilmicin, kanamycin, streptomycin, neomycin, and the other members of the family – are aminosugars joined in glycosidic linkage to cyclohexane rings with hydroxy-, amino- or guanidino-groups as substituents. In almost all aminoglycoside antibiotics, 2-deoxystreptamine is usually in the central position. Streptomycin has streptamine, an aminocyclitol (Fig. 2). A concise review of their pharmacology, toxicology and therapeutic uses was published by Sande and Mandell (1990). Although the aminoglycoside antibiotics are considerably bulkier than the polyamines, the structural similarity between these two groups of natural polycations is nevertheless so obvious that Umezawa (1983) called the aminoglycosides "antibacterial polyamines".

Both the aminoglycosides and the polyamines have amino groups arranged along flexible aliphatic carbon chains. Under physiological conditions the amino groups are nearly completely protonated (properties and metabolism of the natural polyamines were recently reviewed (Seiler, 1991; 1994)). Their polycationic nature allows the aminoglycosides, as well as the polyamines, to interact electrostatically with a great variety of anionic sites of macromolecules, but of course also with small anions. In general, the affinity to anionic binding sites increases with the number of positive charges of the polycations. In the case of the natural polyamines spermine is usually more potent than spermidine. The binding affinity of putrescine is in most cases too low for physiological function as a modulator of enzymes and receptors unrelated to polyamine metabolism, especially since the cellular concentration of putrescine in tissues of vertebrates (disregarding prostate and other exocrine glands) is of the order of 5–50 nmol/g. Spermidine and spermine are found at much higher concentra-

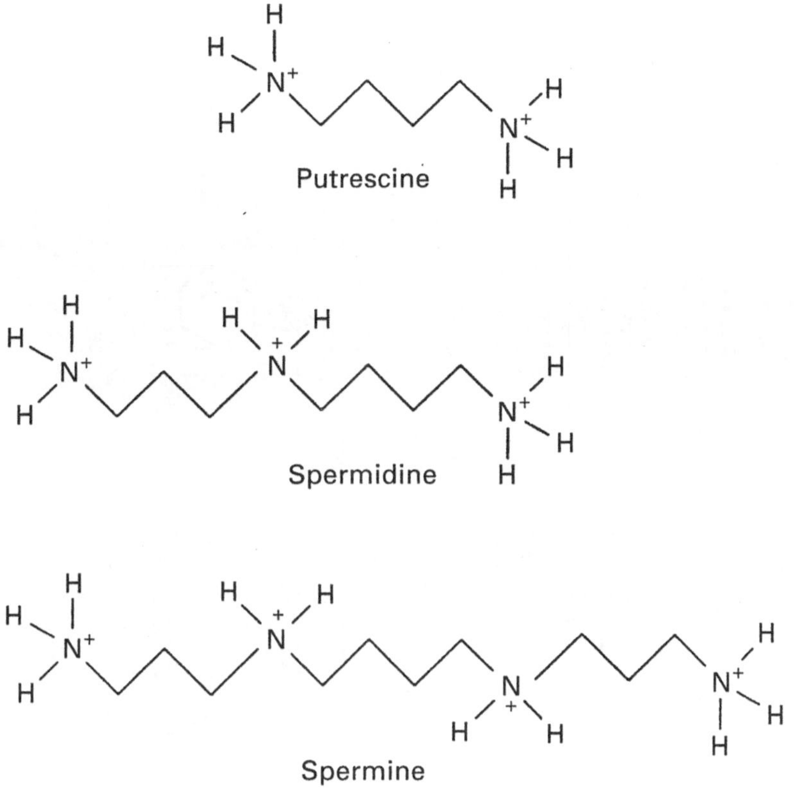

Fig. 1
The structures of putrescine, spermidine and spermine

tions (70–1500 nmol/g) (Seiler, 1992). Since, however interactions may occur at cell surfaces as well as within various intracellular compartments, the knowledge of local free concentrations would be necessary to allow one to estimate the probability of physiologically relevant effects from *in vitro* determined binding affinities. In spite of the limitations in interpreting many of the available data, it seems nevertheless important to evaluate them with an open mind.

In recent years considerable evidence has accumulated in favor of common targets in eukaryotes of aminoglycosides and polyamines. These observations are reviewed in order to show that a coherent picture of the actions of the two groups of natural polycations exists. A better under-

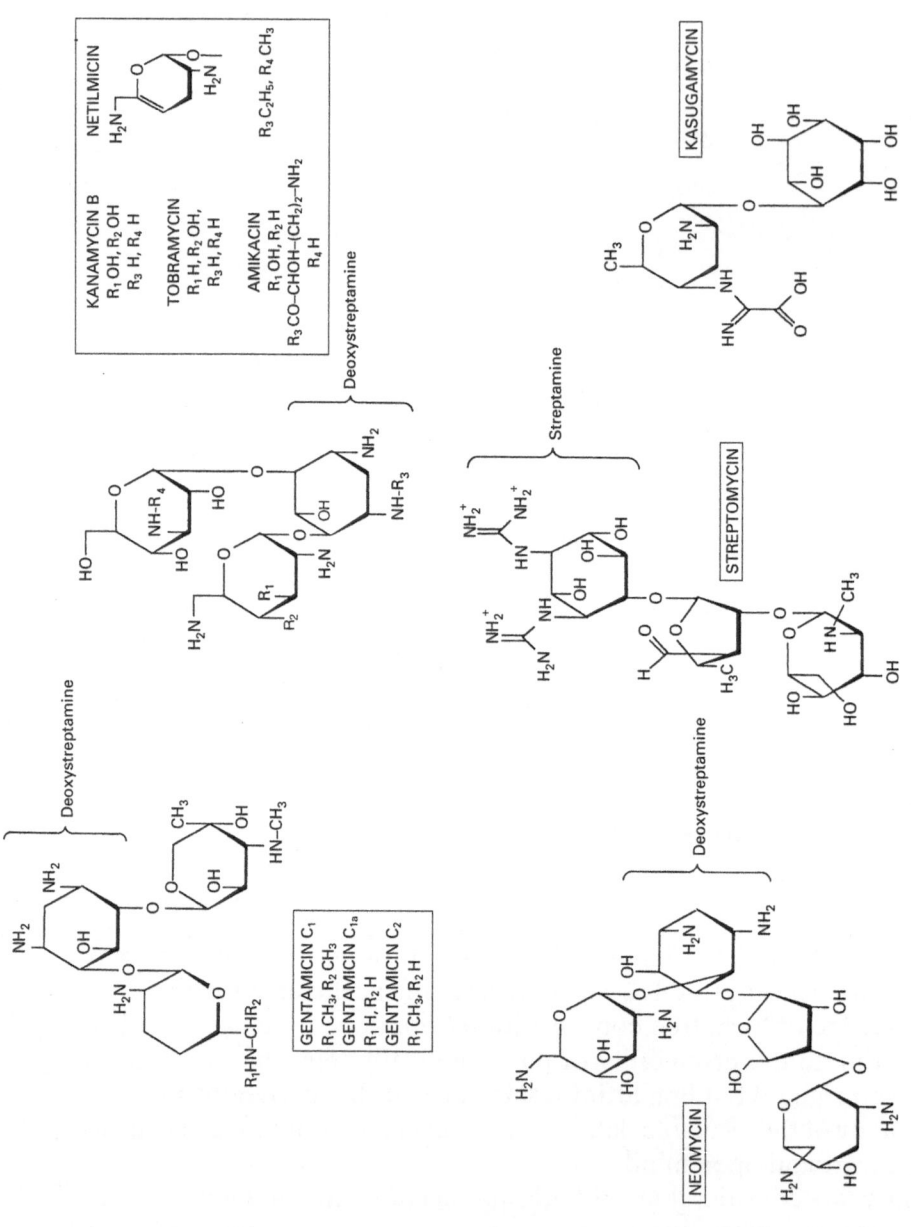

Fig. 2
Structural formulae of the major aminoglycoside antibiotics

standing of the relationships between the two groups of polycations may stimulate the use of aminoglycoside antibiotics as tools in experiments directed towards the elucidation of physiological functions of the polyamines, and it is presumed that the pharmacology and toxicology of the two groups of compounds will be better understood. Perhaps even new applications of the aminoglycosides will be found, based on our understanding of polyamine functions.

2   Bacterial protein synthesis, a function for the polyamines and a target for antimicrobial actions of the aminoglycosides

Gram-negative bacteria are the major targets for the aminoglycoside antibiotics. They enter the periplasmic space of the bacteria by diffusion through the outer membrane (Nakae and Nakae, 1982). Through the cytoplasmic membrane they are transported by an energy requiring process (Bryan and Kwan, 1983; Mates et al., 1983). This inducible transport system is assumed to be shared by putrescine and spermidine (Höltje, 1978), although there is substantial evidence against this notion (Bryan and Kwan, 1983).

As the primary intracellular site of antimicrobial action of aminoglycosides the 30S ribosomal subunit has been identified (Bryan and Kwan, 1983, Davies, 1988). It consists of 21 proteins and a single molecule of 16S RNA. At least three of these proteins, and perhaps also the ribosomal RNA, contribute to aminoglycoside binding, as was shown for streptomycin (Stöffler and Tischendorf, 1975; Cundlieffe, 1989). Streptomycin interferes with the initiation of protein synthesis (Zierhut et al., 1979). This leads to the accumulation of abnormal initiation complexes. Binding of aminoglycosides to the 30S ribosomal subunit has been shown to cause misreading of the mRNA template and consequently the incorrect incorporation of amino acids into the growing peptide chain (Tai et al., 1978; Zierhut et al., 1979; Algranati and Goldemberg, 1989). There is strong correlation between the bactericidal activity of the aminoglycoside antibiotics and their ability to induce misreading (Hummel and Böck, 1989). The polyamines affect protein synthesis virtually at every step, both in bacteria and eukaryotes. The early work has been critically reviewed by Cohen (1973). More recent reviews were published by Loftfield et al. (1981a), Barbiroli et al. (1989) and Algranati and Goldemberg (1977a; 1989). Since no comparable effects of the aminoglycosides on eukaryotic protein synthesis seem to exist, as were described for the bacterial systems, the rather numerous *in vitro* observations on polyamine effects on eukaryotic protein synthesis are not discussed in this review; however, one should bear in mind that the first sign of functional impairment during gradual depletion of intracellular putrescine and spermidine in cells is a change in the polyribosome profile with less ribosomes in polyribosomes, and a decrease in protein synthetic activity (Rudkin et al., 1984; Höltta, 1985).

As far as bacterial ribosomes are concerned, there is multiple evidence for the promotion of association of the 30S and 50S particles by the natural polyamines. The first pertinent observations have been made by Cohen and Lichtenstein (1960). Spermidine binds first to the 30S subunit which renders it fit to associate with the 50S particle. Two different polyamine binding sites were identified on the 30S subunit, but only one gave a complex suited for the formation of the 30S-50S unit (Algranati and Goldemberg, 1989; Garcia-Patrone and Algranati, 1976) The findings that polyamines are essential for the correct assembly of ribosomal subunits have been extended and confirmed by Igarashi et al. (1981a,b; 1982a).

Using natural mRNA as template, cell-free extracts from polyamine deficient mutants of *E. coli* were grown in the presence or absence of putrescine. Supplementation with polyamines showed an increased capacity of this *in vitro* translation system for initiation of polypeptide synthesis (Algranati and Goldemberg, 1977b; 1981; Sander et al., 1978), demonstrating the importance of polyamines in this step of protein synthesis. Loftfield et al. (1981a) and Algranati and Goldemberg (1989) have also reviewed evidence in favor of a role of the polyamines in the fidelity of translation of the message. The effect is mainly due to a decrease of tRNA misacetylation and an improvement of the discrimination during the initial binding of the aminoacyl-tRNA to the ribosomes (Igarashi et al., 1982b; Loftfield et al., 1981; Thompson et al., 1982).

From the work quoted above, and other observations, it is evident that the natural polyamines are essential in those steps of bacterial protein synthesis, which are targets for the antimicrobial actions of the aminoglycosides. Endogenous polyamines of *E. coli* mutants appear to modulate the aminoglycoside action on polypeptide synthesis (Goldemberg and Algranati, 1981). In polyamine-deficient mutants a marked inhibition of protein synthesis was seen only in the polyamine-supplemented cells, while putrescine-deprived cells behaved as cells phenotypically resistant to the antibiotic. A relationship between polyamine function and the effects of the acitivity of the antibiotics on miscoding was postulated, because those aminoglycosides which increase mistranslation (streptomycin, neomycin, kanamycin) required the presence of polyamines for inhibition of protein synthesis, whereas spectinomycin, which has no effect on the fidelity of translation, was inhibitory, irrespective of the presence or absence of putrescine. There are, however, exceptions to this rule. Probably because of multiple sites of interaction on both ribosomal subunits, gentamicin was inhibitory in the presence and in the absence of putrescine, although it enhances miscoding. Another exception is kasugamycin: although not affecting the accuracy of translation, its effect on protein synthesis was polyamine-dependent. This was explained by the undermethylation of the 16S ribosomal RNA of polyamine-deficient bacteria (Igarashi et al., 1979), indicating that the 30S ribosomal subunit formed in polyamine-starved cells is not an appropriate target for aminoglycosides. More recently, Nastri et al. (1993) observed that mistranslation in the presence of streptomycin causes in the polyamine requiring mutants the formation of more basic coat proteins than the normal MS2 coat protein. However, this happened only if putrescine was added to the culture medium. It is not excluded that the formation of these basic coat proteins is of toxicological importance.

A further aspect of the interaction between the antibiotics and bacteria was discussed by Kashiwagi et al. (1992). The sensitivity to aminoglycoside antibiotics increased if the polyamine-induced oligopeptide-binding protein was expressed in *E. coli*. In contrast with polyamines, the aminoglycoside antibiotics were not capable to stimulate the synthesis of this protein. If the gene for the oligopeptide-binding protein was deleted, sensitivity to aminoglycosides was greatly diminished, obviously due to a lack in transport of the antibiotics. Although spermidine is transported by the oligopeptide-binding protein, and the binding site for isepamicin overlaps with that of spermidine, the ordinary spermidine uptake system is not shared by the aminoglycosides.

There are several obvious molecular targets for aminoglycoside antibiotics in bacteria which are not available in mammalian cells. All these targets are interrelated with polyamine functions. However, direct competitions for specific binding sites between polyamines and aminoglycosides seem to be, if existing, the exception, not the rule in the antimicrobial actions of these drugs.

3   Toxic effects of polyamines and aminoglycosides

3.1   Nephrotoxicity

Nephrotoxicity is one of the most important pathogenic effects of the aminoglycosides. In some species it may be gender-related (Goodrich and Hottendorf, 1995). Although in most cases reversible, it limitates the long-term administration of aminoglycoside antibiotics (Sande and Mandell, 1990). Polyamines, which enter the vertebrate organism by a non-natural route, i.e. polyamines which are not formed intracellularly by *de novo* synthesis or are taken up from the gastro-intestinal tract, produce numerous toxic effects (Seiler, 1991). Among these nephrotoxicity was the first to be observed and studied in some detail (Fisher and Rosenthal, 1954; Rosenthal and Tabor, 1956). These works mark the beginning of the systematic exploration of the biochemistry and physiology of the polyamines.

The toxicity of the aminoglycosides is apparently a result of their accumulation and retention in the proximal tubular cells (Pastoriza-Munoz et al., 1979; Aronoff et al., 1983; Lietmann and Smith, 1983). From there they are released gradually in the course of days.

Repeated administration of spermine to rats also causes its accumulation in kidney cortex (Rosenthal and Tabor, 1956), and its gradual release is of about the same rate (Siimes, 1967) as that of aminoglycosides (Luft and Kleit, 1974; Fabre et al., 1976). Transport across the apical and basolateral membrane appears to involve binding of aminoglycosides to the plasma membrane (Hancock, 1981; Takano et al., 1994). Just and Habermann (1977) observed that binding of a cationic peptide, aprotinin, to the brush border of the proximal tubule of the rat kidney was antagonized by several aminoglycoside antibiotics, but also by about the same concentration of spermine, indicating a comparable affinity of spermine and aminoglycosides for the plasma membrane. The observation of Lipsky et al. (1980), who found that spermine inhibited binding and uptake of gentamicin by brush border membrane vesicles, indicates into the same direction, especially since Sastrasinh et al. (1982) identified an "aminoglycoside receptor" of renal brush border membranes. *In vivo* the accumulation of [^{3}H]gentamicin in renal cortex was competitively inhibited by other aminoglycosides and by spermine. The order of potency was:

neomycin = spermine > netilmicin > amikacin > tobramycin,

and paralleled the net positive charges of the molecules, as determined by titration (Josepovitz et al., 1982).

In a recent study on the uptake of gentamicin by a kidney epithelial cell line it was concluded that the aminoglycoside antibiotics bind electrostatically to the apical membrane and are subsequently taken up by endocytosis (Takano et al., 1994). That endocytosis is an important mechanism of aminoglycoside uptake by kidney cortex has long been evidenced (Just et al., 1977; Silverblatt and Kuehn, 1979). Their prolonged administration causes a reduction in the capillary ultrafiltration coefficient (Bayliss et al., 1977) due to interaction with the atrial natriuretic polypeptide receptors (Hori et al., 1989), and related receptors. Morphologically a decrease of the number of endothelial fenestrations was observed (Luft and Evans, 1980).

Binding to anionic sites of phospholipid-constituents of the plasma membrane is the prerequisite for endocytosis and for the formation of multilamellar phospholipid structures, called myeloid bodies. These were found both in animals and man as a consequence of prolonged administration of aminoglycosides (Aubert-Tulkens et al., 1979; Feldman et al., 1982). Myeloid bodies indicate that the pinocytosed drugs are trapped in liposomes and prepared for extrusion into the urine (Aronoff et al., 1983; Silverblatt, 1982).

Binding to anionic sites of membranes is a characteristic feature of spermidine and spermine and the basis of many of their interactions with cells (Schuber, 1989). It may, therefore, not surprise that spermine, the polyamine with the highest positive net charge, and consequently the compound which binds most tightly to anionic binding sites, is not only the most toxic among the polyamines, but that the pathophysiology of its nephrotoxicity resembles strikingly that of the aminoglycosides. In rats exposed to daily injections of 40 mg spermine tetrahydrochloride myeloid bodies are formed in glomerular capillary endothelial cells of the vacuolar type. Free-floating myeloid bodies have been identified in the proximal tubular lumen, in the interstitial space beneath the tubular basement membrane, the lumina of the blood vessels and in the uriniferous space of the Malphigian corpuscle (Campbell et al., 1983).

These observations suggest identical pathogenic mechanisms of aminoglycosides and the polyamines in the kidney, including the primary site of action, namely the binding sites on the plasma membrane. One has to emphasize, however, that these binding sites are not selective, but capable of binding various compounds of cationic nature. A natural substrate for this uptake system seems not to be known. It is of practical importance that the aminoglycoside and polyamine binding sites can bind calcium as well, so that elevated dietary calcium levels compete with aminoglycosides and thus protect against their nephrotoxic effects (Humes et al., 1984).

3.2　　Uptake by mammalian cells and ototoxicity

Several different polyamine uptake systems with differing substrate profiles and kinetic properties have been described for mammalian cells (Seiler and Dezeure, 1990). Some of these transport systems are not highly selective for the natural polyamines but are capable to transport polyamine derivatives (e.g. N^1,N^{12}-diethylspermine (Bergeron et al., 1989)), and even some related structures, such as methylglyoxal-bis(guanylhydra-zone) (MGBG) and paraquat (Byers et al., 1987). In Lewis lung carcinoma cells putrescine uptake is inhibited by neomycin and streptomycin, but aminoglycosides have no effect on the uptake of putrescine by red blood cells (A. Hardy, unpublished observations). In a study on the mechanism of putrescine transport in human pulmonary artery endothelial cells (Sokol et al., 1993) the following rank order of inhibition was determined: MGBG > spermine > spermidine > gentamicin. Similarly putrescine uptake by intestinal epithelial cells (IEC-6) was inhibited by several non-absorbable aminoglycoside antibiotics (Osborne and Seidel, 1989). The fact that putrescine uptake by mammalian cells is competitively inhibited by aminoglycoside antibiotics is a better indicator for the structural similarity of polyamines and aminoglycosides than the nephrotoxic effects of these compounds.

Ototoxicity is the result of progressive destruction of vestibular or cochlear sensory cells (Brummett and Fox, 1982) due to the progressive accumulation of aminoglycoside antibiotics (Desrochers and Schacht, 1982; Huy et al., 1983; Beaubien et al., 1995) or of spermine (Yung and Wright, 1987). An "aminoglycoside receptor" was isolated from inner ear tissues (Schacht, 1979) and active transport systems of the inner ear for aminoglycoside antibiotics were demonstrated (Schacht and Van De Water, 1986). The characteristics of gentamicin uptake by isolated crista ampullaris of the inner ear of guinea pigs were studied with the following results (Williams et al., 1987): Gentamicin was transported against a concentration gradient in an energy-dependent manner. The uptake system had a high affinity site (K_D = 39 nM) and a low affinity site (K_D 16 µM); the latter had, however, a 55-times higher capacity than the high affinity site. Competition for uptake was observed both for other aminoglycosides (netilmicin, neomycin, tobramycin) and the polyamines spermine, spermidine and putrescine.

With increasing dosage and time of exposure, damage progresses from the base of the cochlea, where high-frequency sounds are processed, to the apex, which is necessary for the perception of low frequencies. The degree of permanent dysfunction correlates with the number of destroyed or altered sensory hair cells (Sande and Mandell, 1990). The toxicity of aminoglycoside antibiotics and of spermine on hair cells was recently studied *in vitro* using cochlear cultures prepared from the early postnatal mouse (Kotecha and Richardson, 1994). Damage was assessed by scanning and transmission electron microscopy. The following ranking of toxicity was obtained: poly-L-lysine > neomycin > gentamicin > dihydrostreptomycin > spermine > amikacin > neamine > spectinomycin. All toxic polycations formed within the apical surface lesion whorls of tightly packed membrane, resembling myelin. Spermine caused in addition a dramatic increase in cytoplasm of material with a high electron density, and condensation of nuclear chromatin, while poly-L-lysine induced necrosis of the cells.

Developing animals are more sensitive to aminoglycoside ototoxicity than adults (Henley and Rybak, 1995). Maximum sensitivity coincides with the anatomical and functional maturation of the cochlea (Pujol, 1986). Early changes induced by aminoglycosides are reversible, however, once sensory cells are lost, retrograde degeneration of the auditory nerve follows, resulting in irreversible hearing loss (Lietman, 1990).

The pathogenetic mechanisms involved in aminoglycoside ototoxicity are not well understood, although several hypotheses have been suggested (Sande. and Mandell, 1990; Schacht, 1986). A first hint to the potential involvement of the polyamines came from clinical observations: In patients receiving large doses of 2-(difluoromethyl)ornithine (DFMO), a selective inactivator of ornithine decarboxylase (ODC), reversible hearing loss was observed as a side effect of the treatment (Schechter et al., 1987). The critical period of DFMO-induced ototoxicity in developing rats was found to be identical with the critical period of aminoglycoside toxicity (Henley et al., 1990, Henley and Rybak, 1995), and it turned out that aminoglycoside antibiotics are inhibitors of ODC, both from kidney and cochlea (Henley et al., 1987, 1988; Lyos et al., 1992). The kinetic analysis showed that inhibition was uncompetitive, in contrast with putrescine, which is a competitive inhibitor of ODC with a $K_i = 1.7 \pm 1.4$ mM. K_i values of the aminoglycosides ranged from 1.3 ± 0.1 mM (neomycin) to 1.9 ± 0.2 mM (kanamycin) for the renal enzyme and from $K_i = 50$ µM (neomycin) to $K_i = 99$ µM (kanamycin) for the cochlear ODC.

Evidently the aminoglycosides do not compete with putrescine for the active site of the enzyme. Whether they compete with pyridoxal 5-phosphate has not been entirely clarified, but seems unlikely, because of the opposite charges of aminoglycosides and pyridoxal 5-phosphate, and the low inclination of these compounds to interact hydrophobically. In kidney two forms of ODC were found, one with a low, the other with a high affinity for pyridoxal 5-phosphate. Neomycin inhibited both forms with similar inhibitor constants ($K_i = 1.5 \pm 0.3$ and 1.8 ± 0.4 mM). Since the affinity of the aminoglycosides for ODC is low, considerable accumulation of the drugs is a prerequisite, however, as was discussed above, accumulation of the aminoglycosides in the cochlea occurs if plasma values are high.

It is well documented that polyamines are involved in a great variety of fundamental processes of cell biology, including growth and differentiation (Bachrach and Heimer, 1988), and it was mentioned before that impairment of protein synthesis is an early event following depletion of intracellular spermidine due to inhibition of ODC (Rudkin et al., 1984; Hölttä, 1985). It is, therefore, conceivable that impairment of the synthesis of specific proteins is an important step in the ototoxic effect of aminoglycosides, especially in developing animals. However, inhibition of ODC may only be one of many effects of the aminoglycosides.

4   Aminoglycosides, polyamines and inositol phosphates

Ever since Hokin and Hokin (1953) demonstrated that the stimulation of pancreas by acetylcholine enhances the incorporation of ^{32}P from $(\gamma^{32}P)ATP$ into phospholipids, it became more and more apparent that polyphosphoinositides play a paramount role in transmembrane signal transduction of many neurotransmitters and hormones. It was later shown that inositol-1,4,5 triphosphate and 1,2-diacylglycerol are two interacting second messengers which are formed by hydrolysis from inositol 4,5-diphosphate. They are intimately involved in the control of intracellular Ca^{2+} levels and through the control of Ca^{2+} in the regulation of secretory processes, and of cell proliferation via the control of DNA synthesis (Berridge, 1987a). The events leading to cell proliferation may be summarized briefly as follows (Berridge, 1987b): Mitogens stimulate the hydrolysis of phosphatidylinositol 4,5-diphosphate to form inositol 1,4,5-triphosphate and 1,2-diacylglycerol, initiating a bifurcating signal pathway. The water-soluble inositol 1,4,5-triphosphate diffuses into the cytosol to mobilize Ca^{2+}. This explains the increase of intracellular Ca^{2+} which occurs when cells are stimulated to grow. Diacylglycerol remains within the plane of the membrane and stimulates protein kinase C, which then activates a number of cellular processes, particularly the increase in intracellular pH. Another function of this signal pathway, which might be linked to the changes in intracellular Ca^{2+} and pH, is to initiate the transcription of specific genes such as myc and fos which pave the way for the subsequent DNA synthesis. In Fig. 3 the major metabolic pathways and the presumed functions of diacylglycerol and the inositol phosphates are illustrated.

Since the polyamines are constituents of all cells, the events summarized in Fig. 3 take place in their presence, although this fact is usually not mentioned in pertinent reviews of the signal transduction pathways. In numerous reports the possibility has been suggested that the natural polyamines affect several processes involved in voltage-dependent and receptor-mediated signal transduction pathways, Ca^{2+} mobilization, and phosphatidylinositol metabolism. A compilation of pertinent observations has been published (Seiler, 1991). Aminoglycoside antibiotics are known to influence the inositolphosphate signal transduction pathway at different levels. These observations are discussed in the following.

4.1   Binding to phosphatidylinositols

Ca^{2+} is considered a natural counterion of polyphosphoinositids in biological systems (Hendricksson and Reinertsen, 1971). Cytoplasmic free Ca^{2+} concentrations are only 100–200 nM (Rasmussen and Barrett, 1984). The concentration of free cytoplasmic polyamines of mammalian cells is not precisely known, but there is evidence that they are of the order of 40–60 μM (spermidine) and 3–4 μM (spermine) (Brosnan and Hu, 1985). Since these values are well above those of Ca^{2+}, it is conceivable that the polyamines effectively compete with Ca^{2+} to form salts (or ion pairs) with phosphatidylinositols. In any case, if phospholipid bilayers are exposed to polyamines (Tadolini and Varani, 1986; Yung and Green, 1986) or aminoglycoside antibiotics (Schacht, 1976; Gabev et al., 1989) they show strong binding. The strongest ionic interactions occurs with the phosphoinositide with the highest number of negative charges, i.e. with phosphatidylinositol 4,5-diphosphate. High-affinity binding of spermine to polyphosphoinositides was observed even in the presence of physiological concentrations of Mg^{2+} (Toner et al., 1988). No evidence was found for a significant contribution to the binding energy of hydrophobic interactions. The strong binding to phosphatidylinositol 4,5-diphosphate is presumably a key event in the pathogenetic mechanisms of aminoglycosides. Since binding of the polycations to phosphatidylinositol 4,5-diphosphate changes the surface charge, the reduction of their electrophoretic mobility after exposure to aminoglycosides (Langford et al., 1982), respectively the aminoglycoside actions on monomolecular films of polyphosphoinositides (Lodhi et al., 1980) were considered as *in vitro* models suitable for the evaluation of the toxicity of these antibiotics.

4.1.1   Functional consequences of interactions of the polyacations with phosphatidylinositol 4,5-diphosphate

It has been mentioned above that formation of inositol 1,4,5-triphosphate and diacylglycerol from polyphosphoinositides is catalyzed by phospholipase C. The activity of this enzyme is dependent on a number of factors, among which the Ca^{2+} concentration seems most important. In several early reports the inhibition of phospholipase C by neomycin due to bind-

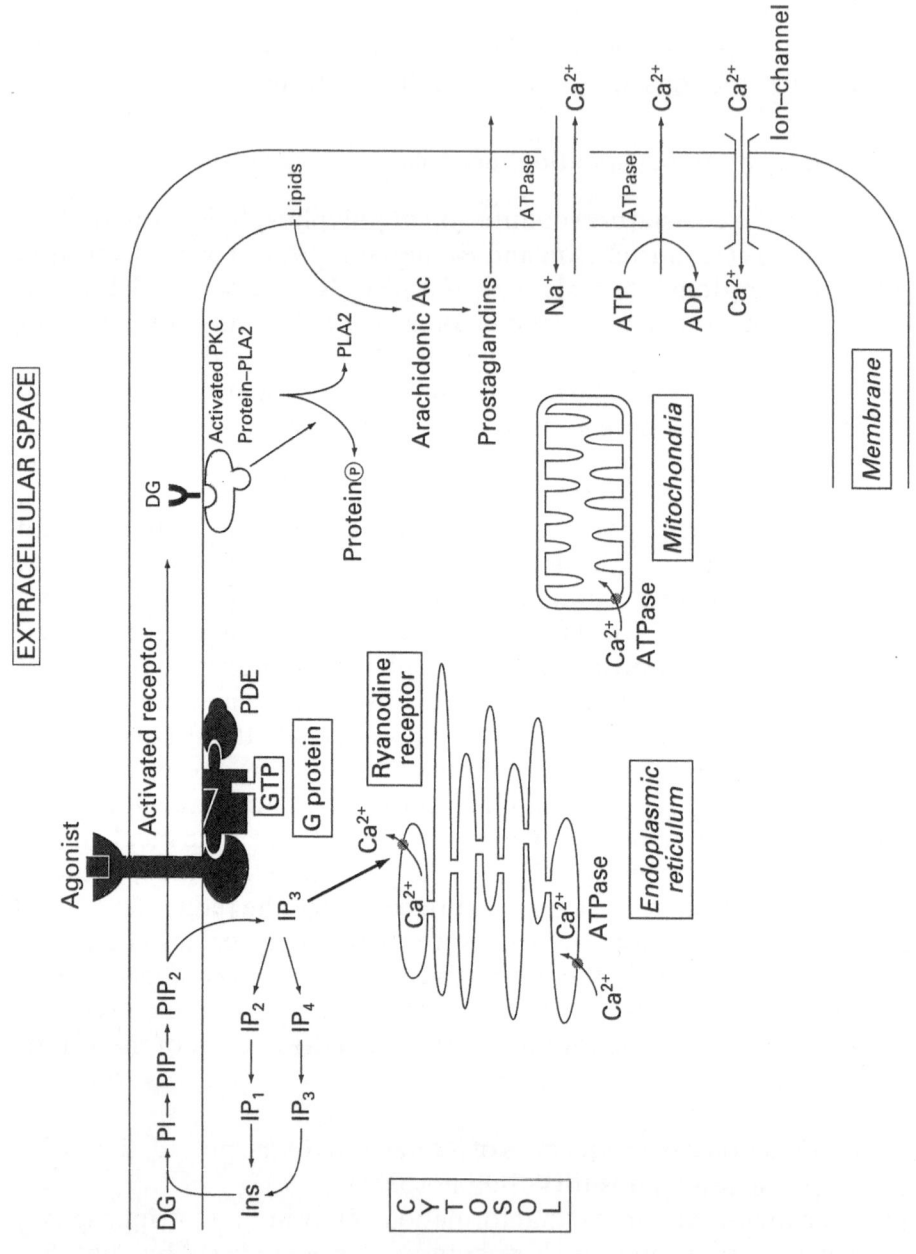

Fig. 3

ing of the aminoglycoside to inositol phospholipids, the substrates of phospholipase C, was postulated (Schacht, 1976; Lohdi et al., 1979; Van Rooijen and Agranoff, 1985). Subsequently evidence was presented by many workers that aminoglycosides inhibit functional consequences of phospholipase C catalyzed reactions, and neomycin became a standard tool as "inhibitor of phospholipase C". Most frequently the impairment of neurotransmitter- or hormone-stimulated formation of inositol 1,4,5-triphosphate by neomycin was demonstrated. Examples are the vasopressin- (Kondo et al., 1989) and the endothelin-stimulated (Little et al., 1992) generation of inositol 1,4,5-triphosphate and the subsequent influx of extracellular Ca^{2+} in aortic smooth muscle cells. The prevention of thrombin-induced inositol phosphate formation in human platelets by neomycin (Siess and Lapetina, 1986) is presumably not a direct consequence of the action of neomycin on phospholipid metabolism, but apparently the result of the inhibition of thrombin binding to its receptor by the polycations (Tysnes et al., 1991). Neomycin reduces the release of arachidonic acid from rat brain cortical membranes (Strosznajder and Samochocki, 1991) and from permeabilized myometrial cells (Khouja and Jones, 1993). (For the pathway of this reaction see Fig. 3.) However, not only metabolic, but also functional consequences of the stimulation of the inositol phsophate pathway are blocked by neomycin. For example, the proliferative stimulus in calvarial bone cells to mechanical strain is prevented by neomycin, i.e. neomycin not only blocked the accumulation of inositol 1,4,5-triphosphate but also the increase in DNA synthesis (Brighton et al., 1992). The

---

Fig. 3

The role of inositol lipid hydrolysis in transmembrane signal transduction

Agonists acting on specific receptors use G protein to stimulate phosphodiesterase, which cleaves phosphatidylinositol 1,4-diphosphate to diacylglycerol and inositol 1,3,5-triphosphate. The latter acts to release Ca^{2+} from the endoplasmic reticulum. Diacylglycerol stimulates protein kinase C. Protein kinase C has several functions: activation of Na^+-H^+ exchange, phosphorylation of lipocortin (protein-PLA_2), resulting in the activation of phospholipase A_2 (cleaving off the arachidonic acid for prostaglandin formation), initiation of the translation of specific genes (e.g. myc and fos), and others.

Abbreviations: DG diacylglycerol; PI phosphatidylinositol; PIP phosphatidylinositol 4-phosphate; PIP_2 phosphatidylinositol 4,5-diphosphate; IP_1 Inositol 4-phosphate; IP_2 inositol 1,4-diphosphate; IP_3 inositol 1,4,5-triphosphate; IP_4 inositol 1,3,4,5-tetraphosphate; PLA_2 phospholipase A_2; GTP guanosine triphosphate; G protein guanosine triphosphate binding protein; PDE phosphodiesterase; PKC protein kinase C; ATPase adenosine triphosphatase; ATP adenosine triphosphate; ADP adenosine diphosphate.

dose-dependent (1–5 mM) inhibition of hormone-stimulated smooth muscle contraction by neomycin (Phillippe, 1994) demonstrates the ability of aminoglycosides to interrupt functions of the phosphatidylinositol signaling pathway not only at the cellular level. Using two near-physiological smooth muscle preparations in which receptor coupling was retained, it was shown that α-adrenergic (phenylephrine) and muscarinic (carbamoyl cholin) agonists, as well as caffeine and inositol 1,4,5-triphosphate caused contractions mediated by Ca^{2+} release. Neomycin blocked only the Ca^{2+} release induced by carbamoyl choline, but not by caffeine (an agonist of the ryanodyne receptor). It was, therefore, concluded that inositol 1,4,5-triphosphate is the major physiological messenger of the Ca^{2+} release component of pharmacomechanical coupling, but not of the components which are mediated by Ca^{2+} influx (Kobayashi et al., 1989). In a recent paper the improvement by neomycin (15 mg/kg i.v.) of the metabolic and neurologic outcome following traumatic brain injury in rats was reported (Golding and Vink, 1994). This observation suggests the possibility that aminoglycoside antibiotics interfere in signal transduction pathways *in vivo*.

Spermine and spermidine are known to inhibit a phospholipase C-dependent hydrolysis of phosphoinositides in rat brain (Eichberg et al., 1981), and in blood platelets (Nahas and Graff, 1982). Inhibition is usually non-competitive with respect to Ca^{2+} and competitive with phosphatidylinositol. Cooper and Holz (1993) found that in chromaffin cells spermine concentrations > 1 mM selectively inhibit the formation of inositol 4,5-diphosphate without, however, affecting the Ca^{2+}-stimulated formation of inositol 1,4,5-triphosphate. In contrast, neomycin at a concentration > 0.1 mM was found to inhibit both Ca^{2+}-stimulated formation of inositol 4,5-diphosphate and inositol 1,4,5-triphosphate. These results appear to disagree with a report by Vergera et al. (1985) who observed that spermine was able to induce the blockage of the Ca^{2+}-signals in electrically stimulated muscle fibers. He explained his findings by assuming that spermine interfered with the formation of inositol 1,4,5-triphosphate. Das et al. (1987) reported the inhibitory action of 10 µM spermidine on formyl-methionine-leucyl-phenylalanine-stimulated production of inositol phosphate in human neutrophils, a known model of phosphatidylinositol 4,5-diphosphate hydrolysis (Cockcroft et al., 1985). Although aware of the antagonistic action of spermidine on phospholipase C, these authors assume, based on the low concentration of spermidine necessary to produce the maximal effect, that the site of action of spermidine is at the cell surface. Cell surface binding sites of the polyamines have indeed been described (Quemener et al., 1992, Hashimoto and London, 1994), but their physiological role has not yet been established, if we disregard the N-methyl-D-aspartate (NMDA) and some other well-characterized receptors which are known to bind polyamines (Schoemaker et al., 1994).

Presumably the most convincing example for a role of the polyamines at various sites of the signal transduction pathway is that described by Sjöholm (1992) and Sjöholm et al. (1993). These authors studied the role of polyamines in insulin production, metabolism and secretion in a model of pancreatic β-cells. For this purpose RINm5F insulinoma cells were partially depleted of putrescine and spermidine by inhibition of ODC with DFMO. This led to an increase of cellular insulin and ATP. K^+-induced depolarization revealed the enhanced secretion of insulin and an increase of intracellular free Ca^{2+}. Since these events were paralleled by increased voltage-activated Ca^{2+} currents, an enhanced Ca^{2+}-channel activity is likely to be a consequence of putrescine and spermidine depletion. In this regard it is important to remember that the polyamines are capable of modulating voltage and ligand-activated Ca^{2+}-channel-mediated currents, presumably due to interaction with a Ca^{2+}-binding site of the channel (Scott et al., 1992; 1994). Polyamine depletion also rendered phospholipase C more sensitive to a muscarinic agonist, as was evidenced by the enhanced generation of inositol phosphates.

Unfortunately the relationships between phospholipase C activity and polycations are complex, because their effect may not only be exerted via binding to inositol phosphates but also by direct interaction with the enzyme. Haber et al. (1991) studied the kinetic properties of phospholipase C delta from rat liver, and found that the enzyme was activated by neomycin, optimally at 10 µM of the antibiotic. Half maximum activation by spermine was observed at 150 µM, maximum activation at 200–500 µM, but activation with spermine was greater than with neomycin. Concentrations of spermine > 500 µM were inhibitory. For activation by spermidine six times higher concentrations were required than of spermine, and putrescine was effective only at 6 mM. Inhibition at low, and activation at high concentrations of spermine were also observed for a phosphatidylinositol-specific phospholipase C, which is dependent on an effective concentration of substrate and Ca^{2+} (Sagawa et al., 1983). The subtle modulation of this enzyme, depending on the polyamine/Ca^{2+}-ratio was, therefore, postulated. Three multiple forms of phosphatidylinositol-specific phospholipase C from bovine aorta were able to hydrolyze phosphatidylinositol as well as phosphatidylinositol 4-phosphate and phosphatidylinositol 4,5-diphosphate. Spermine and spermidine stimulated form I and II, but neomycin inhibited all three subtypes (Spath et al., 1991).

From these and related observations it is obvious that it is not possible to identify precisely the mechanisms by which the natural polycations exert their effects on phospholipase C activity under physiological conditions. Among other reasons this is due to the fact that the multiple forms of this enzyme show vastly varying sensitivity to polycations and the effects on enzyme activity can be opposite, depending on the potency of the drug and its concentrations. But there is little doubt that phospholipase C is an important target for the natural polycations.

Experiments with permeabilized cells have revealed that very different concentrations of neomycin are required to affect inositol phospholipid turnover. In platelets only 10 μM was required (Rock and Jackowski, 1987) whereas in mast cells 1 mM was necessary to inhibit the antagonist-induced breakdown of phosphatidylinositol 4,5-diphosphate (Cockcroft et al., 1987). In addition to the above-mentioned difficulties in interpreting mechanistically the observations made with polycations on inositol phosphate formation and metabolism, a further difficulty arises from the fact that the polycations are not only interacting with acidic phospholipids and enzymes, but are also capable of direct interaction with inositol phosphates and ATP (Prentki et al., 1986). By these interactions they reduce the "free" pool of these metabolites. The specificity and the mechanism of the inhibitory effect of neomycin on phosphatidylinositol metabolism has, therefore, been a matter of debate (Gabev et al., 1989).

4.1.2 Phosphatidylinositol turnover and exocytosis

The maintenance of the pools of phosphatidylinositol 4-phosphate and phosphatidylinositol 4,5-diphosphate in the plasma membrane is necessary in order to secure the formation of inositol 1,4,5-triphosphate and thus the functioning of transmembrane signalling and Ca^{2+} mobilization. The phosphorylation of phoshatidylinositol and of phosphatidylinositol 4-phosphate is catalyzed by kinases bound to the inner surface of the plasma membrane. These kinases are activated by polycations, including spermidine and spermine, as is documented by several publications (Vogel and Hoppe, 1986; Lundberg et al., 1986; Kurosawa et al., 1990; Yang and Boss, 1994). The extent of activation depends on the concentration of Mg^{2+} (Lundberg et al., 1986; Cochet and Chambaz, 1986). The presence of 2 mM spermine decreased the EC_{50} for Mg^{2+} from 5 mM to 0.5 mM, indicating that Mg^{2+} and the polyamines activate inositol phospholipid kinases most probably by the same mechanism. In contrast with phosphorylation, the hydrolysis of inositol phosphates seems preferentially inhibited by the polycations. This is at least the case for a phosphatidylinositol 4-phosphate specific phosphomonoesterase (Smith and Wells, 1984). One role of the polyamines is obviously to ensure optimum reaction conditions in the presence of physiological concentrations of Mg^{2+} for the maintenance of inositolphosphate pools (Smith and Snyderman, 1988).

In digitonin-permeabilized rat anterior pituitary tumor cells [^{3}H]polyphosphoinositide breakdown and [^{3}H]inositol phosphate production are stimulated by guanosin 5'-(γ-thio)triphosphate (GTPγS), a GTP analog resistant to hydrolysis, and by Ca^{2+}. Spermine (IC_{50} 0.25 mM) and spermidine (IC_{50} 2 mM) antagonized the stimulatory effects of 10 µM GTPγS on [^{3}H]inositolphosphate formation. At a higher concentration (2.5 mM) spermine reversed the GTPγS-induced decrease in [^{3}H]polyphosphoinositide levels. The corresponding effects of the polyamines on Ca^{2+}-stimulated inositol phosphate metabolism were considerably weaker (Wojcikiewicz and Fain, 1988). Comparable results were obtained for spermine with SH-SY5Y human neuroblastoma cells electrically permeabilized (Wojcikiewicz et al., 1990). In contrast, spermidine and spermine enhanced the GTPγS-stimulated phosphoinositide turnover (EC_{50} 100 µM and 50 µM) if rat brain membranes prelabelled with [^{3}H]inositol were used (Periyasami et al., 1994). Neomycin inhibited the GTPγS- and Ca^{2+}-stimulated hydrolysis of phosphatidylinositol (Wojcikiewicz and Nahorsky, 1989). Furthermore GTPγS-stimulated inositol 1,4,5-triphopshate-formation was observed by a membrane fraction from heart ventricles prelabelled with [^{3}H]inositol. Again, neomycin proved to be an inhibitor of GTPγS stimulated breakdown of polyphosphoinositides (Renard and Poggioli, 1990). From the fact that in these experiments the formation of inositol 1,4,5-triphosphate was stimulated by the GTP analog one has to conclude that the phosphatidylinositol specific phospholipase isoenzyme C involved in the reaction is regulated in the different cells by guanine nucleotide binding proteins (G proteins) (Fig. 3). Further evidence to this notion is that the GTPγS-stimulated reactions were antagonized by other nucleotides. Evidence will be presented further below in favor of the enhanced binding of ligands to their respective G protein-coupled receptors due to interaction with polyamines and aminoglycosides.

In agreement with these observations is the early work of Schacht (1976) and Schibeci and Schacht (1977), who observed a decrease in the turnover of polyphosphoinositides *in vivo* by treatment with neomycin. The decreased incorporation of ^{32}P from ($γ^{32}$ATP) due to chronic administration of neomycin was exclusive for the formation of phosphatidylinositol 4,5-diphosphate. Incorporation of radioactive phosphate into other lipids remained unaffected by exposure to the antibiotic. Impairment of polyphosphoinositide labelling in inner ear tissue by aminoglycosides has also been reported (Orsulakova et al., 1975).

By inhibiting phosphatidylinositol breakdown and activating phosphorylation, the polyamines promote the accumulation of polyphosphoinositides in biological systems. Eberhard et al. (1990) suggested that the poly-phosphoinositides are not only needed for the regulation of inositolphosphate metabolism, but also for exocytosis. This assumption was based on the fact that the secretory response of chromaffin cells was found to correlate with the endogenous polyphosphoinositide levels. It turned out (Cooper and Holz, 1993) that spermine and neomycin had nearly identical effects on both secretion of catecholamines and on phosphoinositide levels. Both polycations were able to maintain secretion in the absence of ATP, but had no effect in the presence of ATP. Furthermore, spermine and neomycin inhibited Ca^{2+}-stimulated catecholamine secretion. One may conclude from these results that the maintenance of the polyphosphoinositide level is indeed important for secretion, especially since, as was mentioned above, the effect of spermine and neomycin on Ca^{2+}-stimulated formation of inositol 1,4,5-triphosphate differed in the chromaffin cells: spermine was ineffective whereas neomycin was inhibitory (Cooper and Holz, 1993).

4.2   Membrane permeability

The involvement of polyphosphoinositides in changes of membrane permeability has long been suspected. The following two test systems were used to study effects of aminoglycoside antibiotics on membrane permeability (Van Bambeke et al., 1993): release of Mn^{2+} from large unilamellar vesicles, and influx of Ca^{2+} into cultured macrophages. Streptomycin and isepamicin markedly increased membrane permeability, whereas gentamicin and others had no effect. Compounds which caused membrane fusion were also ineffective. In computer-aided conformational analysis of mixed monolayers between phosphatidylinositol and the aminoglycosides it was found that those compounds which induce an increase in membrane permeability adopted an orientation perpendicular to the interface, whereas those with no or moderate effect were placed in parallel orientiation on the interface. It was concluded that the perpendicular orientiation might cause a local condition of disorder.

In the light of the above results it is surprising that neomycin was able to antagonize the mastoparan-induced release of lactate dehydrogenase, and the accumulation of ethidium bromide in MDCK cells (Eng and Lo, 1993). Mastoparan is a polycationic tetradecapeptide from wasp venom, which impairs the integrity of the plasma membrane. The authors of this work assume that neomycin competes with mastoparan for binding to polyphos-phoinositides.

Although polyamines bind to a variety of membrane constitutents and affect numerous membrane bound enzymes, an effect analogous to that found on membrane permeability with streptomycin and isepamicin is not known. On the contrary, polyamines stabilize bacterial, mitochondrial and erythrocyte membranes (for review see Schuber, 1989). The fact that the natural polyamines are stabilizing, not destabilizing cell membranes is in support of the above considerations, that cell membranes are destabilized only by aminoglycosides with specific structural features. The fact that the polyamines efficiently induce membrane fusion (Schuber, 1989), together with the above-mentioned observation, that compounds capable to induce membrane fusion did not affect membrane permeability in two models, is also in favor of the absence of impairments of membrane permeability by the polyamines.

4.3 Inhibition of membrane-associated ATPases

Membrane-associated ATPases are key regulatory units of intracellular concentrations of K^+, Na^+, Ca^{2+} and Mg^{2+}. It has been known since more than 20 years that spermine, and to a lesser extent spermidine, affect the activity of different ATPases in a concentration-dependent manner (De Meis and Paula, 1967; Nagai et al., 1969; Peter et al., 1973; Heinrich-Hirsch et al., 1977; Rilo and Stoppani, 1993). It was also clear from the early work that the effect was indirect.

Membrane-associated ATPases are dependent of their lipid environment. Purified plasma-membrane Ca^{2+}-transporting (Ca^{2+}/Mg^{2+}) ATPase was inactive in the absence of lipids, but could be reactivated by adding phos-pholipids. The stimulatory effect increased when phosphatidylinositol 4-phosphate, and especially phosphatidylinositol 4,5-diphosphate partially replaced phosphatidylcholine and phosphatidylinositol in the lipid bilayer. Spermine in 1–10 mM concentrations decreased the activity of the plasma membrane (Ca^{2+}/Mg^{2+}) ATPase, without affecting the stimulation of the enzyme by phosphatidylinositol 4-phosphate. Neomycin exerted similar effects as spermine at ten times lower concentrations (Missiaen et al., 1989). These results are in agreement with the notion that the inhibitory effect of the polycations on phosphatidylinositol phosphate-stimulated ATPases is due to changes of the lipid environment of the enzymes brought about by electrostatic interactions of the polycations with the polyphosphoinositides. It is of interest to note that the ATPase associated with pig liver ribosomes is insensitive to neomycin, whereas the corresponding yeast enzyme is sensitive. The lacking inhibition by neomycin on translation by pig liver ribosomes appears directly correlated with the absence of an effect of neomycin on the ribosomal ATPase (Kovalchuke and Chakraburtty, 1994). It has been proposed that the aminoglycosides may exert in part their nephrotoxic effect by inhibiting reactions of plasmalemma-bound $[Na^+,K^+]$ ATPase (Quarfoth et al., 1978; Williams et al., 1984). In agreement with this suggestion the activities of the Mg^{2+}-dependent and the Mg^{2+}-dependent, HCO_3^--stimulated ATPase of the kidney cortex decrease after repeated administration of neomycin (Suzuki et al., 1994). Daily 10 mg/kg of the aminoglycoside injected subcutaneously for 7 days produced a significant decrease of the enzyme in rat kidney cortex, but even 80 mg/kg per day of neomycin did not produce an analogous loss of ATPase activity in mice, indicating a considerable species difference in the sensitivity to aminoglycosides.

4.4   Agonist-binding of G-protein-coupled receptors

Mg^{2+} and other divalent cations induce a conversion of many G protein-coupled receptors from a low-affinity to a high affinity agonist binding state. Mg^{2+} also increases the binding affinity of G proteins for GTP, and it is required for GTPase activity.

The inflammatory response of neutrophils, macrophages and differentiated human leukemia (HL 60) cells to chemotactic factors, such as the tripeptide N-formylmethionine-leucyl-phenylalanine (fMet-Leu-Phe) requires the activation of phosphatidylinositol specific phospholipase C. Using HL 60 cells Herrmann et al. (1989) demonstrated that binding of fMet-Leu-Phe to its receptor site was enhanced by mM concentrations of neomycin, gentamicin and streptomycin. The aminoglycosides were as potent in this regard as Mg^{2+}, but neomycin had no effect on GTP binding and GTPase activity. Analogous effects were observed for isoproterenol-binding to G protein-coupled β-adrenoreceptors of guinea pig lung membranes (Herrmann et al., 1987). More recently Walters et al. (1992) reported that spermidine and putrescine in concentrations ranging from 50 μM to 1 mM significantly enhanced fMet-Leu-Phe-induced Ca^{2+}-mobilization in HL 60 cells, an effect which was associated with the inhibition of Ca^{2+}-efflux and the prolongation of the association of protein kinase C translocation. Conversion of adenosin A_1 receptors into a high affinity state by spermine ($EC_{50} = 100$ μM) (Wasserkort et al., 1991), the inhibition of $[^{125}I]$FSH binding to membranes from bovine testes by endogenous polyamines, and inhibition of $[^{125}I]$omega conotoxin GVIA binding to neuronal membranes are further examples for the ability of the polyamines and aminoglycosides to mimick Mg^{2+} effects on the binding of effectors to their respective binding sites of G-protein coupled receptors.

Since cationic amphiphilic peptides, such as mastoparan, substance P and bradykinin have been shown to interact directly with G-proteins (Aridor et al., 1990; Higashijima et al., 1990; Bueb et al., 1990) it was speculated that polyamines may interact directly with G-proteins as well. It was shown that the release of histamine from mast cells by polyamines correlated directly with their ability to inhibit purified GTPase of G-proteins, which was reconstituted in phospholipid vesicles, and to produce inositol phosphates in mast cells. The electrostatic character of the interaction of the polyamines with GTPase is evident from the order of potency: spermine > spermidine > putrescine = cadaverine > tyramine (Bueb et al., 1991; 1992). Surprisingly neomycin does not seem to affect GTPase activity (Herrmann et al., 1989), as was already mentioned.

4.5   Metabolism of inositol phosphates and interaction with the sarcoplasmic Ca^{2+}-release channels.

Ca^{2+} is the ubiquitous intracellular messenger (Rasmussen and Barrett, 1984) involved in the control of numerous functions, including secretion and cell proliferation. Its careful control is, therefore, of vital importance for the cells. The sarcoplasmic reticulum is the major structure for the sequestration of intracellular Ca^{2+}. Uptake by a Ca^{2+} ATPase, and release via specific ion channels are the major regulatory units for the control of intracellular Ca^{2+} levels. Ca^{2+} movements are mediated by the so-called ryanodyne and inositol-1,4,5-triphosphate receptors. Ryanodyne receptors are tetramers; the C-terminal regions of each subunit probably form the Ca^{2+} channel (Berridge, 1993).

While phospholipase C isoenzymes control the formation of inositol 1,4,5-triphosphate from phosphatidylinositol 4,5-diphosphate, inositol 1,4,5-triphosphate 5-phosphatase metabolizes the second messenger into the inactive inositol 1,4-diphosphate and thus terminates its action on sarcoplasmic Ca^{2+}-mobilization. Thus this plasma membrane-associated enzyme controls a key catabolic reaction of the transmembrane signal transduction pathway. Seyfred et al. (1984) found that inositol 1,4,5-triphosphate 5-phosphatase was blocked by concentrations of spermine corresponding to its intracellular concentration. This blockade should affect the turnover rate of inositol 1,4,5-triphosphate.

Inositol 1,4,5-triphosphate binds to the ryanodine receptors (see Fig. 3) which are part of the Ca^{2+}-release channels of the endoplasmic reticulum as has been mentioned above. Several lines of evidence suggest that Mg^{2+} and the polycations are modulators of the ryanodine receptors. Inositol 1,4,5-triphosphate-induced release of Ca^{2+} from rat cerebellar microsomes can be inhibited by spermine with an $IC_{50} = 1$ mM. Neomycin was even more efficacious ($IC_{50} = 0.4$ mM), whereas spermidine and putrescine were less potent antagonists of inositol 1,4,5-triphosphate (Sayers and Michelangeli, 1993). These observations may suggest the allosteric modulation of effector binding. Since Mg^{2+} is an efficient inhibitor of sarcoplasmic Ca^{2+} release, it is likely that the polycations compete with Mg^{2+} for its binding site.

The effects of polyamines and neomycin on the binding of [^{3}H]ryanodyne to the Ca^{2+}-release channel receptors have been characterized in sarcoplasmic reticulum of heart an skeletal muscle by several groups (Zimanyi and Pessah, 1991; Mack et al., 1992; Zarka and Shoshan-Barmatz, 1992). The polyamines and neomycin enhance binding of [^{3}H]ryanodine to the sarcoplasmic Ca^{2+}-release channel receptor, both by increasing the apparent affinity for the receptor, and by decreasing the rate of dissociation from the binding site. For half-maximal stimulation 3.5 mM spermine was required; spermidine and putrescine also stimulated ryanodine binding, but they were about 12-fold less potent. The polyamines had no effect on the Ca^{2+}-concentration dependency of ryanodine binding. Since the effects on ryanodyne binding require higher polycation concentrations than the blockade of caffeine-induced Ca^{2+}-release, it is debated whether the polyamine effects are due to modulation of ryanodyne binding in the first place. Palade (1987) was the first to demonstrate the blockade of caffeine-induced release of Ca^{2+} from sarcoplasmic reticulum by low concentrations of spermine ($IC_{50} = 22$ µM) and spermidine ($IC_{50} = 64$ µM). The sensitivity of Ca^{2+}-release channels to activators and inhibitors depends very much on the source of the sarcoplasmic reticulum. Neomycin was 100-times more potent in preparations of sarcoplasmic reticulum from skeletal than from cardiac muscle (Mack et al., 1992), whereas the activators caffeine and daunorubicin were significantly more potent towards the cardiac receptor (Zimanyi and Pessah, 1991). In a medium allowing active Ca^{2+}-loading of heavy sarcoplasmic-reticulum vesicles from skeletal muscle show not only induction of Ca^{2+}-release into the medium by the ryanodine receptor activator caffeine, but also oscillations in Ca^{2+}-concentrations. Ca^{2+}-releasing compounds with different structures, such as adenosine nucleotides and calmodulin antagonists do not induce this effect. By blocking the ryanodine receptor with neomycin and Mg^{2+} it was demonstrated that the ryanodine-Ca^{2+}-channels were involved in the oscillation mechanism (Wyskovsky, 1994).

It is known that the polyamines associate with inositol 1,4,5-triphosphate, although more weakly than with polyphosphoinositides (Tadoloni and Varani, 1986). Therefore, they decrease the concentration of "free" inositol 1,4,5-triphosphate. The available observations are nevertheless more likely to be a consequence of the direct interaction of the polyamines with an anionic regulatory site of the inositol 1,4,5-triphosphate receptor, and not by the formation of the inositol 1,4,5-triphosphate-spermine complexes. Along this line is the suggestion (Mack et al., 1992) that aminoglycoside-induced muscle paralysis may be mediated by direct block of pre- and postsynaptic Ca^{2+}-release channels of the endoplasmic reticulum.

Blockade of Ca^{2+} release from the sarcoplasmic reticulum by neomycin and gentamicin, and by spermine, were also reported by Brunder et al. (1992). In these experiments it was observed that much higher concentrations of the polycations were required to inhibit the contraction of skeletal muscles associated with the release of Ca^{2+} than the inhibition of Ca^{2+}-release from the sarcoplasmic reticulum. (This finding is similar to the abovementioned results of Vergara et al., 1985.) In contrast, the release of Ca^{2+} from the sarcoplasmic reticulum due to depolarization of transverse tubules of the skeletal muscle was blocked by nM concentrations of neomycin. This observation induced the authors to suggest that the high affinity binding of neomycin to the inositol 1,4,5-triphosphate receptor leads to the specific blockade of the signal transmission from T-tubules to the sarcoplasmic reticulum (Yano et al., 1994). Another example suggesting the blockade of receptors by polycations was reported by Faddis and Brown (1993): Heparin is thought to inhibit inositol 1,4,5-triphosphate binding to its sarcoplasmic receptors. It was shown that intracellular injections of spermine and neomycin into Limulus ventral photoreceptors mimicked the effect of heparin injections, i.e. the light-induced increase of cytoplasmic Ca^{2+} was antagonized. The authors of this work believe that the predominant effect of the polycations was the blockade of inositol 1,4,5-triphosphate formation due to inhibition of phospholipase C activity. However, based on the fact that the polycations are capable of interacting directly with the inositol 1,4,5-triphosphate receptor, the latter possibility cannot be excluded.

5   Mitochondrial Ca^{2+} storage

Mitochondria seem to play a minor role in the control of cytosolic Ca^{2+} under physiological conditions, but they have the capacity to accumulate considerable amounts of Ca^{2+} by deposits of hydroxyapaptite. This capacity is important when noxious agents interfere with the permeability of the plasma membrane, and intracellular Ca^{2+} concentrations rise. Under these conditions the mitochondria are able to store away the excess Ca^{2+} and antagonize the development of a cytotoxic cascade (Rasmussen and Barrett, 1984; Carafoli, 1987). The activation of Ca^{2+}-uptake by the polyamines (Akerman, 1977; Nicchitta and Williamson, 1984; Jensen et al., 1987) is, therefore, presumably of considerable pathophysiological importance. A considerable work has been devoted to the study of polyamine uptake by mitochondria (Toninello et al., 1992; Tassani et al., 1995) and especially to the effect of polyamines on mitochondrial Ca^{2+} storage. It is evident that the activation of mitochondrial Ca^{2+} transport results from the allosteric modulation of the Ca^{2+}-transporter, which increases its affinity for Ca^{2+} due to polyamine binding (Kröner, 1988; Jensen et al., 1989a,b; Rottenberg and Marbach, 1990; Lenzen and Rustenbeck, 1991; Lenzen et al., 1992; Rustenbeck et al., 1993). Polyamines may also affect Ca^{2+}-efflux from mitochondria by decreasing the apparent K_m for efflux (Nicchitta and Williamson, 1984).

Similar to the natural polyamines, the aminoglycosides are capable of activating mitochondrial Ca^{2+}-uptake. At 2 µM Ca^{2+}, and in the presence of 1 mM Mg^{2+}, a sixfold activation of uptake was achieved by 20 µM neomycin. Gentamicin, kanamycin and streptomycin require higher concentrations to achieve a comparable effect (Kröner, 1990). Most probably the mode of action of the aminoglycosides is analogous to that of spermine.

6   Calmodulin

Calmodulin, an ubiquitous small protein ($M_r = 16800$) undergoes conformational changes upon binding of Ca^{2+} and permits it to interact with a great variety of proteins, peptides (melittin, mastoparan) and drugs (phenothiazines). Calmodulin regulates very numerous Ca^{2+}-dependent, but also some Ca^{2+}-independent target proteins, including plasmalemma Ca^{2+}-ATPase, cyclic nucleotide phosphodiesterase, adenylate cyclase and many protein kinases (Johnson and Mills, 1986). An example is the activation of inositol 1,4,5-triphosphate kinase: Ca^{2+} released from the sarcoplasmic reticulum may bind to calmodulin, which activates the phoshorylation of inositol 1,4,5-triphosphate to inositol 1,3,4,5-tetraphosphate (Fig. 3). The tetraphosphate cannot release Ca^{2+} from the sarcoplasmic reticulum; thus calmodulin mediates the inactivation of inositol 1,4,5-triphosphate.

It has been found that spermine binds to calmodulin to five Ca^{2+}-independent binding sites, which are presumably different from the hydrophobic drug binding sites. Binding of spermine antagonized the activation by calmodulin of two phosphatases, cyclic nucleotide phosphodiesterase and calcineurin (Walters and Johnson, 1988). Since the affinity of spermine to calmodulin was low (K_i = 1.1 mM) one may question a physiological relevance of these observations, which nevertheless indicate the possibility of the regulation of a great variety of calmodulin-dependent reactions by spermine. In this regard it is important to note that calmodulin antagonists (phenothiazines, melittin etc.) inhibit polyamine uptake by tumor cells and cells of the gastrointestinal tract (Heston and Charles, 1988; Khan et al., 1993; Scemama et al., 1994), as well as by isolated intestines (Dumontier et al., 1992). Evidence was presented that during the transport process calmodulin was recruited towards the plasma membrane (Khan et al., 1993).

The direct interaction of aminoglycoside antibiotics with calmodulin seems not to have been studied.

7 Protein kinases and the polycations

In addition to inositol 1,4,5-triphosphate, diacylglycerol is formed by hydrolysis of inositol 4,5-diphosphate, as has been mentioned above (Fig. 3). Diacylglycerol, phosphatidylserine and Ca^{2+} are necessary for the activation of protein kinase C (Hannun et al., 1986); inositol 4.5-diphosphate is also an activator of this enzyme; the activation process is inhibited by neomycin (Chauhan, 1990; Chauhan et al., 1990).

7.1 Protein kinase C

The activation of protein kinase C causes a number of events, among others the initiation of the transcription of specific genes. Protein kinase C is, therefore, a centrally important protein phosphorylating enzyme in signal transduction, cell metabolism, and cell growth, but also in tumor promotion (Nishizuka, 1986). All activators act by translocation of protein kinase C from a soluble to a membrane-bound state, and they increase its affinity for Ca^{2+}. Spermine inhibits translocation and phorbolester binding to protein kinase C (Moruzzi et al., 1987; 1990). (Phorbolesters, such as tetradecanoyl-phorbol-13-acetate mimick the effects of diacylglycerol. Long-term exposure to phorbol esters leads to a gradual loss of protein kinase C activity due to translocation into the membrane. The fact that protein kinase C mediates practically all effects of phorbolesters, which are potent tumor promoters, is evidence for a role of protein kinase C in cell growth and proliferation.)

Protein kinase C has been demonstrated to exhibit two membrane-bound states: one is Ca^{2+}-dependent, the other is Ca^{2+}-independent. It has the characteristics of an intrinsic membrane protein, i.e. the enzyme is inserted into the cell membrane (Bazzi and Nelsestuen, 1988). Although phosphatidylserine and inositol phosphates are activators, they inactivate protein kinase C at µM concentrations in the absence of Ca^{2+} in a time dependent manner. It was recently found that spermine prevents this inactivation, most probably by preventing the insertion of the enzyme into the membrane (Monti et al., 1994; Singh et al., 1994). It is believed that the protection of protein kinase C against inactivation by inositol 4,5-diphosphate is a physiological function of spermine.

Neomycin at a concentration of 0.1 M inhibits by 65% the phospholipid-dependent phosphorylation of a renal 88 kDa protein by protein kinase at a pH of 5–7; inhibition decreases if the pH is elevated above 7 (Hagiwara et al., 1988). Since a series of other aminoglycoside antibiotics (tobramycin, gentamicin, kanamycin and amikacin) were also capable of inhibiting this reaction, although weaker, in correlation with the number of amino groups, it was suggested that the inhibition of protein kinase C-catalyzed phosphorylation of the renal protein is part of the nephrotoxic effect of neomycin.

7.2   Messenger-independent protein kinases

Interaction of polycations with messenger-independent protein kinases seems a general phenomenon. Not only the natural polyamines (Ahmed et al., 1985; 1986; Jacob et al., 1981; Cochet and Chambaz, 1983; Hathaway and Traugh, 1984 a,b) and in millimolar concentrations the aminoglycosides (gentamicin, neomycin, streptomycin, tobramycin, kanamycin, amikacin) (Ahmed et al., 1988), but even $Co[NH_3]_6^{3+}$ (Ahmed et al., 1983) and many other polycations may affect certain phosphorylation reactions by messenger-independent protein kinases. In most cases activations of phosphorylation reactions were reported (Ahmed et al., 1986; Cochet and Chambaz, 1983; Feige et al., 1985; Khan et al., 1990), but inhibitions of protein kinase-catalyzed reactions by polyamines are also known (Ahmed et al., 1986; Qi et al., 1983). Sarno et al. (1993) reported, for example, that the polylysine-triggered phosphorylation of calmodulin by casein kinase-2 is prevented by spermine. There are also examples demonstrating no effect on phosphorylation reactions. Thus, at concentrations up to 0.1 mM neomycin seems to affect little, or not at all cyclic GMP-dependent protein kinase, cyclic AMP-dependent protein kinase, casein kinase-1, casein kinase-2, and Ca^{2+}-calmodulin-dependent myosin light chain kinase (Hagiwara et al., 1988), but it may well be that the concentrations of amino-glycosides used in this work were too low to produce an effect (see Ahmed et al., 1988). The insulin-dependent phosphorylation of calmodulin by the insulin receptor tyrosine kinase seems also unaffected by the natural poly-amines, although this reaction requires the presence of histones or other polybasic peptides (Laurino et al., 1988).

Two major mechanisms of action of the polycations were proposed: alter-ations of the conformation of protein substrates by non-covalent interac-tions so as to facilitate access to serine or threonine with protein substrates (Ahmed et al., 1985), and binding of the polycations to one or two func-tional Mg^{2+} binding sites of the enzyme (Hathaway and Traugh, 1984a, b). The most profound experiments were carried out with casein kinase-2, a serine-threonine protein kinase, found in both nuclear and cytoplasmic cell compartments (Pinna, 1990). The following observations suggest func-tional interrelationships between polyamines and this enzyme: casein kinase-2 is markedly activated by µM concentrations of the natural poly-amines, spermine being the most potent (Feige et al., 1985; Cochet and Chambaz, 1983). The uptake of casein kinase-2 by cell nuclei as well as its binding to double stranded DNA is enhanced in the presence of poly-amines (Filhol et al., 1990a, b), and there is a temporal relationship between the accumulation of casein kinase-2 in cell nuclei, and the increase in intra-cellular polyamines of adrenocortical cells exposed to ACTH (Filhol et al., 1991b) These observations recommend the polyamines as intracellu-lar messengers in the regulation of the subcellular distribution and activ-ity of protein kinases in response to stimulation by hormones and trophic factors. It has been demonstrated that [^{3}H]spermine binds to the β-sub-unit of casein kinase-2 with a K_D in the µM range (Filhol et al., 1991a). The high affinity of the polyamines to casein kinase-2 support the view of a physiological interaction.

8   Interactions with receptors

Until recently the polyamines were not attractive to pharmacologists (Seiler, 1991). The situation changed profoundly when the allosteric mod-ulation of a subtype of glutamate receptors, the N-methyl-D-aspartate receptor, by spermine and other polycations became apparent (Ransom and Stec, 1988). Although more complex, allosteric regulations of recep-tors are in principle not different from the regulation of the activity of membrane-bound enzymes by allosteric effectors. In fact the allosteric modification of enzymes by polyamines has long been known, the first thoroughly studied example was the modulation of the catalytic properties of membrane-bound acetylcholine esterase by µM concentrations of spermine and spermidine (Kossorotow et al., 1974).

A great number of publications appeared within a few years giving evidence for direct interactions of the polyamines with a variety of receptors and ion channels, and the electrophysiology of polyamines was studied by several groups. Much of this work is summarized in various chapters of a monography (Shaw, 1994; Romano and Williams, 1994; Schoemaker et al., 1994; Hashimoto and London, 1994; Usherwood and Blagbrough, 1994; Scott et al., 1994; Carter, 1994). In the following some of the most pertinent observations on the effects of the polyamines on ligand binding are summarized. For electrophysiological studies the reader is referred to the reviews by Usherwood and Blagbrough (1994) and Scott et al. (1993; 1994) and original works quoted in these papers.

8.1   N-Methyl-D-aspartate receptor

The N-methyl-D-aspartate (NMDA) receptor is a major subtype of the glutamate receptor family, widely distributed on neurons. The observation that the natural polyamines increased the affinity of the NMDA receptor for MK-801 ((+)-5-methyl-10,11-dihydro-5H-dibenzo(a,d)cyclohepten-5,10-imine) at a binding site distinct from that of glutamate (Ransom and Stec, 1988) was the first to evidence allosteric modulation of a receptor by polyamine binding. Rat and human receptor are very similar in this regard (Subramaniam et al., 1994). Most of the work on polyamine-NMDA receptor complex interactions has recently been reviewed (Seiler, 1991; Williams et al., 1991; Romano and Williams, 1994; Macdonald and Rock, 1995). The present considerations will be restricted to the comparisons of polyamine and aminoglycoside effects.

In Fig. 4 the sites of interaction of a variety of agonists and antagonists with the NMDA receptor are illustrated. Glutamate is the physiological agonist. Glycine has been shown to enhance the effects of glutamate, and there appears to be a requirement for glycine in order to open the channel (Kleckner and Dingledine, 1988). Thus glycine can be considered a coagonist.

Polyamines interact with the NMDA receptor at several sites. Since they enhance binding of MK-801 and TCP (N-[1-(2-thienyl)cyclohexyl]piperidine), both in the virtual absence of glutamate and glycine, as well as in the presence of optimally effective concentrations of these amino acids (Ransom and Stec, 1988), it is evident that the stimulatory site of the polyamines is different from the glycine and glutamate recognition sites. Spermine and glutamate increase the rates of association and dissociation of

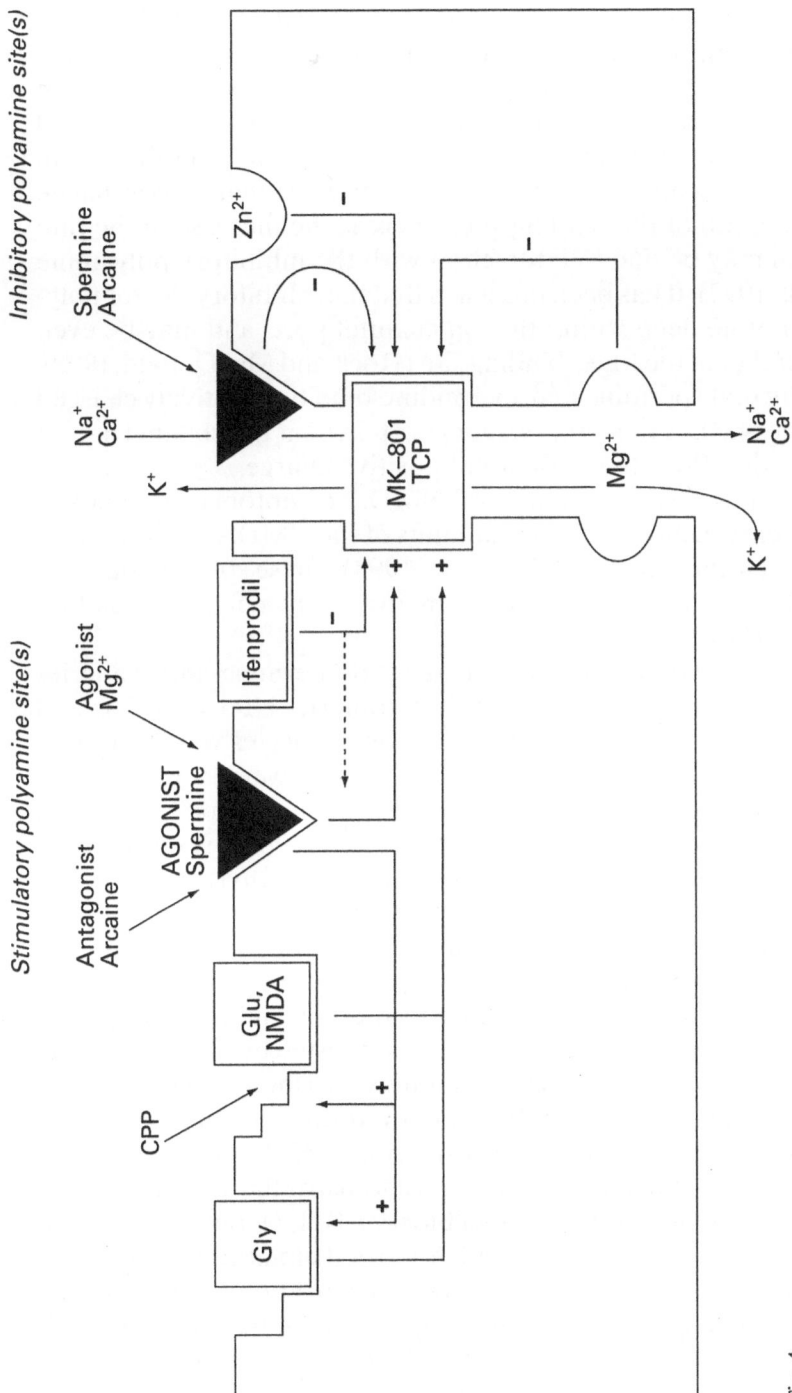

Fig. 4

Major agonist and antagonist binding sites of the NMDA receptor: their interrelationships with the polyamine sites.

Abbreviations: Gly glycine; Glu glutamate; Arcaine 1,4-diguanidinobutane; CPP 2-(2-carboxypiperazin-4-yl)propyl-1-phosphonic acid; Ifenprodil α-(4-hydroxyphenyl)-β-methyl-4-benzyl-1-piperidineethanol; MK-801 (+)-5-methyl-10,11 -dihydro-5H-dibenzo(a,d)cyclo-hepten-5,10-imine; TCP N-[1-(2-thienyl)cyclohexyl]piperidine.

According to Romano and Williams (1994) (modified).

MK-801 binding. This was interpreted as an increased accessibility of the ion channel binding site for this antagonist (Reynolds and Miller, 1989; Bonhaus and McNamara,1988; Kloog et al.,1988). However, the effect of spermine may be mediated by two separate sites. Evidence was presented by Reynolds (1990; 1992) that the spermine effect may be due to an increase in the association of binding of MK-801, presumably by a change in the conformation of the binding site, whereas the increase in the rate of dissociation may be due to interaction with the inhibitory polyamine site (Reynolds, 1992). It has been proposed that the inhibitory site for poly-amines does not lie deep within the ion channel pore, and may be even more peripheral than the Mg^{2+} binding site (Rock and MacDonald,1992). Thus it is likely that spermine and spermidine bind to negatively charged residues on the NMDA receptor-channel protein near the channel mouth and impede cation flow due to their net positive charge.

The subunit composition of the natural NMDA receptors is not known. Howewer, several cDNAs encoding subunits of the NMDA receptor have been isolated (Hollmann and Heinemann, 1994). These splice variants of the NMDA receptor allow to identify domains involved in the regulation by polyamines (Durand et al., 1993).

In a recent work the voltage-dependent effects of spermine, and of a series of N^α,N^ω-bis(ethyl) polyamines on heteromeric NR1A/NR2A and NRR1A/NR1 B receptors, expressed in Xenopus oocytes were reported. Most of the bis(ethyl)spermine homologs and analogs were, similar to sper-mine, potent antagonists, especially at oocytes voltage clamped at –80 mV. Potentiating responses to glutamate required higher concentrations than did inhibition. The effects of penta-amines and bis(ethyl)penta-amines were maximal only at –100 mV, suggesting that the mechanisms of inhi-bition of NMDA receptors by penta-amines is different from that of sper-mine (Igarashi and Williams, 1995).

The structural requirements for binding to the polyamine binding sites of the NMDA receptor are not stringent, as is suggested by the great variety of diamines and polyamines which can mimick spermine and spermidine effects (Romano and Williams, 1994). It is, therefore, not surprising, that aminoglycoside antibiotics are interacting with NMDA receptors. Pullan et al. (1992) found that neomycin was a full agonist at the site where poly-amines enhance binding of the channel blocker TCP. Neomycin, gentam-icin, kanamycin, spermidine and spermine showed biphasic concentration curves, enhancing [^{3}H]TCP binding at low concentrations with decreases at higher concentrations. Arcain and ifenprodil inhibited the neomycin and spermidine-induced enhancement of TCP binding. Using [^{3}H]dizo-cilpine for binding, it was possible to distinguish the major polyamine sites.

Ifenprodil affected both sites, but it had a lower affinity for the inhibitory site. This was also the case for the polyamines and neomycin, which produced only partial inhibition of dizocilpine equilibrium binding (Marvizon and Baudry, 1994). It should be pointed out that specific binding of [^{3}H]Ifenprodil is potently inhibited not only by the polyamines spermidine and spermine, but also by neomycin (Hashimoto et al., 1994). In a recent autoradiographic study on the regional distribution of polyamine-sensitive [^{3}H]Ifenprodil binding sites in rat brain it was confirmed that high- and low-affinity ifenprodil sites are sensitive to polyamines, but also to neomycin, gentamicin and kanamycin (Nicolas and Carter, 1994).

Evidence for the interaction of spermidine and spermine with the glutamate binding site (Fig. 4) was obtained by showing that polyamines enhance the binding of the competitive glutamate antagonists CPP (2-(carboxypiperazine-4-yl)propyl-1-phosphonic acid), and decrease the binding of glutamate (Carter et al., 1989; Pullan and Powel, 1991). In contrast to the other polyamine sites the glutamate binding site is not affected in the same sense by neomycin and the other aminoglycosides, as by the polyamines; at concentrations up to 1 mM they do not enhance, but rather weakly inhibit CPP binding (Pullan et al., 1992).

NMDA receptors are involved in a great variety of physiological processes in the central nervous system, including the generation of long-term potentiation (Nicoll et al., 1988), neuronal development (Brewer et al., 1989) and pain inhibition (Jacquet, 1988), but also in excitotoxic damage which appears to involve endogenous polyamines (Carter, 1994). Exogenous polyamines exacerbate neurotoxic effects of NMDA (Munir et al., 1993). In view of the agonist properties of the aminoglycoside antibiotics at polyamine regulatory sites of the NMDA receptor, neurotoxic effects of these compounds can be expected in situations where the blood brain barrier function is impaired. It is, therefore, quite surprising that neomycin improved the neurologic and functional outcome after traumatic brain injury (Golding and Vink, 1994). This example is indicative for the difficulties to interpret *in vivo* effects on the basis of observations on a molecular level of multifunctional molecules, such as the polyamines, and their analogs.

8.2   Transmitter-independent, voltage-dependent Ca^{2+} channels, inwardly rectifying K$^+$ channels and receptors other than MDA receptors

A possible role of polyamines in effector-mediated and transmitter-independent, voltage-dependent Ca^{2+}-fluxes has been evidenced by the work of H. Koenig and his colleagues. A compilation of the major results was

Table 1.
Effect of polyamines and aminoglycosides on ligand binding to various receptors and binding sites

Receptor	Ligand	Polycation	Conc.	Effect on binding etc.	Reference
Ca²⁺ ion channels					
L-type Ca^{2+} channel	[^{3}H]Diltiazem [^{3}H]Nitrendipin [^{3}H]Verapamil	Spm; Spd; Put	μM	Full inhibition	Schoemaker 1992
	[^{3}H]Diltiazem [^{3}H]Desmethoxy-verapamil	Neomycin	μM	No effect	Knaus et al. 1987; Wagner et al. 1988
N-type Ca^{2+} channel	[^{125}I]ω–Conotoxin	Spm	0.03–0.3 μM >0.3 μM 100 μM	stimulation inhibition displacement	Pullan et al. 1990
		Spd	0.1–3 μM >0.3 μM 1 mM	stimulation inhibition displacement	
		Put	10–100 μM	stimulation	
	[^{125}I]ω–Conotoxin GVIA	Spm Neomycin, Gentamicin	IC$_{50}$ 14 μM μM	inhibition inhibition	Scott et al. 1992 Knaus et al. 1987, Wagner et al. 1988, Feigenbaum et al. 1988
	[^{125}I]ω–Conotoxin MVIIA	Spm; Spd	μM	inhibition	Stoehr and Dooley, 1993
Glutamate receptors					
NMDA receptor					
Glutamate site	[^{3}H]Glutamate [^{3}H]CPP	Spm; Spd Spm; Spd		inhibition stimulation	Pullan and Powel 1991 Carter et al. 1989; Pullan et al. 1992; Williams et al. 1992; Pullan et al. 1992
	[^{3}H]CPP	Neomycin Gentamicin Kanamycin	100–1000 μM 10–50 μM	weak inhibition antagonism of Spm	Oblin et al. 1992
	[^{3}H]CGP39653	Spm	μM	no effect	Oblin et al. 1992
Glycine site	[^{3}H]Glycine	Spm	μM	enhancement of affinity	Sacaan and Johnson 1989; Ransom 1991
	Ifenprodil	Spm	μM	decrease of inhibition	Ransom 1991
	[^{3}H]5,7-Dichloro-kynurenate	Spm	IC$_{50}$ 7.3 μM	inhibition	Oblin et al. 1994

Target	Ligand	Polyamine	Concentration	Effect	Reference
Channel blocker domain	[3H]MK-801	Spm;Spd		enhancement of affinity	
	[3H]TCP	Neomycin Gentamicin Kanamycin	EC50 2 μM	stimulation	Pullan et al. 1992
Nicotinic ACh receptors	α[125I]Bungarotoxin	Spm	IC50 30 μM	inhibition	Anis et al. 1990
	[3H]Perhydrohistrio-nicotoxin	Spd	IC50 110 μM	inhibition	Anis et al. 1990
	[125I]PhTX derivatives	Spm; Spd	μM	inhibition	
		Spm	IC50 38 μM	inhibition	Goodnow et al. 1991
GABA receptors	[3H]Diazepam	Put	EC50 4.5 μM	potentiation	Morgan and Stone 1983
		Spm	EC50 80 μM	potentiation	Gilad et al. 1992
		Spd	IC50 12 μM	potentiation	
	[3H]Gabapentin	Spm	IC50 15 μM	inhibition	Suman-Chauhan 1993
		Spd		inhibition	
Ryanodine receptor	[3H]Ryanodyne	Spm	EC50 3 μM	stimulation	Zarka and Shoshan-Barmatz 1992; Zimanyi and Pessah 1991
G-Protein coupled receptors					
Muscarinic ACh receptors	[3H]Scopolamine	Spm	μM	No effect	Hu et al. 1992
Adenosine A1 receptors	Adenosin	Spm	μM	enhancement of affinity	Wasserkort et al. 1991
Follicle stimulating hormone receptors	[125I]FSH	Spm; Spd	μM	inhibition	Dias et al. 1983; Swift and Dias 1986
Insulin receptors	tyrosin-A14[125I]insulin	Spm		enhancement	Pedersen et al. 1989 Pettersson et al. 1984 Filetti et al. 1981
		Spm		inhibition	
Sigma receptors	[3H](+)3 PPP	Spm	IC50 9.2 μM	inhibition	Paul et al. 1990
		Spd	IC50 70 μM		
		Spm; Spd	μM	no effect	Contreras et al. 1990
Peripheral benzo-diazepine sites	[3H]PK 11195	Spm; Spd	100 μM	partial inhibition	Gilad et al. 1992
Dopamine transporter	[3H]Cocaine	Spm	μM	inhibition	Ritz et al. 1994

presented by the authors (Koenig et al., 1988a) and in a previous volume of this series (Seiler, 1991). More recently, in numerous reports evidence was presented for the ability of the natural polyamines to antagonize the binding of specific ligands to a variety of receptors. In some instances aminoglycosides were included in these studies. In Table 1 effects of aminoglycosides and polyamines on receptor-ligand interactions are summarized. Effects of aminoglycosides on inward rectifying K^+ channels have not yet been studied, however, it appears that the natural polyamines could function as physiological gating molecules of these channels. Inward rectifier K^+ channels are open at hyperpolarized membrane potentials, i.e. they behave opposite to what is expected from the K^+ gradient between the intra- and extracellular space. Their role is the maintenance of stable resting potentials and the modulation and control of excitability of a great variety of neuronal and non-neuronal cells. It has been shown by patch clamp studies that 10 nM spermine and 1 μM spermidine, by entering the K^+ channel from the intracellular compartment, were sufficient to mimick the time-dependence of inwardly rectified K^+ currents of cells (Lopatin et al., 1994; Ficker et al., 1994; Wible et al., 1994). These concentrations are well within the range of calculated free intracellular polyamine concentrations (spermidine: 40–60 μM; spermine: 3–4 μM (Brosnan and Hu, 1985)). Since the gating mechanism of inwardly rectifying K^+ channels by Mg^{2+} and the polyamines does not require additional assumptions for a physiological function, such as modulation of polyamine concentrations in small, local pools or their regulated release into the extracellular space, it is highly probable that the "long pore blockade" is a general physiological function of spermidine and spermine in the control of cellular excitability. Since the effects of putrescine are similar to those of Mg^{2+}, its role in the rectification of inward K^+-currents is not likely.

Numerous electrophysiological studies of polyamine-receptor interactions were stimulated by the discovery that amides of the polyamines which are found as constituents in arthropod toxins (the first example being described already in 1957 by Fischer and Bohn) interact with the polyamine binding sites of various receptors. Usually the polyamine amides are more potent, both as agonists and antagonists, than the parent compounds. This interesting work is, however, beyond the scope of this review. The reader is referred to recent reviews (Usherwood and Blagbrough, 1991; 1994; Moya and Blagbrough, 1994).

From the ability of the natural polyamines to interact with a variety of receptors it is evident that the structural requirements of many receptors for binding small cationic molecules are not stringent, as has already been mentioned. In view of the ubiquity of the polyamines, specific functions at certain receptors types, with the exception of inward rectifier K^+ channels, appear more unlikely than likely. In order to achieve rapid modifications of receptor properties one has to postulate either a very high affinity, together with an appropriate mechanism for the termination of the interaction, or specific mechanisms which locally, i.e. in the immediate vicinity of the receptor, regulate small polyamine pools. Since receptor binding sites are usually extracellular, controlled release of polyamines into the extracellular space, and their reuptake by neurones or glia could be a suitable mechanism. Indeed polyamine release has been repeatedly shown *in vitro* from brain slices and cells, and *in vivo* by microdialysis (Shaw, 1994). However, the polyamine release as determined by microdialysis under a variety of conditions (Speciale et al., 1992a, b; Fage et al., 1992; 1993a) is presumably considerably affected by the traumatic processes induced by the implanation of the dialysis probes (Fage et al., 1993b).

9   Aminoglycosides, polyamines and cancer therapy

Since cancer patients have a compromised immune defense they constitute a group with additional hazards. Various antibiotics, including aminoglycoside antibiotics were, therefore, suggested to be used prophylactically against bacterial infections of cancer patients (Rolston and Bodev, 1992; Rolston et al., 1993). A new clinical application of non-resorbable aminoglycoside antibiotics may arise from the observations which are discussed in the following.

It is well established that inhibition of ODC by DFMO prevents proliferation of tumor cells in culture, but even large daily doses of DFMO had only relatively marginal effects on the growth of tumor cell grafts in experimental animals (Sunkara et al., 1987; Sarhan et al., 1989), and on human tumors (Schechter et al., 1987; Seiler, 1991). The failure of tumor growth inhibition *in vivo* can be explained by the fact that a tumor growing in a mammalian organism has access to two major polyamine sources (Sarhan et al., 1989):

a) *De novo* synthesis
b) Uptake from the blood

Uptake is enhanced if intracellular polyamines are depleted, e.g. by treatment with DFMO (Seiler and Dezeure, 1990).

Circulating polyamines may originate from tissues due to phsyiological release or due to cell death, and from the gastrointestinal tract. Cachexia developing in the course of the growth of tumors causes the release of enormous amounts of polyamines from muscle which may be utilized by the tumor. Gastrointestinal polyamines derive from gut bacteria and from the alimentation. Most foodstuffs contain considerable amounts of polyamines (Bardocz et al., 1993).

It was shown in several studies that a variety of solid tumors [Lewis lung carcinoma (Sarhan et al., 1989; Seiler et al., 1990; Hessels et al., 1991), glioblastoma (Moulinoux et al., 1991; Sarhan et al., 1991), fibrosarcoma (Hessels et al., 1991), prostatic adenocarcinoma (Moulinoux et al., 1991) and ascitic L1210 leukemia cells (Hessels et al., 1989)] can be very considerably inhibited in their growth if the administration of DFMO is combined with the partial or complete decontamination of the gastrointestinal tract by aminoglycoside antibiotics. In fact, even in the absence of a polyamine biosynthesis inhibitor, decontamination of the gastrointestinal tract has already a significant antitumoral effect, as was shown by the administration of a polyamine deficient diet, which contained 200 mg neomycin and 3.4 mg metronidazol per 100 g. It had the same inhibitory effect on the growth of Lewis lung carcinoma in mice, as the same diet, containing instead of the antibiotics 3 g of DFMO (Sarhan et al., 1992). Although neomycin is an inhibitor of ODC (Henley et al., 1988), the growth inhibitory effect of neomycin could not be explained by depletion of tumor polyamines, since the difference in tumor polyamine contents between animals receiving the polyamine deficient diet alone, and those receiving in addition the antibiotic was not significant, whereas the presence of DFMO in the diet depleted putrescine and spermidine contents by 75% and 46%, respectively. It is, therefore, likely that the reduction of gastrointestinal polyamines by the impairment of bacterial growth caused the neomycin effect.

The oral administration of neomycin and of related non-absorbable aminoglycoside antibiotics does not seem to cause major problems; its long-term administration is clinical routine in inflammatory bowel disease. The development of a malabsorption syndrome caused by neomycin is known (Venho, 1986). However, this may even be used to advantage in hypercholesteraemic patients (Vanhanen, 1994). Administration of aminoglycosides in combination with polyamine biosynthesis inhibitors is a new method with potentials in the treatment of various cancers. Therefore, it will be of considerable importance to clarify the mechanisms by which neomycin and other aminoglycoside antibiotics impair tumor growth. Since it has been shown that the dose of cytotoxic drugs can be reduced in combination with polyamine depletion without losing efficacy on tumor growth, but increasing survival time (Quemener et al., 1992) the systematic exploration of the therapeutic potentials of aminoglycoside antibiotics in combination with a low polyamine diet and conventional cytotoxic therapy is a challenge for the coming years.

10   Conclusions

Based on numerous reports which describe effects of the polyamines and the aminoglycoside antibiotics on the same targets, it is possible to compare actions of the two types of natural polycations on a great variety of biological systems of different complexity: enzymes, receptors, metabolic and signalling pathways and cells. In spite of the bulkiness of the aminoglycosides a considerable similarity between polyamines and aminoglycosides is apparent from this work, even when very complex phenomena, such as the development of nephrotoxicity and ototoxicity, are compared. Usually the compounds with the highest number of positive charges are most potent and most toxic at the same time. If the concentration of the less potent members of the two polycation families is sufficiently high, they produce in most cases the same effect as the higher charged members. This is not surprising, since many of the known *in vitro* effects of the polyamines and of the aminoglycosides are even mimicked by cations such as Mg^{2+} and $Co[NH_3]_6^{3+}$, i.e. by cations with point like charges. The specific structural features of the aliphatic polycations, namely the arrangement of positive charges along flexible carbon chains, which in principle would allow to form bridges between two negatively charged structures, and thus hold these structures together in a clamp-like manner, does not seem to be required for most effects of these compounds. That structure-specific interactions of the polycations exist is evident from the inhibition of microbial protein synthesis by the aminoglycosides and the activating effects of the polyamines on the same reactions. In the vertebrate organism specific polycation interactions are difficult to detect, because they are blurred by the presence of large numbers of non-specific anionic binding sites. Specific interactions seem indicated whenever polyamines and aminoglycosides do not produce analogous effects. It was observed, for example, that the aminoglycosides do not affect the glutamate binding site of the NMDA receptor in the same sense as the natural polyamines (Pullan et al., 1992). This and other examples suggest that not only the number of neutralized negative charges, but the specific three-dimensional distribution of the positive charges of the polycation is essential to produce the specific effect. Since spermine and spermidine are the presumed natural effectors in numerous biological systems, the systematic exploration of the capacity of the aminoglycosides with regard to their ability to produce effects qualitatively or quantitatively different from those of the polyamines will assist in detecting specific polyamine-protein interactions. It is, however, important to remember that steric problems may arise from the bulkiness of the aminoglycosides.

Bulkiness may, for example, prevent the aminoglycosides from intruding into narrow channel pores.

Owing to their repetitive structural units the nucleic acids have long been considered to be the preferred general targets for polyamine binding, and likewise the aminoglycosides are known to bind to nucleic acids. Stabilization of specific conformations of ribonucleic acids as well as of deoxyribonucleic acids, regulation of the transition from one conformational state into another (e.g. B to Z transition of DNA), and formation of condensed structures (toroids, chromatin packaging) are the major aspects of polyamine-nucleic acid interactions (Feuerstein and Marton, 1988). Since proteins lack regular patterns of anionic sites along the peptide chains, the interactions of polycations with proteins are more selective than with nucleic acids. They depend on amino acid composition and sequence, and on other specific structural features of the peptide chain, as well as on the secondary and tertiary structure. Therefore, more specific effects can be expected from the binding of polycations to proteins. But not only the conformation of individual proteins can be affected by polycations. Polyamines are also known to play a role in the assembly of globular proteins to complex structures. Examples are the polymerization of tubulin to microtubules (Anderson et al., 1985) and the formation of actin filaments (Oriol-Audit, 1985). Based on these considerations it does not seem daring to speculate that the natural polyamines are involved in the assembly and conformational stabilization of very numerous proteins, including receptors. Polyamines are present in all cells and their contents is normally well regulated (Pegg, 1986; Seiler and Heby, 1988). Under physiological conditions any ligand-induced allosteric effect will occur under the effect of a defined number of bound polyamines, may the target be an enzyme protein, or a membrane-bound receptor complex. If the polyamine concentration deviates from physiological values, the observed effects of a given ligand will change accordingly. This general function does not exclude the existence of specific modulatory functions at some receptors, or second messenger functions, as has been repeatedly postulated, based on a variety of observations, among others by Feige et al. (1985), Iqbal and Koenig (1985), Koenig et al. (1988a, b), Baudry et al. (1986) and Carter (1994). In fact the systematic comparison of the actions of the natural polyamines with those of the aminoglycosides on a variety of cell types leaves little doubt about the involvement of the polyamines in Ca^{2+}-signalling, an aspect that has nearly completely been neglected in the pertinent literature, in spite of increasing evidence in favor of this idea. The observations reported in this review demonstrate that the polyamines are capable of interacting in principle with nearly all receptors, enzymes and other complex structures, as well as with small molecules, which play a major role in signal transduction mechanisms and the control of Ca^{2+}-homeostasis. The fact that it is not possible to pinpoint the sites at which the polyamines exert specific or even only prominent effects is not an argument against their importance Since they are basically multifunctional molecules, they act most probably at many sites of the transmembrane signalling cascade. An even more general function in cell physiology is indicated by their presumed function as gating molecules of inward K^+ rectifier channels, a function that is likely to become the first firmly proven role of the natural polyamines in a process unrelated (or more precisely only indirectly related) to cell growth.

Polyamines bind very tightly to certain membranes, such as the membrane of nerve endings (Seiler and Deckardt, 1976). Since many of the observations reported in this review, especially most receptor binding studies, were performed with crude tissue preparations (e.g. "washed" membranes) the polyamine content of the preparations was in most cases ill defined. This uncertainty may have contributed to differences in effective concentrations found by different groups, and it may even explain some contradictory results reported in this review. It will be imperative in the future to include a more careful control of the polyamine content of the experimental systems, whenever their potential functions are studied. There is no doubt that in well-designed experiments the systematic exploration of the effects of the aminoglycosides in the mammalian cells, but also in the whole mammalian organism, will improve our knowledge of polyamine functions.

From the study of the sources of polyamines which may contribute to tumor growth a new therapeutic application of the aminoglycosides became apparent. As is indicated by animal experiments, the careful administration of the toxic aminoglycosides in combination with treatments suitable to deplete endogenous polyamines has considerable cytostatic effects. In view of the severity of cancer diseases, minor, reversible side effects seem tolerable and the use of aminoglycosides in cancer therapy justified. For their extended application the knowledge of all major aspects and hazards of the aminoglycosides seems imperative. It is hoped that this review will contribute to their better understanding.

References

Ahmed, K. Goueli, S.A., and Williams-Ashman, H.G. (1983) Polyamine-like effects of cobalt(III)hexammine on various cyclic nucleotide-independent phosphokinase reactions. Biochem. Biophys. Res. Commun. *112*, 139–146.

Ahmed, K. Goueli, S.A. and Williams-Ashman, H.G. (1985) Characteristics of polyamine stimulation of cyclic nucleotide-independent protein kinase reactions. Biochem.J. *232*, 767–771.

Ahmed, K., Goueli, S.A. and Williams-Ashman, H.G. (1986) Mechanism and significance of polyamine stimulation of various protein kinase reactions. Adv. Enzyme Regul. *25*, 173–175.

Ahmed, K., Goueli, S.A. and Williams-Ashman, H.G. (1988) Polyamine-like effects of aminoglycosides on various messenger-independent protein kinase reactions. Biochim. Biophys. Acta *966*, 384–389.

Akerman, K.E.O. (1977) Effect of Mg^{2+} and spermine on the kinetics of Ca^{2+} transport in rat liver mitochondria. J. Bioenerg. Biomembranes *9*, 65–72.

Algranati, I.D. and Goldemberg, S.H. (1977a) Polyamines and their role in protein synthesis. Trends Biochem. Sci. *2*, 272–275.

Algranati, I.D. and Goldemberg, S.H. (1977b) Translation of natural mRNA in cell-free systems from a polyamine-requiring mutant of *Escherichia coli*. Biochem. Biophys. Res. Commun. *75*, 1045–1051.

Algranati, I.D. and Goldemberg, S.H. (1981) Initiation, elongation and termination of polypeptide synthesis in cell-free systems from polyamine-deficient bacteria. Biochem. Biophys. Res. Commun. *103*, 8–15.

Algranati, I.D. and Goldemberg, S.H. (1989) Effects of polyamines and antibiotics on the structure and function of ribosomes. in: The Physiology of Polyamines. (Bachrach, U. and Heimer, Y.M., eds.) pp. 143–156, CRC Press, Boca Raton.

Anderson, P, Bardocz, C., Campos, R. and Brown, D.L. (1985) The effect of polyamines on tubulin assembly. Biochem. Biophys. Res. Commun. *132*, 147–154.

Anis, N., Sherby, S., Goodnow, R.Jr., Niwa, M., Konno, K., Kallimopoulos, T., Bukownik, R., Nakanishi, K., Usherwood, P. and Eldefrawi, A. (1990) Structure-activity relationships of philanthotoxin analogs and polyamines on N-methyl-D-aspartate and nicotinic acetylcholine receptors. J. Pharmacol. Exp. Ther. *254*, 764–773.

Aridor, M., Traub, L.M. and Sagi-Eisenberg, R. (1990) Exocytosis in mast cells by basic secretagogues: evidence for direct activation of GTP-binding proteins. J. Cell Biol. *111*, 909–917.

Aronoff, G.R., Pottratz, S.T., Brier, M.E., Walker, M.E., Fineberg, N.S., Glant, M.D., and Luft, F.C. (1983) Aminoglycoside accumulation kinetics in rat renal parenchyma. Antimicrob. Agents Chemother. *23*, 74–78.

Aubert-Tulkens, G., Van Hoof, F. and Tulkens, P. (1979) Gentamicin-induced lysosomal phospholipidosis in cultured rat fibroblasts. Quantitative ultrastructural and biochemical study. Lab. Invest. *40*, 481–491.

Bachrach, U. and Heimer, Y.M. (eds.) (1988) The Physiology of Polyamines, two volumes, CRC Press, Boca Raton.

Barbiroli, B., Mezzetti, G. and Moruzzi, M.S. (1989) Polyamines and initiation of protein synthesis in eukaryotes. In: The Physiology of Polyamines, Vol.1 (Bachrach U. and Heimer, Y.M., eds) pp. 125–132, CRC Press, Boca Raton.

Bardocz, S., Grant, G., Brown, D.S., Ralph, A. and Pusztai, A. (1993) Polyamines in food. Implications for growth and health. J. Nutr. Biochem. *4*, 66–71.

Baudry, M., Lynch, G. and Gall, C. (1986) Induction of ornithine decarboxylase as a possible mediator of seizure-elicited changes in genomic expression in rat hippocampus. J. Neurosci. *6*, 3430–3454.

Bayliss, C., Rennke, H.R. and Brenner, B.M. (1977) Mechanism of the defect in glomerular ultrafiltration associated with gentamicin administration. Kidney Int. *12*, 344–353.

Bazzi, M.D. and Nelsestuen, G.L. (1988) Properties of membrane-inserted protein kinase C. Biochemistry *27*, 7589–7593.

Beaubien, A.R., Karpinski, K. and Ormsby, E. (1995) Toxicodynamics and toxicokinetics of amikacin in the guinea pig cochlea. Hear. Res. *83*, 62–79.

Bergeron, R.J., Hawthorne, T.R., Vinson, J.R., Beck, D.E. Jr. and Ingeno, M.J. (1989) Role of the methylene backbone in the antiproliferative activity of polyamine analogues on L1210 cells. Cancer Res. *49*, 2959–2964.

Berridge, M.J. (1987a) Inositol triphosphate and diacylglycerol: two interacting second messengers. Ann. Rev. Biochem. *56*, 159–193.

Berridge, M.J. (1987b) Inositol lipids and cell proliferation. Biochim. Biophys. Acta *907*, 33–45.

Berridge, M.J. (1993) Inositol triphosphate and calcium signalling. Nature *361*, 315–325.

Bonhaus, D.W. and McNamara, J.O. (1988) N-Methyl-D-aspartate receptor regulation and uncompetitive antagonist binding in rat brain membranes: kinetic analysis. Mol. Pharmacol. *34*, 250–255.

Brewer, G.J. and Cotman, C.W. (1989) NMDA receptor regulation of neuronal morphology in cultured hippocampal neurons. Neurosci. Lett. *99*, 268–273.

Brighton, C.T., Sennet, B.J., Farmer, J.C., Ianotti, J.P., Hansen, C.A., Williams, J.L. and Williamson, J. (1992) The inositol phosphate pathway as a mediator in the proliferative response of rat calvarial bone cells to cyclical biaxial mechanical strain. J. Orthop. Res. *10*, 385–393.

Brosnan, M.E. and Hu, Y.W. (1985) Synthesis and function of polyamines in mammary gland during lactation. In: Recent Progress in Polyamine Research. (Selmeci, L., Brosnan, M.E. and Seiler, N., eds.) pp.169–180; Akademiai Kiado, Budapest.

Brummett, R.E. and Fox, K.E. (1982) Studies of aminoglycoside ototoxicity in animal models. In: The Aminoglycosides: Microbiology, Clinical Use and Toxicity (Whelton, A. and Neu, H.G., eds.) pp. 419–451, Marcel Dekker, New York.

Brunder, D.G., Györke, S., Dettbarn, C. and Palade, P. (1992) Involvement of sarcoplasmic reticulum "Ca^{2+} release channels" in excitation-contraction coupling in vertebrate skeletal muscle. J. Physiol. London *445*, 759–778.

Bryan, L.E. and Kwan, S. (1983) Roles of ribosomal binding, membrane potential and electron transport in bacterial uptake of streptomycin and gentamicin. Antimicrob. Agents Chemother. *23*, 835–845.

Bueb, J.L., Mousli, M., Bronner, C., Rouot, B. and Landry, Y. (1990) Activation of G-like proteins, a receptor-independent effect of kinins in mast cells. Mol. Pharmacol. *38*, 816–822.

Bueb, J.L., Mousli, M. and Landry, Y. (1991) Molecular basis for cellular effects of naturally occurring polyamines. Agents and Actions *33*, 84–87.

Bueb, J.L., Da Silva, A., Mousli, M. and Landry, Y. (1992) Natural polyamines stimulate G proteins. Biochem. J. *282*, 545–550.

Byers, T.L., Kameji, R., Rannels, D.F., and Pegg, A.E. (1987) Multiple pathways for uptake of paraquat, MGBG and polyamines. Am. J. Physiol. *252*, 663–669.

Campbell, R.A., LaBerge, T., Campbell-Boswell, M., Brooks, R.E. and Talwalkar, Y.B. (1983) Myeloid body formation under conditions of polyamine stress. In: Advances in Polyamine Research, Vol. 4. (Bachrach, U., Kaye, A. and Chayen, R., eds.) pp. 107–125, Raven Press, New York.

Carafoli, E. (1987) Intracellular calcium homeostasis. Ann. Rev. Biochem. *56*, 359-433.

Carter, C. (1994) Brain polyamines: intra- and intercellular messengers and neurotoxins? in: The Neuropharmacology of Polyamines (Carter, C., ed.) pp. 255–296, Academic Press, London.

Carter, C., Rivy, J.P., Thuret, F., Lloyd, K.G. and Scatton, B. (1989) Ifenprodil and SL 82.0715 are antagonists at the polyamine site of the N-methyl-D-aspartate receptor complex. Eur. J. Pharmacol. *164*, 611–612.

Chauhan, V.P. (1990) Phosphatidylinositol 4, 5-biphosphate stimulates protein kinase C-mediated phosphorylation of brain proteins. Inhibition by neomycin. FEBS Lett. *272*, 99–102.

Chauhan, V.P.S., Chauhan, A., Desmukh, D.S. and Brockerhoff, H. (1990) Lipid activators of protein kinase C. Life Sci. *47*, 981–986.

Cochet, C. and Chambaz, E.M. (1983) Polyamines and Protein kinases. Mol. Cell. Endocrinol. *30*, 247–266.

Cochet, C. and Chambaz, E.M. (1986) Catalytic properties of a purified phosphatidylinositol 4-phosphate kinase from rat brain. Biochem. J. *237*, 25–31.

Cockcroft, S., Barrowman, M.M. and Gomperts, B.D. (1985) Breakdown and synthesis of polyphosphoinositides in fMetLeuPhe-stimulated neutrophils. FEBS Lett. *181*, 259–263.

Cockcroft, S., Howell, T.W., Gomperts, B.D. (1987) Two G-proteins act in series to control stimulus secretion coupling in mast cells; use of neomycin to distinguish between G-proteins controlling polyphosphoinositide phosphodiesterase and exocytosis. J. Cell Biol. *105*, 2745–2750.

Cohen, S.S. (1973) Introduction to the Polyamines, Prentice-Hall Inc. Englewood Cliffs.

Cohen, S.S. and Lichtenstein, J. (1960) Polyamines and ribosome structure. J. Biol. Chem. *235*, 2112–2116.

Contreras, P.C., Bremer, M.E. and Gray, N.M. (1990) Ifenprodil and SL 82.0715 potently inhibit binding of [^{3}H](+)3-PPP to sigma binding sites in rat brain. Neurosci. Lett. *116*, 190–193.

Cooper, C.L. and Holz, R.W. (1993) Neomycin and spermine have similar effects on secretion and phosphoinositide metabolism in ATP-depleted permeabilized adrenal chromaffin cells. Biochem. Biophys. Res. Commun. *194*, 1135–1142.

Cundlieffe, E. (1989) Methylation of RNA and resistance to antibiotics. In: Microbial Resistance to Drugs (Bryan, L.E., ed.) Handbook of Experimental Pharmacology, Vol. 91, pp. 291–312, Springer-Verlag, Berlin.

Das, I., de Belleroche, J. and Hirsch, S. (1987) Inhibitory action of spermidine on formyl-methionine-leucyl-phenylalanine stimulated inositol phosphate production in human neutrophils. Life Sci. *41*, 1037–1041.

Davies, B.D. (1988) The lethal action of aminoglycosides. J. Antimicrob. Chemother. *22*, 1–3.

De Meis, L. and de Paula, H.J. (1967) Polyamines and muscle relaxation. Inhibition of actomyosin ATPase by spermine and spermidine. Arch. Biochem. Biophys. *119*, 16–21.

Desrochers, C.S. and Schacht, J. (1982) Neomycin concentrations in inner ear tissues and other organs of the guinea pig after chronic drug administration. Acta Otolaryngol. *93*, 233–236.

Dias, J.A., Treble, D.H. and Reichert, L.E. Jr. (1983) Effect of bacitracin and polyamines on follicle-stimulating hormone binding to membrane-bound and detergent-solubilized bovine calf testis receptor. Endocrinology *113*, 2029–2034.

Dumontier, A.M., Brachet, P. Huneau, J.F. and Tome, D. (1992) Transport of putrescine in the isolated rabbit intestine. Pflügers Arch. *420*, 329–335.

Durand, G.M. Bennett, M.V. and Zukin, R.S. (1993) Splice variants of the N-methyl-D-aspartate receptor NR1 identify domains involved in regulation by polyamines and protein kinase C. Proc. Natl. Acad. Sci. USA, *90*, 6731–6735.

Eberhard, D.A., Cooper, C.L. and Holz, R.W. (1990) Evidence that the inositol phospholipids are necessary for exocytosis. Loss of inositol phospholipids and inhibition of secretion in permeabilized cells caused by bacterial phospholipase and removal of ATP. Biochem. J. *268*, 14–25.

Eichberg, J., Zetusky, W.J., Bell, M.E. and Cavanagh, E. (1981) Effects of polyamines on calcium-dependent rat brain phosphatidylinositol phosphodiesterase. J. Neurochem. *36*, 1868–1871.

Eng, S.P. and Lo, C.S. (1993) Neomycin inhibits mastoparan-induced lactate dehydrogenase release, ethidium bromide accumulation and intracellular fluorescein depletion in MDCK cells. Cell Biol. Toxicol. *6*, 95–104.

Fabre, J., Rudhart, M., Blanchard, P. and Regamay, C. (1976) Persistence of sisomicin and gentamicin in renal cortex and medulla compared with other organs and serum of rats. Kidney Int. 10, 444–449.

Faddis, M.N., and Brown, J.E. (1993) Intracellular injection of heparin and polyamines. Effects on phototransduction in Limulus ventral photoreceptors. J. Gen. Physiol. *101*, 909–931.

Fage, D., Voltz, C. Scatton, B. and Carter, C. (1992) Selective release of spermine and spermidine from rat striatum by N-methyl-D-aspartate receptor activation *in vivo*. J. Neurochem. *58*, 2170–2175.

Fage, D., Voltz, C. and Carter, C. (1993a) Ouabain releases striatal polyamines *in vivo* independently of N-methyl-D-aspartate receptor activation. J. Neurochem. *61*, 261–265.

Fage, D., Carboni, S., Voltz, C., Scatton, B. and Carter, C. (1993b) Ornithine decarboxylase inhibition or NMDA receptor antagonism reduce cortical polyamine efflux associated with dialysis probe implantation. Neurosci. Lett. *149*, 173–176.

Feige, J.J., Cochet, C. and Chambaz, E.M. (1985) Potential role of polyamines as intracellular messengers in hormonal regulation and cellular activity. In: Recent Progress in Polyamine Research, (Selmeci, L., Brosnan, M.E. and Seiler, N., eds.) pp. 181–201, Akademiai Kiado, Budapest.

Feigenbaum, P., Garcia, M.L. and Kaczorowski, G.J. (1988) Evidence for distinct sites coupled to high affinity omega-conotoxin receptors in rat brain synaptic plasma membrane vesicles. Biochem. Biophys. Res. Commun. *154*, 298–305.

Feldman, S., Wang, M. and Kaloyanides, G.J. (1982) Aminoglycosides induce a phospholipidosis in the renal cortex of the rat. J. Pharmacol. Exp. Ther. *220*, 514–520.

Feuerstein, B.G. and Marton, L.J. (1988) Polyamines and the structure of nucleic acids. in: The Physiology of Polyamines (Bachrach, U. and Heimer, Y.M., eds.) Vol. 1, pp. 109–124, CRC Press, Boca Raton.

Ficker, E., Taglialatela, M., Wible, B.A., Henley, C.M. and Brown, A.M. (1994) Spermine and spermidine as gating molecules for inward rectifier K^+ channels. Science 1068–1072.

Filetti, S., Takai, N.A. and Rapoport, B. (1981) Insulin receptor down-regulation, prevention at post-receptor site. Endocrinology *108*, 2409–2411.

Filhol, O., Cochet, C. and Chambaz, E.M. (1990a) Cytoplasmic and nuclear distribution of casein kinase II: characterization of the enzyme uptake by bovine adrenocortical nuclear preparation. Biochemistry 29, 9928–9936.

Filhol, O,. Cochet, C. and Chambaz, E.M. (1990b) DNA binding activity of casein kinase II. Biochem. Biophys. Res. Commun. 173, 862–871.

Filhol, O., Cochet, E., Delagoutte, T. and Chambaz, E.M. (1991a) Polyamine binding activity of casein kinase II. Biochem. Biophys. Res. Commun. 180, 945–952.

Filhol, O., Loue-Mackenbach, P., Cochet, C. and Chambaz, E.M. (1991b) Casein kinase II and polyamines may interact in the response of adrenocortical cells to their trophic hormone. Biochem. Biophys. Res. Commun. 180, 623–630.

Fischer, F.G. and Bohn, H. (1957) Die Giftsekrete der Vogelspinnen. Liebigs Ann. Chem. 603, 232–250.

Fisher, E.R. and Rosenthal, S.M. (1954) Pathology and pathogenesis of spermine-induced renal disease. Arch. Pathol. 57, 244–253.

Forray, C. and el Fakahany, E.E. (1992) Complex allosteric modulation of cardiac muscarinic receptors by protamine: potential model for putative endogenous ligands. Mol. Pharmacol. 42, 311–321.

Gabev, E., Kasianowicz, J. Abbott, T. and McLaughlin, S. (1989) Binding of neomycin to phosphatidylinositol 4, 5-biphosphate (PIP2). Biochim. Biophys. Acta 979, 105–112.

Garcia-Patrone, M. and Algranati, I.D. (1976) Association of ribosomal subunits: studies on the binding of polyamines to 30S and 50S particles. FEBS Lett. 66, 39–43.

Gilad, G.M., Gilad, V.H. and Wyatt, R.J. (1992) Polyamines modulate the binding of $GABA_A$-benzodiazepine receptor ligands in membranes from the rat forebrain. Neuropharmacology 31, 895–989.

Goldemberg, S.H. and Algranati, I.D. (1981) Polyamine requirement for streptomycin action on protein synthesis in bacteria. Eur. J. Biochem. 117, 251–255.

Golding, E.M. and Vink, R. (1994) Inhibition of phospholipase C with neomycin improves metabolic and neurologic outcome following traumatic brain injury. Brain Res. 668, 46–53.

Goodnow, R.A. Jr., Bukownik, R., Nakanishi, K., Usherwood, P.N., Eldefrawi, A.T., Anis, N.A. and Eldefrawi, M.E. (1991) Synthesis and binding of [125I] philanthotoxin-343, [125I]philanthotoxin-343-lysine, and [125I]philanthotoxin-343-arginine to rat brain membranes. J. Med. Chem. 34, 2389–2394.

Goodrich, J.A. and Hottendorf, G.H. (1995) Tobramycin, gender-related nephrotoxicity in Fischer but not Sprague-Dawley rats. Toxicol. Lett. 75, 127–131.

Haber, M.T., Fukui, T. and Lowenstein, J.M. (1991) Activation of phosphoinositide-specific phospholipase C delta from rat liver by polyamines and basic proteins. Arch. Biochem. Biophys. 288, 243–249.

Hagiwara, M., Inagaki, M., Kanamura, K., Ohta, H. and Hidaka, H. (1988) Inhibitory effects of aminoglycosides on renal protein phosphorylation by protein kinase C. J. Pharmacol. Exp. Ther. 244, 355–360.

Hancock, R.E.W. (1981) Aminoglycoside uptake and mode of action – with special reference to streptomycin and gentamicin. I. Antagonists and mutants. J. Antimicrob. Chemother. 8, 249–276.

Hannun, Y.A., Loomis, C.R. and Bell, R.M. (1986) Protein kinase C activation in mixed micelles. Mechanistic implications of phospholipid, diacylglycerol and calcium. J. Biol. Chem. 261, 7184–7190.

Hashimoto, K. and London, E.D. (1994) Specific binding sites for polyamines in the brain. In: The Neuropharmacology of Polyamines (Carter C., ed.) pp. 155–165, Academic Press, London.

Hashimoto, K., Mantione, C.R., Spada, M.R., Neumeyer, J.L. and London, E.D. (1994) Further characterization of [^{3}H]ifenprodil binding in rat brain. Eur. J. Pharmacol. *266*, 67–77.

Hathaway, G.M. and Traugh, J.A. (1984a) Interaction of polyamines and magnesium with casein kinase II. Arch. Biochem. Biophys. *233*, 133–138.

Hathaway, G.M. and Traugh, J.A. (1984b) Kinetics of activation of casein kinase II by polyamines and reversal of 2,3-biphosphoglycerate inhibition. J. Biol. Chem. *259*, 7011–7015.

Heinrich-Hirsch, B., Ahlers, J. and Peter, H.W. (1977) Inhibition of Na, KATPase from chick brain by polyamines. Enzyme *22*, 235–241.

Hendrickson, H.S. and Reinertsen, J.L. (1971) Phosphoinositide interconversion: a model for control of Na$^+$ and K$^+$ permeability in the nerve axon membrane. Biochem. Biophys. Res. Commun. *44*, 1258–1264.

Henley, C.M. and Rybak, L.P. (1995) Ototoxicity in developing mammals. Brain Res. Rev. *20*, 689–90.

Henley, C.M. III, Gerhardt, H.J. and Schacht, J. (1987) Inhibition of inner ear ornithine decarboxylase by neomycin *in vitro*. Brain Res. Bull. *19*, 695–698.

Henley, C.M. III, Mahran, L.G. and Schacht, J. (1988) Inhibition of renal ornithine decarboxylase by aminoglycoside antibiotics *in vitro*. Biochem.Pharmacol.*37*,1679–1682.

Henley, C.M., Atkins, J., Martin, G., and Lonsbury-Martin, B. (1990) Critical period for alpha-difluoromethylornithine (DFMO) ototoxicity in the developing rat. J. Cell Biochem. *14F* (Suppl.) 22.

Herrmann, E., Gierschik, P. and Jakobs, K.H. (1989) Neomycin induces high-affinity agonist binding of G protein-coupled receptors. Eur. J. Biochem. *185*, 677–683.

Hessels, J., Kingma, A.W., Ferwerda, H., Keij, J., van den Berg, G.A., and Muskiet, F.A.J. (1989) Microbial flora in the gastrointestinal tract abolishes cytostatic effects of α-difluoromethylornithine *in vivo*. Int. J. Cancer *43*, 1155–1164.

Hessels, J., Kingma, A.W., Muskiet, F.A.J., Sarhan, S. and Seiler, N. (1991) Growth inhibition of two solid tumors in mice, caused by polyamine depletion, is not attended by alterations in cell-cycle phase distribution. Int. J. Cancer *48*, 697–703.

Heston, W.D.W. and Charles, M. (1988) Calmodulin antagonists inhibition of polyamine transport in prostatic cancer cells *in vitro*. Biochem. Pharmacol. *37*, 2511–2514.

Higashijima, T., Burnier, J. and Ross, E.M. (1990) Regulation of Gi and Go by mastoparan, related amphiphilic peptides, and hydrophobic amines. Mechanism and structural determinant of activity. J. Biol. Chem. *265*, 14176–14186.

Höltje, V.E. (1978) Streptomycin uptake via an inducible polyamine transport system in *Escherichia coli*. Eur. J. Biochem. *86*, 345–351.

Höltta, E. (1985) Polyamine requirement for polysome formation and protein synthesis in human lymphocytes. in: Recent Progress in Polyamine Research. (Selmeci, L., Brosnan, M.E. and Seiler, N., eds.) pp. 137–150, Akademiai Kiado, Budapest.

Hokin, M.R. and Hokin, L.E. (1953) Enzyme secretion and the incorporation of ^{32}P into phospholipids of pancreas slices. J. Biol. Chem. *203*, 967–977.

Hollmann, M. and Heinemann, S. (1994) Cloned glutamate receptors. Ann. Rev. Neurosci. *17*, 31–108.

Hori, R., Saito, H., Iwata, T. and Inui, K. (1989) Interaction of gentamicin with atrial natriuretic polypeptide receptors in renal cells. Biochem. Pharmacol. *38*, 1359–1361.

Hu, J., Wang, S.Z., Forray, C. and el Fakahany, E.E. (1992) Complex allosteric modulation of cardiac muscarinic receptors by protamine: potential model for putative endogenous ligands. Mol. Pharmacol. *42*, 311–321.

Humes, H.D., Sastrasinh, M. and Weinberg, J.M. (1984) Calcium is a competitive inhibitor of gentamicin-renal membrane binding interactions, and dietary calcium supplementation protects against gentamicin nephrotoxicity. J. Clin. Invest. *73*, 143–147.

Hummel, H. and Böck, A. (1989) Ribosomal changes resulting in antibiotic resistance. In: Microbial Resistance to Drugs. (Bryan, L.E., ed.); Handbook of Experimental Pharmacology, Vol. 91. pp. 235–262, Springer-Verlag, Berlin.

Huy, P.T.B., Meulemans, A., Wassef, M., Manuel, C., Sterkers, O. and Amiel, C. (1983) Gentamicin persistence in rat endolymph and perilymph after a two-day constant infusion. Antimicrob. Agents Chemother. *23*, 344–346.

Igarashi, K. and Williams, K. (1995) Antagonist properties of polyamines and bis(ethyl)polyamines at N-methyl-D-aspartate receptors. J. Pharmacol. Exp. Ther. *272*, 1101–1109.

Igarashi, K., Kashiwagi, K., Kishida, K., Watanabe, Y., Kogo, A. and Hirose, S. (1979) Defect in the split proteins of 30S ribosomal subunits and undermethylation of 16S ribosomal RNA in a polyamine-requiring mutant of *Escherichia coli* grown in the absence of polyamines. Eur. J. Biochem. *93*, 345–353.

Igarashi, K., Kashiwagi, K., Kishida, K., Kakegawa, T. and Hirose, S. (1981a) Decrease in the S1 protein of 30S ribosomal subunits in polyamine-requiring mutants of *Escherichia coli* grown in the absence of polyamines. Eur. J. Biochem. *114*, 127–131.

Igarashi, K., Kishida, K., Kashiwagi, K., Tatokoro, I., Kakegawa, T. and Hirose, S. (1981b) Relationship between methylation of adenine near the 3' end of 16S ribosomal RNA and the activity of 30S ribosomal subunits. Eur. J. Biochem. *113*, 587–593.

Igarashi, K. Kakegawa, T. and Hirose, S. (1982a) Stabilization of 30S ribosomal subunits of *Bacillus subtilis* W168 by spermidine and magnesium ions. Biochim. Biophys. Acta *697*, 185–192.

Igarashi, K., Hashimoto, S., Miyake, A., Kashiwagi, K. and Hirose, S. (1982b) Increase of fidelity of polypeptide synthesis in eukaryotic cell-free systems. Eur. J. Biochem. *128*, 597–604.

Iqbal, Z. and Koenig, H. (1985) Polyamines appear to be second messengers in mediated Ca^{2+}-fluxes and neurotransmitter release in potassium-depolarized synaptosomes. Biochem. Biophys. Res. Commun. *133*, 563–573.

Jacob, S.T., Duceman, B.W. and Rose, K.M. (1981) Spermin-mediated phosphorylation of RNA polymerase I and its effect on transcription. Biol. Med. *59*, 381–388.

Jacquet, Y.F. (1988) The NMDA receptor: central role in pain inhibition in rat periaqueductal gray. Eur. J. Pharmacol. *154*, 271–276.

Jensen, J.R., Lynch, G.R. and Baudry, M. (1987) Polyamines stimulate mitochondrial calcium transport in rat brain. J. Neurochem. *48*, 765–772.

Jensen, J.R., Lynch, G.R. and Baudry, M. (1989a) Allosteric activation of brain mitochondrial calcium uptake by spermine and by calcium: Developmental changes. J. Neurochem. *53*, 1173–1181.

Jensen, J.R., Lynch, G.R. and Baudry M. (1989b) Allosteric activation of brain mitochondrial calcium uptake by spermine and by calcium: Brain regional differences. J. Neurochem. *53*, 1182–1187.

Johnson, J.D. and Mills, J.S. (1986) Calmodulin. Med. Res. Rev. *6*, 341–363.

Josepovitz, C., Pastoriza-Munoz, E., Timmerman, D., Scott, M., Feldman, S. and Kaloyanides, G.J. (1982) Inhibition of gentamicin uptake in rat renal cortex *in vivo* by aminoglycosides and organic polycations. J. Pharmacol. Exp. Ther. *223*, 314–321.

Just, M., Erdmann, G. and Habermann, E. (1977) The renal handling of polybasic drugs. 1. Gentamicin and aprotinin in intact animals. Naunyn-Schmiedeberg's Arch. Pharmacol. 300, 57–66.

Just, M. and Habermann, E. (1977) The renal handling of polybasic drugs. 2. *In vitro* studies with brush border and lysosomal preparations. Naunyn-Schmiedeberg's Arch. Pharmacol. *300*, 57–66.

Kashiwagi, K., Miyaji, A., Ikeda, S., Tobe, T., Sasakawa, C. and Igarashi, K. (1992) Increase of sensitivity to aminoglycoside antibiotics by polyamine-induced protein (oligopeptide-binding protein) in *Escherichia coli*. J. Bacteriol. *174*, 4331–4337.

Khan, N.A., Masson, I. Quemener, V., Clari, G., Moret, V. and Moulinoux, J.Ph. (1990) Polyamines and polyamino acids regulation of cytosolic tyrosine protein (Tyr-P) kinase from human erythrocytes. Biochem. Int. *20*, 863–868.

Khan, N.A., Sezan, A., Quemener, V. and Moulinoux, J.P. (1993) Polyamine transport regulation by calcium and calmodulin: role of Ca^{2+}-ATPase. J. Cell Physiol. *157*, 493–501.

Khouja, A. and Jones, C.T. (1993) Phospholipase A2 and arachidonic acid release from permeabilized myometrial cells from guinea pig uterus. J. Dev. Physiol. *19*, 61–66.

Kleckner, N.W. and Dingledine, R. (1988) Requirement for glycine in inactivation of NMDA receptors expressed in Xenopus oocytes. Science *241*, 835–837.

Kloog, Y., Haring, R. and Sokolovsky M. (1988) Kinetic characterization of the phencyclidine-N-methyl-D-aspartate receptor interaction: evidence for a steric blockade of the channel. Biochemistry *27*, 843–848.

Knaus, H.G., Striessnigg, J., Koza, A. and Glossmann, H. (1987) Neurotoxic aminoglycoside antibiotics are potent inhibitors of [^{125}I]-omega-conotoxin GVIA binding to guinea pig cerebral cortex membranes. Naunyn-Schmiedeberg's Arch. Pharmacol. *336*, 583–586.

Kobayashi, S., Kitazawa, T., Somlyo, A.V. and Somlyo, A.P. (1989) Cytosolic heparin inhibits muscarinic and α-adrenergic Ca^{2+} release in smooth muscle. Physiological role of inositol 1,4,5-triphosphate in pharmacomechanical coupling. J. Biol. Chem. *264*, 17997–18004.

Koenig, H., Goldstone, A.D., Lu, C.Y., Iqbal, Z., Fan, C.C. and Trout, J.J. (1988a) Polyamines, hormone receptors, and calcium fluxes. in: The Physiology of Polyamines (Bachrach, U. and Heimer, Y.M., eds.) Vol. 1, pp. 57–81.

Koenig, H., Goldstone, A.D. and Lu C.Y. (1988b) Polyamines are intracellular messengers in the beta-adrenergic regulation of Ca^{2+}-fluxes, $[Ca^{2+}]_i$ and membrane transport in rat heart myocytes. Biochem. Biophys. Res. Commun. *153*, 1179–1185.

Kondo, K. Kozawa, O., Takatsuki, K. and Oiso, Y. (1989) Ca^{2+} influx stimulated by vasopressin is mediated by phosphoinositide hydrolysis in rat smooth muscle cells. Biochem. Biophys. Res. Commun. *161*, 677–682.

Kossorotow, A., Wolf, H.U. and Seiler, N. (1974) Regulatory effects of polyamines on membrane-bound acetylcholinesterase. Biochem. J. *144*, 21–27.

Kotecha, B. and Richardson, G.P. (1994) Ototoxicity *in vitro*: effects of neomycin, gentamicin, dihydrostreptomycin, amikacin, spectinomycin, neamine, spermine and poly-L-lysine. Hear Res. *73*, 173–184.

Kovalchuke, O. and Chakraburtty, K (1994) Comparative analysis of ribosome-associated adenosinetriphosphatase (ATPase) from pig liver and the ATPase of elongation factor 3 from Saccharomyces cerevisiae. Eur. J. Biochem. *226*, 133–140.

Kröner, H. (1988) Spermine, another specific allosteric activator of calcium uptake in rat liver mitochondria. Arch. Biochem. Biophys. *267*, 205–210.

Kröner, H. (1990) Activation of calcium uptake in rat liver mitochondria by aminoglycoside antibiotics. Biochem. Pharmacol. *39*, 891–894.

Kurosawa, M., Uno, D., Hanawa, K. and Kobayashi, S. (1990) Polyamines stimulate the phosphorylation of phosphatidylinositol in rat mast cell granules. Allergy *45*, 262–267.

Langford, P.R., Harpur, E.S., Kayes, J.B. and Gonda, I. (1982) Studies of a potential *in vitro* test for estimation of toxicity of aminoglycoside antibiotics and polyamines. J. Antibiotics *35*, 1387–1393.

Laurino, J.P., Colca, J.R., Pearson, J.D., DeWald, D.B., and McDonald, J.M. (1988) The *in vitro* phosphorylation of calmodulin by the insulin receptor tyrosine kinase. Arch. Biochem. Biophys. *265*, 8–21.

Lenzen, S. and Rustenbeck, I. (1991) Effects of IP_3, spermine, and Mg^{2+} on regulation of Ca^{2+} transport by endoplasmic reticulum and mitochondria in permeabilized pancreatic islets. Diabetes *40*, 323–326.

Lenzen, S., Münster, W. and Rustenbeck, I. (1992) Dual effect of spermine on mitochondrial Ca^{2+} transport. Mol. Cell Biochem. *118*, 141–151.

Lietman, P.S. (1990) Aminoglycosides and spectinomycin: Aminocyclitols. in: Principles and Practice of Infectious Diseases. 3rd ed. (Mandell, G.L., Douglas, R.G. Jr. and Bennett, J.E., eds.) pp. 269–284, Churchill Livingstone, Inc. New York.

Lietman, P.S. and Smith, C.R. (1983) Aminoglycoside nephrotoxicity in humans. J. Infect. Dis. *5* (Suppl. 2) S284–S292.

Lipsky, J.J., Cheng, L., Sacktor, B. and Lietman, P.S. (1980) Gentamicin uptake by renal tubule brush border membrane vesicles. J. Pharmacol. Exp. Ther. *215*, 390–393.

Little, P.J., Neylon, C.B., Tkachuk, V.A. and Bobik, A. (1992) Endothelin-1 and endothelin-3 stimulate calcium mobilization by different mechanisms in vascular smooth muscle. Biochem. Biophys. Res. Commun. *183*, 694–700.

Lodhi, S. Weiner, N.D. and Schacht, J. (1979) Interaction of neomycin with films of polyphosphoinositides and other lipids. Biochim. Biophys. Acta *557*, 1–8.

Lodhi, S., Weiner, N.D., Mechigian, I. and Schacht, J. (1980) Ototoxicity of aminoglycosides correlates with their action on monomolecular films of polyphosphoinositides. Biochem. Pharmacol. *29*, 597–601.

Loftfield, R.B., Eigner, E.A. and Pastuszyn, A. (1981a) Polyamines and protein synthesis. In: Polyamines in Biology and Medicine (Morris, D.R. and Marton, L.J., eds.). pp. 207–221, Marcel Dekker, NewYork.

Loftfield, R.B., Eigner, E.A. and Pastuszyn, A. (1981b) The role of spermine in preventing misacylation by phenylalanine-tRNA synthetase. J.Biol.Chem. *256*, 6729–6735.

Lopatin, A.N., Makhina, E.N. and Nichols, C.G. (1994) Potassium channel block by cytoplasmic polyamines as the mechanism of intrinsic rectification. Nature *372*, 366–369.

Luft, F.C. and Evans, A.P. (1980) Comparative effects of tobramycin and gentamicin on glomerular ultrastructure. J. Infect. Dis. *142*, 910–914.

Luft, F.C. and Kleit, S.A. (1974) Renal parenchymal accumulation of aminoglycoside antibiotics in rats. J. Infect. Dis. *130*, 656–659.

Lundberg, G.A., Jergil, B.A. and Sundler, R. (1986) Phosphatidylinositol 4-phosphate kinase from rat brain. Activation by polyamines and inhibition by phosphatidylinositol 4, 5-diphosphate. Eur. J. Biochem. *161*, 257–262.

Lyos, A.T., Winter, W.E. and Henley, C.M. III (1992) Kanamycin inhibits cochlear-renal ODC in neonatal rats. Otolaryngol. Head Neck Surg. *107*, 501–510.

Macdonald, R.L. and Rock, D.M. (1995) Polyamine regulation of N-methyl-D-aspartate receptor. Ann. Rev. Pharmacol. Toxicol. *35*, 463–482.

Mack, W.M. Zimanyi, I. and Pessah, I.N. (1992) Discrimination of multiple binding sites for antagonists of the calcium release channel complex of skeletal and cardiac sarcoplasmic reticulum. J. Pharmacol. Exp. Ther. *262*, 1028–1037.

Marvizon, J.C. and Baudry, M. (1994) [^{3}H]Dizocilpine association kinetics distinguish stimulatory and inhibitory polyamine sites of N-Methyl-D-aspartate receptors. J. Neurochem. *63*, 963–971.

Mates, S.M., Patel, L., Kaback, H.R. and Miller, M.H. (1983) Membrane potential in anaerobically growing *Staphylococcus aureus* and its relationship to gentamicin uptake. Antimicrob. Agents Chemother. *23*, 526–530.

Missiaen, L., Wuytack, F., Raeymaekers, L., De Smedt, H. and Casteels, R. (1989) Polyamines and neomycin inhibit the purified plasma-membrane Ca^{2+} pump by interacting with associated polyphosphoinositides. Biochem. J. *261*, 1055–1058.

Monti, M.G., Marverti, G., Ghiaroni, S., Piccinini, G., Pernecco, L. and Moruzzi, M.S. (1994) Spermine protects protein kinase C from phospholipid-induced inactivation. Experientia *50*, 953–957.

Morgan, P.F. and Stone, T.W. (1983) Structure-activity studies on the potentiation of benzodiazepin receptor binding by ethylenediamine analogues and derivatives. Br. J Pharmacol. *79*, 973–978.

Moruzzi, M., Barbiroli, B., Monti, M.G., Tadolini, B., Hakim, G., and Mezzetti, G. (1987) Inhibitory action of polyamines on protein kinase C association to membranes. Biochem. J. *247*, 175–180.

Moruzzi, M., Monti, M.G., Piccinini, G., Marverti, G. and Tadolini, B. (1990) Effect of spermine on association of protein kinase C with phospholipid vesicles. Life Sci. *47*, 1475–1482.

Moulinoux, J.P., Darcel, F., Quemener, V., Havouis, R. and Seiler, N. (1991) Inhibition of the growth of U-251 human glioblastoma in nude mice by polyamine deprivation. Anticancer Res. *11*, 175–180.

Moulinoux, J.P., Quemener, V., Cipolla, B., Guille, F., Havouis, R., Martin, C., Lobel, B. and Seiler, N. (1991) The growth of MAT-LyLu rat prostatic adenocarcinoma can be prevented *in vivo* by polyamine deprivation. J. Urol. *146*, 1408–1412.

Moya, E. and Blagbrough, I.S. (1994) Syntheses and neuropharmacological properties of arthropod polyamine amide toxins. In: The Neuropharmacology of Polyamines (Carter, C., ed.) pp. 167–184.

Munir, M., Subramanian, S. and McGonigle, P. (1993) Polyamines modulate the neurotoxic effects of NMDA *in vivo*. Brain Res. *616*, 163–170.

Nagai, T., Takauji, M. and Takahashi, S. (1969) Aliphatic polyamines as interaction inhibitors of actomyosin systems. Am. J. Physiol. *217*, 743–746.

Nahas, N. and Graff, G. (1982) Inhibitory activity of polyamines on phospholipase C from human platelets. Biochem. Biophys. Res. Commun. *109*, 1035–1040.

Nakae, R. and Nakae, T. (1982) Diffusion of aminoglycoside antibiotics accross the outer membrane of *Escherichia coli*. Antimicrob. Agents Chemother. *22*, 554–559.

Nastri, H.G. and Algranati, I.D. (1988) Inhibition of protein synthesis by aminoglycoside antibiotics in polyamine-requiring bacteria. Biochem. Biophys. Res. Commun. *150*, 947–954.

Nastri, H.G., Fastame, I.G. and Algranati, I.D. (1993) Polyamines modulate streptomycin-induced mistranslation in *Escherichia coli*. Biochim. Biophys. Acta *1216*, 455–459.

Nicchitta, C.V. and Williamson, J.R. (1984) Spermine: A regulator of mitochondrial calcium cycling. J. Biol. Chem. *21*, 12978–12983.

Nicolas, C. and Carter, C. (1994) Autoradiographic distribution and characteristics of high- and low-affinity polyamine-sensitive [^{3}H]ifenprodil sites in the rat brain: possible relationship to NMDAR2B receptors and calmodulin. J. Neurochem. *63*, 2248–2258.

Nicoll, R.A., Kauer, J.A. and Malenka, R.C. (1988) The current excitement in long-term potentiation. Neuron *1*, 97–103.

Nishizuka, Y. (1986) Studies and perspectives of protein kinase C. Science 233, 305–312.

Oblin, A., Bidet, S. and Schoemaker, H. (1992) Polyamines modulate the binding of the NMDA antagonist [³H]CGP 39653 via the glycine site. Br. J. Pharmacol. 105, 182P.

Oblin, A., Carter, C. and Schoemaker, H. (1994) Pharmacological characterisation of the binding of the glycine antagonist [³H]5,7-dichlorokynurenate and its modulation by spermine. Br. J. Pharmacol. 112, 355P.

Oriol-Audit, C. (1985) Actin and polyamines: a further approach to the cytokinesis mechanism. in:Recent Progress in Polyamine Research (Selmeci, L., Brosnan, M.E. and Seiler, N., eds.) pp. 151–160. Akademiai Kiado, Budapest.

Orsulakova, A., Stockhorst, E. and Schacht, J. (1975) Effect of neomycin on phosphoinositide labelling and calcium binding in guinea pig inner ear tissues *in vivo* and *in vitro*. J. Neurochem. 26, 285–290.

Osborne, D.L. and Seidel, E.R. (1989) Microflora-derived polyamines modulate obstruction-induced colonic mucosal hypertrophy. Am. J. Physiol. 256, G 1049–G 1057.

Palade, P. (1987) Drug-induced Ca^{2+}-release from isolated sarcoplasmic reticulum. III. Block of Ca^{2+}-induced Ca^{2+}-releasebyorganicpolyamines. J. Biol. Chem. 262, 6149–6154.

Pastoriza-Munoz, E., Bowman, R.L. and Kaloyanides, G.J. (1979) Renal tubular transport of gentamicin in the rat. Kidney Int. 16, 440–450.

Paul, I.A., Kuypers, G., Youdim, M., and Skolnick, B. (1990) Polyamines noncompetitively inhibit [³H]3-PPP binding to sigma receptors. Eur. J. Pharmacol. 184, 203–204.

Pedersen, S.B., Hougard, D.M. and Richelsen, B. (1989) Polyamines in rat adipocytes: their localization and their effects on insulin receptor binding. Mol Cell. Endocrinol. 62, 161–166.

Pegg, A.E. (1986) Recent advances in the biochemistry of polyamines in eukaryotes. Biochem. J. 234, 249–262.

Periyasami, S., Kothapalli, M.R. and Hoss, W. (1994) Regulation of the phosphoinositide cascade by polyamines in brain. J. Neurochem. 63, 1319–1327.

Peter, H.W., Wolf, U. and Seiler, N. (1973) Influence of polyamines on two bivalent-cation-activated ATPases. Hoppe-Seyler's Z. Physiol. Chem. 354, 1146–1148.

Pettersson, K., Koivula, T. and Kokko, E. (1984) Binding of tyrosin A[¹²⁵I]monoiodoinsulin to human erythrocytes. Scand. Clin. Lab. Invest. 44, 393–400.

Phillippe, M. (1994) Neomycin inhibition of hormone-stimulated smooth muscle contractions in myometrial tissue. Biochem. Biophys. Res. Commun. 205, 245–250.

Pinna, L.A. (1990) Casein kinase 2: an "eminence grise" in cellular regulation? Biochim. Biophys. Acta 1054, 267–284.

Prentki, M., Deeney, J., Matschinsky, F.M. and Joseph, S.K. (1986) Neomycin a specific drug to study the inositol-phospholipid signalling system? FEBS Lett. 197, 285–288.

Pujol, R. (1986) Periods of sensitivity to antibiotic treatment. Acta Otolaryngol. 249, 29–33.

Pullan, L.M. and Powel, R.J. (1991) Spermine reciprocally changes the affinity of NMDA receptor agonists and antagonists. Eur. J. Pharmacol. 207, 173–174.

Pullan, L.M., Keith, R.A., LaMonte, D., Stumpo, R.J. and Salama, A.I. (1990) The polyamine spermine affects omega-conotoxin binding and function at N-type voltage-sensitive calcium channels. J. Auton. Pharmacol. 10, 213–219.

Pullan, L.M., Stumpo, R.J., Powel, R.J., Paschetto, K.A. and Britt, M. (1992) Neomycin is an agonist at a polyamine site on the N-methyl-D-aspartate receptor. J. Neurochem. 59, 2087–2093.

Quarfoth, G., Ahmed, K. and Foster, D. (1978) Effects of polyamines on partial reactions of membrane (Na⁺, K⁺)ATPase. Biochim. Biophys. Acta 526, 580–590.

Qi, D.F., Schatzmann, R.C., Mazzei, G.J., Turner, R.S., Raynor, R.L. Liao, S. and Kuo, J.F. (1983) Polyamines inhibit phospholipid-sensitive and calmodulin-sensitive Ca^{2+}-dependent protein kinases. J. Biochem. *213*, 281–288.

Queener, S.F., Luft, F.C. and Hamel, F.G. (1983) Effect of gentamicin treatment on adenylate cyclase and Na^+, K^+-ATPase activity in renal tissues of rats. Antimicrob. Agents Chemother. *24*, 815–818.

Quemener, V., Moulinoux, J.P., Khan, N.A. and Seiler, N. (1990) Effects of a series of homologous α,ω-dimethylaminoalkanes on cell proliferation, and binding and uptake of putrescine by a human glioblastoma cell line (U251) in culture. Biol. Cell. *70*, 133–137.

Quemener, V., Moulinoux, J.P., Havouis, R. and Seiler, N. (1992) Polyamine deprivation enhances antitumoral efficacy of chemotherapy. Anticancer Res. *12*, 1447–1454.

Ransom, R.W. (1991) Polyamine and ifenprodil interactions with the NMDA receptor's glycine site. Eur. J. Pharmacol. *208*, 67–71.

Ransom, R.W. and Stec, N.L. (1988) Cooperative modulation of [^{3}H]MK801 binding to the N-methyl-D-aspartate receptor-ion channel complex by L-glutamate, glycine and polyamines. J. Neurochem. *51*, 830–836.

Rasmussen, H. and Barrett, P.Q. (1984) Calcium messenger system: an integrated view. Physiol. Rev. *64*, 938–984.

Renard, D. and Poggioli, J. (1990) Mediation by GTP(γS) and Ca^{2+} of inositol triphosphate generation in rat heart membranes. J. Mol. Cell. Cardiol. *22*, 13–22.

Reynolds, I.J. (1990) Arcaine uncovers dual interactions of polyamines with the N-methyl-D-aspartate receptor. J. Pharmacol. Exp. Ther. *255*, 1001–1007.

Reynolds, I.J. (1992) 1,5-(Diethylamino)piperidine, a novel spermidine analogue that more specifically activates the N-methyl-D-aspartate receptor-associated polyamine site. Mol. Pharmacol. *41*, 989–992

Reynolds, I.J. and Miller, R.J. (1989) Ifenprodil is a novel type of N-methyl-D-aspartate receptor antagonist: interaction with polyamines. Mol. Pharmacol. *36*, 758–765.

Rilo, M.C. and Stoppani, A.O.M. (1993) Effect of polyamines on mitochondrial F-ATPase from *Crithidia fasciculata* and *Trypanosoma cruzi*. Biochem. Int. *29*, 131–139.

Ritz, M.C., Mantione, C.R. and London, E.D. (1994) Spermine interacts with cocaine binding sites on dopamine transporters. Psychopharmacology *114*, 47–52.

Rock, D.M. and Macdonald, R.L. (1992) Spermine and related polyamines produce a voltage-dependent reduction of N-methyl-D-aspartate receptor single-channel conductance. Mol. Pharmacol. *42*, 157–164.

Rock, C.O. and Jackowski, S. (1987) Thrombin- and nucleotide-activated phophatidylinositol 4,5-bisphosphate phospholipase C in human platelet membranes. J. Biol. Chem. *262*, 5492–5498.

Rolston, K.V. and Bodev, G.P. (1992) Pseudomonas aeruginosa infection in cancer patients. Cancer Invest. *10*, 43–49.

Rolston, K.V., Ho, D.H., LeBlanc, B. and Bodev, G.P. (1993) *In vitro* activities of antimicrobial agents against clinical isolates of *Flavimonas oryzihabitans* obtained from patients with cancer. Antimicrob. Agents Chemother. *37*, 2504–2505.

Romano, C. and Williams, K. (1994) Modulation of NMDA receptors by polyamines. in: The Neuropharmacology of Polyamines (Carter, C., ed.) pp. 81–106. Academic Press, London.

Rosenthal, S.M. and Tabor, C.W. (1956) The pharmacology of spermine and spermidine. Distribution and excretion. J. Pharmacol. Exptl. Therap. *116*, 131–138.

Rosenthal, S.M., Fisher, E.R. and Stohlmann, E.F. (1952) Nephrotoxic action of spermine. Proc. Soc. Exp. Biol. Med. *80*, 432–434.

Rottenberg, H. and Marbach, M. (1990) Regulation of Ca^{2+} transport in brain mitochondria I. The mechanism of spermine enhancement of Ca^{2+} uptake and retention. Biochim. Biophys. Acta *1016*, 77–86.

Rudkin, B.S., Mamont, P.S. and Seiler, N. (1984) Decreased protein-synthetic activity is an early consequence of spermidine depletion in rat hepatoma tissue culture cells. Biochem. J. *217*, 731–741.

Rustenbeck, I., Eggers, G., Münster, W. and Lenzen, S. (1993) Effect of spermine on mitochondrial matrix calcium in relation to its enhancement of mitochondrial calcium uptake. Biochem. Biophys. Res. Commun. *194*, 1261–1268.

Sacaan, A.I. and Johnson, K.M. (1989) Spermine enhances binding to the glycine site associated with the N-methyl-D-aspartate receptor complex. Mol. Pharmacol. *36*, 836–839.

Sagawa, N., Bleasdale, J.F. and DiRenzo, G.C. (1983) The effects of polyamines and aminoglycosides on phosphatidylinositol-specific phospholipase C from human amnion. Biochim. Biophys. Acta *752*, 153–161.

Sande, M.A. and Mandell, G.L. (1990) Antimicrobial agents. The Aminoglycosides. In: The Pharmacological Basis of Therapies (Goodman Gilman, A., Rall, T.W., Nies, A.S., and Taylor, P., eds.), 8th ed. pp. 1098–1115, Pergamon Press, New York.

Sander, G., Parlato, G. Crechet, J.B., Nagel, K. and Parmeggiani, A. (1978) Regulation of turnover GTPase activity of elongation factor G: The 30S-coupled and 30S-uncoupled reaction. Coordinated effects of cations, pH and polyamines. Eur. J. Biochem. *86*, 555–563.

Sarhan, S., Knödgen, B., and Seiler, N. (1989) The gastrointestinal tract as polyamine source for tumor growth. Anticancer Res. *9*, 215–224.

Sarhan, S., Weibel, M. and Seiler, N. (1991) Effect of polyamine deprivation on the survival of intracranial glioblastoma bearing rats. Anticancer Res. *11*, 987–992.

Sarhan, S., Knödgen, B. and Seiler, N. (1992) Polyamine deprivation, malnutrition and tumor growth. Anticancer Res. *12*, 457–466.

Sarno, S., Marin, O., Meggio, F. and Pinna, L. (1993) Polyamines as negative regulators of casein kinase-2: The phosphorylation of calmodulin triggered by polylysine and by the $\alpha(66-86)$ peptide is prevented by spermine. Biochem. Biophys. Res. Commun. *194*, 83–90.

Sastrasinh, M., Knauss, T.C., Weinberg, J.M. and Humes, H.D. (1982) Identification of the aminoglycoside receptor of renal brush border membranes. J. Pharmacol. Exp. Ther. *222*, 350–358.

Sayers, L.G. and Michelangeli, F. (1993) The inhibition of the inositol 1,4,5-triphosphate receptor from rat cerebellum by spermine and other polyamines. Biochem. Biophys. Res. Commun. *197*, 1203–1208.

Schacht, J. (1976) Inhibition by neomycin of polyphosphoinositide turnover in subcellular fractions of guinea pig cerebral cortex *in vitro*. J. Neurochem. *27*, 1119–1124.

Schacht, J. (1979) Isolation of an aminoglycoside receptor from guinea pig inner ear tissues and kidney. Arch. Othorhinolaryngol. *224*, 129–134.

Schacht, J. (1986) Molecular mechanisms of drug-induced hearing loss. Hear Res. *22*, 297–304.

Schacht, J. and Van De Water, T. (1986) Uptake and accumulation of gentamicin in the developing inner ear of the mouse *in vitro*. Biochem. Pharmacol. *35*, 2843–2845.

Schechter, P.J., Barlow, J.L.R. and Sjoerdsma, A. (1987) Clinical aspects of inhibition of ornithine decarboxylase with emphasis on therapeutic trials of Eflornithine (DFMO) in cancer and protozoan diseases. In: Inhibition of Polyamine Metabolism. (McCann, P.P., Pegg, A.E. and Sjoerdsma, A., eds.) pp. 345–364, Academic Press, Orlando.

Schibeci, A. and Schacht, J. (1977) Action of neomycin on the metabolism of polyphosphoinositides in the guinea pig kidney. Biochem.Pharmacol. 26, 1769–1774.

Schoemaker, H. (1992) Polyamines allosterically modulate [³H]nitrendipine binding to the voltage-sensitive calcium chanel in rat brain. Eur. J. Pharmacol. 225, 167–169.

Schoemaker, H., Pigasse, S., Caboi, F. and Oblin, A. (1994) Polyamine effects on radioligand binding to receptors and recognition sites. In:The Neuropharmacology of Polyamines (Carter, C., ed.) pp. 107–154, Academic Press, London.

Schuber, F. (1989) Influence of polyamines on membrane functions. Biochem. J. 260, 1–10.

Scemama, J.L., Grabie, V. and Seidel, E.R. (1994) Characterization of univectorial polyamine transport in duodenal crypt cell line. Am. J. Physiol. 265, G851–G856.

Scott, R.H., Sweeney, M.I., Kobrinsky, E.M., Pearson, H.A., Timms, G.H., Pullar, I.A., Wedley, S. and Dolphin, A.C. (1992) Actions of arginine polyamine on voltage and ligand-activated whole cell currents recorded from cultured neurones. Br. J. Pharmacol. 106, 199–207.

Scott, R.H., Sutton, K.G. and Dolphin, A.C. (1993) Interactions of polyamines with neuronal ion channels. Trends Neurosci. 16, 153–160.

Scott, R.H., Sutton, K.G. and Dolphin, A.C. (1994) Modulation of neuronal voltage-activated Ca^{2+}-currents by polyamines. In:The Neuropharmacology of Polyamines, pp. 205–222, Academic Press, London.

Seiler, N. (1991) Pharmacological properties of the natural polyamines and their depletion by biosynthesis inhibitors as a therapeutic approach. In: Progress in Drug Research. (Jucker, E., ed.) Vol. 37, pp. 107–159, Birkhäuser Verlag, Basel.

Seiler, N. (1992) The role of polyamines in cell biology. In: Fundamentals of Medical Cell Biology, Vol. 3B, Chemistry of the Living Cell. (Bittar, E.E., ed.) pp. 509–528, Jai Press Inc. Greenwhich, USA.

Seiler, N. (1994) Formation, catabolism and properties of the natural polyamines. In:The Neuropharmacology of Polyamines, (Carter, C., ed.) pp. 1–36, Academic Press, London.

Seiler, N. and Deckardt, K. (1976) Association of putrescine, spermidine, spermine and GABA with structural elements of brain cells. Neurochem. Res. 1, 469–499.

Seiler, N. and Dezeure, F. (1990) Polyamine transport in mammalian cells. Int. J. Biochem. 22, 211–218.

Seiler, N. and Heby, O. (1988) Regulation of cellular polyamines in mammals. Acta Biochim. Biophys. Hung. 23, 1–36.

Seiler, N., Sarhan, S., Grauffel, C., Jones, R., Knödgen, B. and Moulinoux, J.P. (1990) Endogenous and exogenous polyamines in support of tumor growth. Cancer Res. 50, 5077–5083.

Seyfred, M.A., Farell, L.N. and Wells, W.W. (1984) Characterization of D-myo-inositol 1,4,5-triphosphate phosphatase in rat liver plasma membranes. J. Biol. Chem. 259, 13204–13208.

Shaw, G. (1994) Polyamines as neurotransmitters or modulators. In:The Neuropharmacology of Polyamines (Carter, C., ed.) pp. 61–80, Academic Press, London.

Siess, W. and Lapetina, E.G. (1986) Neomycin inhibits inositol phosphate formation in human platelets stimulated by thrombin but not other agonists. FEBS Lett. 207, 53–57.

Siimes, M. (1967) Studies on the metabolism of 1,4-¹⁴C-spermidine and 1,4-¹⁴C-spermine in the rat. Acta Physiol.Scand. (Suppl.) 298, 1–66.

Silverblatt, F.J. (1982) Pathogenesis of nephrotoxicity of cephalosporins and aminoglycosides: a review of current concepts. Rev. Infect. Dis. 4 (Suppl.) S360–S365.

Silverblatt, F.J. and Kuehn, C. (1979) Autoradiography of gentamicin uptake by the rat proximal tubule cell. Kidney Int. *15*, 335–345.

Singh, S.S., Chauhan, A., Brockerhoff, H. and Chauhan, V.P.S. (1994) Interaction of protein kinase C and phosphoinositides: regulation by polyamines. Cell. Signalling *6*, 345–353.

Sjöholm, A. (1992) Intracellular signal transduction pathways that control pancreatic β-cell proliferation. FEBS Lett. *311*, 85–90.

Sjöholm, A., Arkhammar, P., Welsh, N., Bokvist, K., Rorsman, P., Hallberg, A., Nilsson, T., Welsh, M. and Berggren, P.O. (1993) Enhanced stimulus-secretion coupling in polyamine-depleted rat insulinoma cells. An effect involving increased cytoplasmic Ca^{2+}, inositol phosphate generation and phorbol ester sensitivity. J. Cin. Invest. *92*, 1910–1917.

Smith, C.D. and Snyderman, R. (1988) Modulation of inositolphospholipid metabolism by polyamines. Biochem. J. *256*, 125–130.

Smith, C.D. and Wells, W.M. (1984) Characterization of a phosphatidylinositol 4-phosphate-specific phosphomonoesterase in rat liver nuclear envelopes. Arch. Biochem. Biophys. *235*, 529–537.

Sokol, P.P., Longenecker, K.L., Kachel, D.L. and Martin, W.J. (1993) Mechanism of putrescine transport in human pulmonary artery endothelial cells. J. Pharmacol. Exptl. Therap. *265*, 60–66.

Spath, M., Woscholski, R. and Schachtele, C. (1991) Characterization of multiple forms of phosphoinositide-specific phospholipase C from bovine aorta. Cell Signal. *3*, 305–310.

Speciale, C., Marconi, M., Raimondi, L., Bianchetti, A. and Fariello, R.G. (1992a) Extracellular polyamines in quinolinic acid-injected striatum. Ann. Soc. Neurosci. *18*, 84.

Speciale, C., Raimondi, L., Marconi, M., and Fariello, R.G. (1992b) Endogenous polyamines in the central nervous system: intracellular and extracellular compartments. Mol. Neuropharmacol. *2*, 121–123.

Stöffler, G. and Tischendorf, G.W. (1975) Antibiotic receptor sites in *E. coli* ribosomes. in: Drug Receptor Interactions in Antimicrobial Chemotherapy. Vol. 1. Topics in Infectious Diseases. (Drews, J. and Hahn, F.E., eds.) Springer Verlag, New York.

Stoehr, S.J. and Dooley, D.J. (1993) Characteristics of [^{125}I]omega-conotoxin MVIIA binding to rat neocortical membranes. Neurosci. Lett. *161*, 113–116.

Strosznajder, J. and Samochocki, M. (1991) Ca^{2+}-independent, Ca^{2+}-dependent, and carbachol-mediated arachidonic acid release from rat brain cortex membrane. J. Neurochem. *57*, 1198–1206.

Stumpo, R.J., Pullan, L.M. and Salama, A.I. (1991) The inhibition of (^{125}I)omega-conotoxin GVIA binding to neuronal membranes by neomycin may be mediated by a GTP-binding protein. Eur. J. Pharmacol. *206*, 155–158.

Subramaniam, S., O'Connor, M.J., Masulawa, L.M. and McGonigle, P. (1994) Polyamine effects on the NMDA receptor in human brain. Exp. Neurol. *130*, 323–330.

Suman-Chauhan, N., Webdale, L., Hill, D.R. and Woodruff, G.N. (1993) Characterisation of [^{3}H]gabapentin binding to a novel site in rat brain: homogenate binding studies. Eur. J. Pharmacol. *244*, 293–301.

Sunkara, P.S., Baylin, S.B. and Luk, G.D. (1987) Inhibitors of polyamine biosynthesis: Cellular and *in vivo* effects on tumor proliferation. In: Inhibition of Polyamine Metabolism. (McCann, P.P., Pegg, A.E. and Sjoerdsma, A., eds.) pp. 121–140, Academic Press, Orlando.

Suzuki, S., Hatashima, S., Shinzawa, Y., Niwa, O. and Tamatani, R. (1994) Toxicity of neomycin on enzyme activities of kidney and duonenal mucosa *in vivo*: organ specificity and species difference between rats and mice. Comp. Biochem. Physiol. *109*C, 77–92.

Swift, T.A. and Dias, J.A. (1986) Effects of the polyamine spermine on binding of follicle-stimulating hormone to membrane-bound immature bovine testis receptors. Biochim. Biophys. Acta *885*, 221–230.

Tadolini, B. anbd Varani, E. (1986) Interaction of spermine with polyphosphoinositides containing liposomes and myo-inositol 1,4,5-triphosphate. Biochem. Biophys. Res. Commun. *135*, 58–64.

Tai, P.C., Wallace, B.J. and Davies, B.D. (1978) Streptomycin causes misreading of natural messenger by interacting with ribosomes after initiation. Proc. Natl. Acad. Sci. USA *75*, 275–279.

Takano, M., Ohishi, Y., Okuda, M., Yasuhara, M. and Hori, R. (1994) Transport of gentamicin and fluid-phase endocytosis markers in the LLC-PK1 kidney epithelial cell line. J. Pharmacol. Exptl. Therap. *268*, 669–674.

Tassani, V., Ciman, M., Sartorelli, L., Toninello, A. and Siliprandi, D. (1995) Polyamine content and spermine transport in rat brain mitochondria. Neurosci. Res. Commun. *16*, 11–18.

Thompson, R.C. and Karim, A.M. (1982) The accuracy of protein biosynthesis is limited by its speed: High fidelity selection by ribosomes of aminoacyl-tRNA ternary complexes containing GTP(γS). Proc. Natl. Acad. Sci.USA *79*, 4922–4926.

Toner, M., Vaio, G., McLaughlin, A.M. and McLaughlin, S. (1988) Adsorption of cations to phosphatidylinositol 4,5-biphosphate. Biochemistry *27*, 7435–7443.

Toninello, A., Via, L.D., Siliprandi, D. and Garlid, K.D. (1992) Evidence that spermine, spermidine and putrescine are transported electrophoretically in mitochondria by a specific polyamine uniporter. J. Biol. Chem. *267*, 18393–18397.

Tysnes, O.B., Johanessen, E. and Steen, V.M. (1991) Neomycin does not interfere with the inositol phospholipid metabolism, but blocks binding of α-thrombin to intact human platelets. Biochem. J. *273*, 241–243.

Umezawa, H. (1983) Role of amines in the action of antibiotics – bleomycin, spergualin and aminoglycosides. in: Advances in Polyamine Research, Vol. 4 (Bachrach, U., Kaye, A. and Chayen, R., eds.) pp. 1–15, Raven Press, New York.

Usherwood, P.N.R. and Blagbrough, I.S. (1991) Spidertoxins affecting glutamate receptors: Polyamines in therapeutic neurochemistry. Pharmacol. Ther. *52*, 245–268.

Usherwood, P.N.R. and Blagbrough, I.S. (1994) Electrophysiology of polyamines and polyamine amides. In: The Neuropharmacology of Polyamines (Carter, C., ed.) pp. 185–204, Academic Press, London.

Van Bambeke, F., Mingeot-Leclercq, M.P., Schanck, A., Brasseur, R. and Tulkens, P.M. (1993) Alterations in membrane permeability induced by aminoglycoside antibiotics: studies on liposomes and cultured cells. Eur. J. Pharmacol. *247*, 155–168.

Vanhanen, H. (1994) Cholesterol malabsorption caused by sitostanol ester feeding and neomycin in pravastatin-treated hypercholesterolaemic patients. Eur. J. Clin. Pharmacol. *47*, 169–176.

Van Rooijen, L.A.A. and Agranoff, B.W. (1985) Inhibition of phosphoinositide phosphodiesterase by aminoglycoside antibiotics. Neurochem.Res. *8*, 1019–1024.

Venho, V.M.K. (1986) Toxicants in the gastrointestinal tract: Drugs. in Gastrointestinal Toxicology (Rozman, K. and Hännien, O. eds. pp. 363–396, Elsevier Amsterdam.

Vergara, J., Tsien, R.Y. and Delay, M. (1985) Inositol 1,4,5-triphosphate: a possible chemical link in excitation coupling in muscle. Proc. Natl. Acad. Sci. USA *82*, 6352–6356.

Vogel, S. and Hoppe, J. (1986) Polyamines stimulate the phosphorylation of phosphatidylinositol in membranes from A 431 cells. Eur. J. Biochem. *154*, 253–257.

Wagner, J.A., Snowman, A.M., Biswas, A., Olivera, B.M. and Snyder, S.H. (1988) Omega-conotoxin GVIA binding to a high-affinity receptor in brain: characterization, calcium sensitivity, and solubilization. J. Neurosci. *8*, 3354–3359.

Walters, J.D. and Johnson, J.D. (1988) Inhibition of cyclic nucleotide phosphodiesterase and calcineurin by spermine, a calcium-independent calmodulin antagonist. Biochim. Biophys. Acta *957*, 138–142.

Walters, J.D., Sorboro, D.M. and Chapman, K.J. (1992) Polyamines enhance calcium mobilization in fMet-Leu-Phe-stimulated phagocytes. FEBS Lett. *304*, 37–40.

Wasserkort, R., Hoppe, E., Reddington, M. and Schubert, P. (1991) Modulation of A1 adenosine receptor function in rat brain by the polyamine spermine. Neurosci. Lett. *124*, 183–186.

Wible, B.A., Taglialatela, M., Ficker, E. and Brown, A.M. (1994) Gating of inwardly rectifying K$^+$ channels localized to a single negatively charged residue. Nature *371*, 246–249.

Williams, K., Romano, C., Dichter, M.A. and Molinoff, P.B. (1991) Modulation of NMDA receptor by polyamines. Life Sci. *48*, 469–498.

Williams, K., Pullan, L.M., Romano, C., Powel, R., Salama, A. and Molinoff, P. (1992) An antagonist/partial agonist at the polyamine recognition site of the N-methyl-D-aspartate receptor that alters the properties of the glutamate recognition site. J. Pharmacol. Exp. Ther. *262*, 539–544.

Williams, P.D., Trimble, M.E., Crespo, L., Holohan, P.D., Freedman, J.C. and Ross, C.R. (1984) Inhibition of renal Na$^+$/K$^+$-adenosine triphosphatase by gentamicin. J. Pharmacol. Exp. Ther. *231*, 248–253.

Williams, S.E., Smith, D.E. and Schacht, J. (1987) Characteristics of gentamicin uptake in the isolated crista ampullaris of the inner ear of the guinea pig. Biochem. Pharmacol. *36*, 89–95.

Wojcikiewicz, R.J.H. and Fain, J.N. (1988) Polyamines inhibit phopsholipase C-catalysed polyphosphoinositide hydrolysis. Studies with permeabilized GH$_3$ cells. Biochem. J. *255*, 1015–1021.

Wojcikiewicz, R.J.H. and Nahorski, S.R. (1989) Phosphoinositide hydrolysis in permeabilized SH-SY5Y human neuroblastoma cells is inhibited by mastoparan. FEBS Lett. *247*, 341–344.

Wojcikiewicz, R.J.H., Lambert, D.G. and Nahorski, S.R. (1990) Regulation of Muscarinic agonist-induced activation of phosphoinositidase C in electrically permeabilized SH-SY5Y human neuroblastoma cells by guanine nucleotides. J. Neurochem. *54*, 676–685.

Wyskovsky, W. (1994) Caffeine-induced calcium oscillations in heavy sarcoplasmic reticulum vesicles from rabbit skeletal muscle. Eur. J. Biochem. *221*, 317–325.

Yang, W. and Boss, W.F. (1994) Regulation of the plasma membrane type II phosphatidylinositol-4 kinase by positively charged compounds. Arch. Biochem. Biophys. *313*, 112–119.

Yano, M., Elhayek, R., Antoniu, B. and Ikemoto, N. (1994) Neomycin: A novel potent blocker of communication between T-tubule and sarcoplasmic reticulum. FEBS Lett. *351*, 349–352.

Yung, M.W. and Green, C. (1986) The binding of polyamines to phospholipid bilayers. Biochem. Pharmacol. *35*, 4037–4041.

Yung, M.W. and Wright, A. (1987) Cochleotoxic effects of spermine and kanamycin. Ann. Otol. Rhinol. Laryngol. *96*, 455–460.

Zarka, A. and Shoshan-Barmatz, V. (1992) The interaction of spermine with the ryanodine receptor from skeletal muscle. Biochim. Biophys. Acta *1108*, 13–20.

Zierhut, G., Piepersberg, W. and Böck, A. (1979) Comparative analysis of the effect of aminoglycosides on bacterial protein synthesis. Eur. J. Biochem. *98*, 577–583.

Zimanyi, I. and Pessah, I.N. (1991) Comparison of [^{3}H]ryanodine receptors and Ca^{2+}-release from rat cardiac and rabbit skeletal muscle sarcoplasmic reticulum. J. Pharmacol. Exp. Ther. *256*, 938–946.

Progress in Drug Research, Vol. 46 (E. Jucker, Ed.)
© 1996 Birkhäuser Verlag, Basel (Switzerland)

Recent developments in antidepressant agents

By James Claghorn and Michael D. Lesem

Claghorn-Lesem Research Clinic Inc., Houston, Texas, USA

1   Introduction

Major depressive disorder is a common illness in the United States. It has a one-month prevalence of 2.2%, a lifetime prevalence of 5.8% [1], and a 15% mortality rate [2]. It imposes an economic burden of billions of dollars lost as a result of worker absenteeism and disability.

The first effective pharmacotherapy of depression came with the advent of monoamine oxidase inhibitors (MAOI's). After initial observations of a possible antidepressant effect among tuberculosis patients who received iproniazid [3], further investigation by Nathan Kline [4] and others lead to the development of these agents as the first true antidepressant medications. These agents have currently gathered a reputation of being effective for atypical depression [5]. The MAOI's popular in the United States are phenelzine (Nardil) and tranylcypromine (Parnate) (Figure 1). Both are relatively nonselective for the MAO-A and MAO-B subtypes of the MAOI enzymes [6]. Because of dietary restrictions and the risk of tyramine-induced hypertensive crisis, their use has been limited. Also included in this first generation of antidepressant agents are the tricyclic antidepressants (TCA). They were discovered to have antidepressant activity in the late 1950s when imipramine, then being studied as a potential antipsychotic agent, was noted to have mood-elevating effects [7]. From this discovery, a number of antidepressant agents evolved with the tricyclic ring as their common denominator (Figure 2). These agents all share the action of blocking neuronal reuptake of norepinephrine (NE) and serotonin, but in varying degrees [8]. Table 1 illustrates the degrees of reuptake selectivity of biogenic amines by the TCA's, and it demonstrates how the side-effect profiles of these different tricyclics vary, based on each drug's binding affinity for adrenergic, histaminergic, and muscarinic receptors. Typically, the tertiary amines are more serotonergic in their reuptake blockade, as well as more anticholinergic and sedative, than their 2° amine metabolites [9, 10]. Tricyclic antidepressants, although often associated with significant side effects, are still considered the most effective agents for the treatment of moderate to severe depression [11–13].

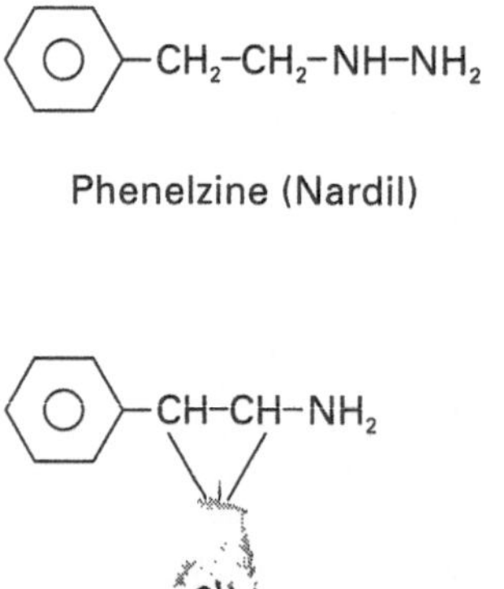

Phenelzine (Nardil)

Tranylcypromine (Parnate)

Fig. 1.

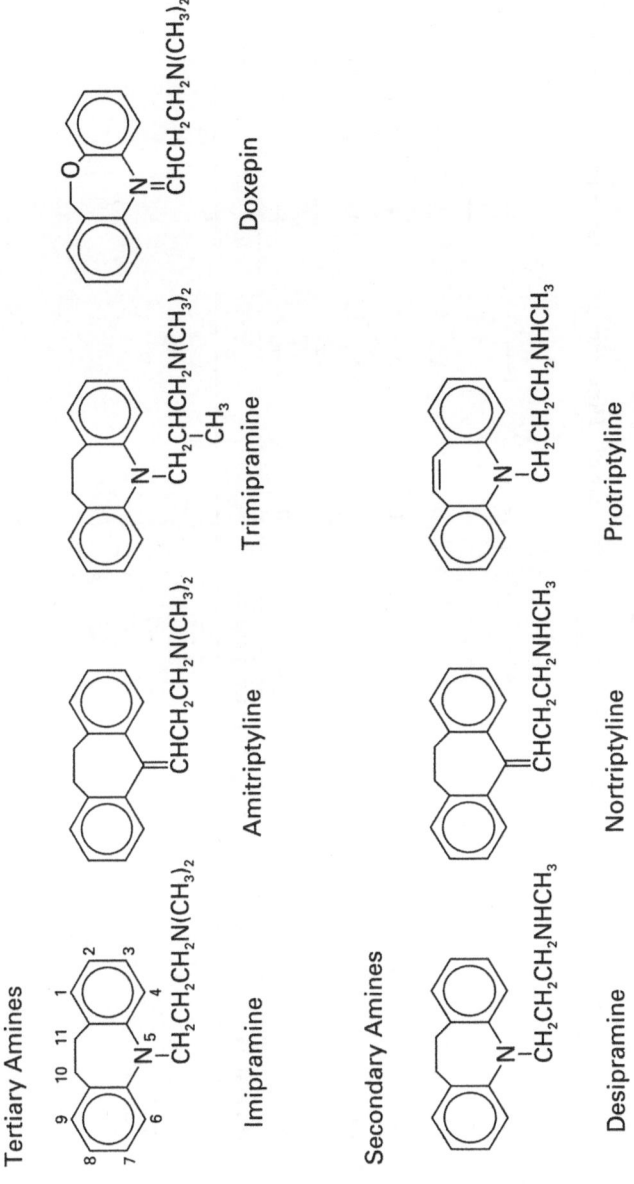

Fig. 2.
Tricyclic antidepressants.

Reprinted with permission from R. Baldessarini: *Chemotherapy in Psychiatry*. Harvard University Press, Cambridge 1985.

Table 1.

	Inhibition of reuptake			Receptor affinity				
	Norepinephrine	Serotonin	Dopamine	Adrenergic	Adrenergic	H₁ Histaminergic	Muscarinic	D₂ Dopaminergic
Older Drugs								
Amitriptyline	±	++	0	+++	±	++++	++++	0
Nortriptyline	++	±	0	+	0	+	++	0
Imipramine	+	+	0	++	0	+	++	0
Desipramine	+++	0	0	+	0	0	+	0
Clomipramine	+	+++	0	++	0	+	++	0
Trimipramine	+	0	0	++	±	+++	++	+
Doxepin	++	+	0	++	0	+++	++	0

Reprinted with permission from W. Potter et al., New Engl. J. Med. 325, 663–642 (1991).

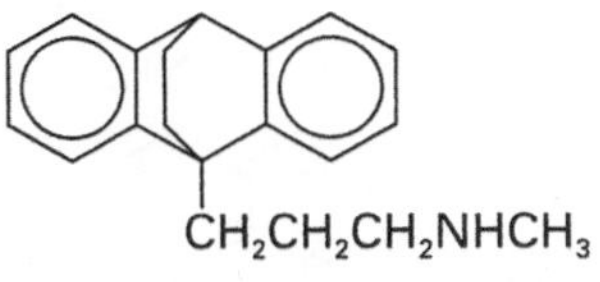

Maprotiline

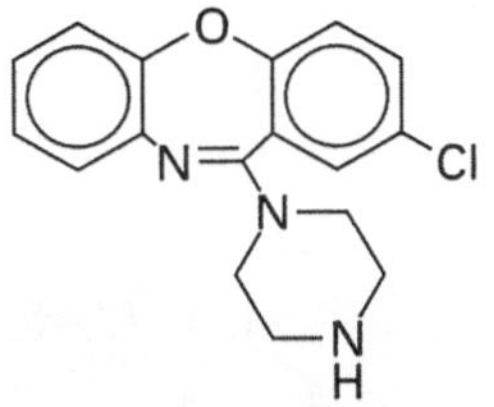

Amoxapine

Atypical agents

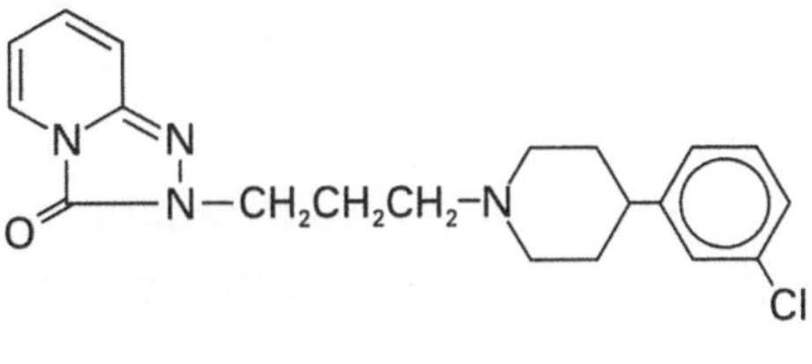

Trazodone

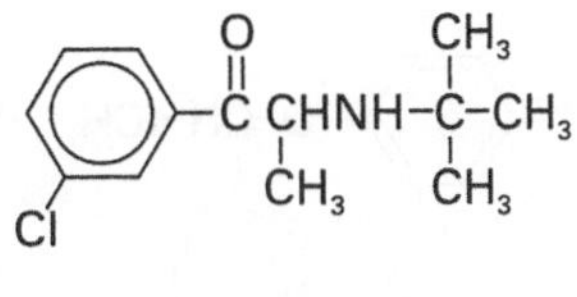

Bupropion

Fig. 3.
Second-generation antidepressant agents.

Reprinted with permission from R. Baldessarini: *Chemotherapy in Psychiatry.* Harvard University Press, Cambridge 1985.

The second-generation antidepressant agents came on the U.S. market in the 1980s. This group typically includes maprotiline, amoxapine, trazodone, and bupropion (Figure 3). Amoxapine and maprotiline are frequently referred to as heterocyclic and tetracyclic, but they are chemically tricyclic [6]. Trazodone and bupropion are chemically dissimilar to tricyclics and do not have a tricyclic ring (Figure 3).

Amoxapine and maprotiline exhibit presynaptic reuptake blockade of serotonin and norepinephrine similar to that of the first-generation tricyclic agents [14]. Trazodone seems to generate its pharmacological effect through the reuptake blockade of serotonin [15], although its active metabolite m-chlorophenyl-piperazine, may also play a role through its effect

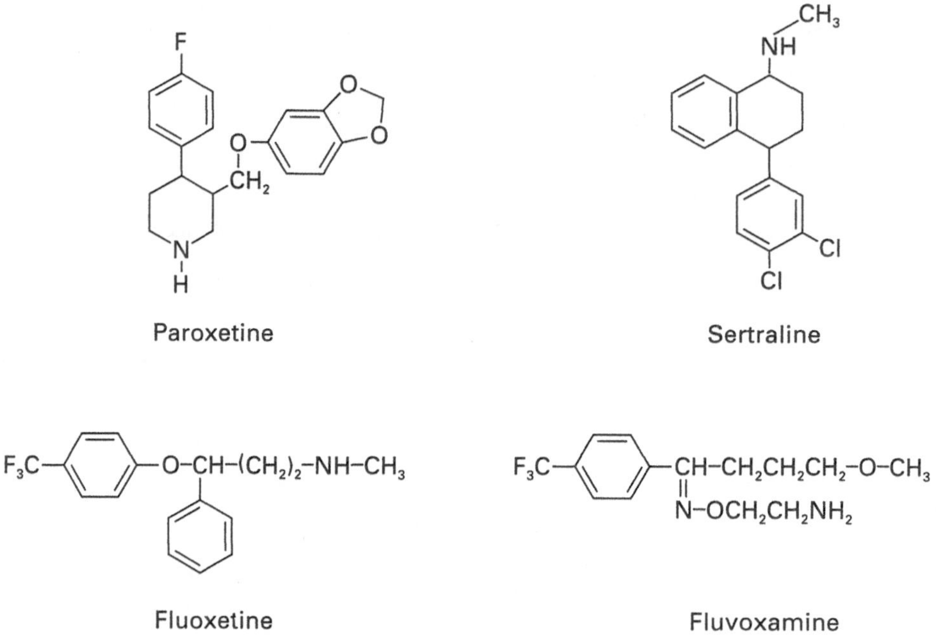

Paroxetine

Sertraline

F_3C—⟨⟩—O-CH-(CH$_2$)$_2$-NH-CH$_3$

Fluoxetine

F_3C—⟨⟩—CH-CH$_2$CH$_2$CH$_2$-O-CH$_3$
∥
N-OCH$_2$CH$_2$NH$_2$

Fluvoxamine

Fig. 4.
The selective serotonin reuptake inhibitors.

Reprinted with permission from S. R. Grimsley and M. W. Jann: Clin. Pharmacol. 2, 930–957 (1992).

on the 5-hydroxy tryptamine-lc (5-HT$_{1c}$) receptor [16]. The mechanism of action of bupropion is unclear. A weak inhibitor of dopamine reuptake, it is metabolized into compounds with stimulant-like effect [17], and it weakly affects NE reuptake [18].

The second-generation medications represent a relatively small share in the clinical use of antidepressants, perhaps because of their side-effect profiles. Amoxapine has been associated with a higher incidence of extrapyramidal effects (EPS) [19]. Maprotiline and bupropion are associated with a higher incidence of seizures [20]. The long-term efficacy of trazodone has been questioned.

Table 2.
Inhibition of [³H]-5-HT and [³H]-NA uptake into rat hypothalamic synaptosomes *in vitro* (after Johnson 1991: Thomas et al. 1987)

Compound	K_i (nmol/l)		K_i ratio
	[³H]-5-HT	[³H]-NA	(NA:5-HT)
Citalopram	2.6	3900	1500
Fluoxetine	25	500	20
Fluvoxamine	6.2	1100	180
Paroxetine	1.1	350	320
Sertraline	7.3	?	190

Abbreviations: 5-HT, 5-hydroxytryptamine (serotonin); NA, noradrenaline (norepinephrine); K_i, inhibitor constant
Reprinted with permission from J. van Harten: Clin. Pharmacokinet. *24*/3, 203–220 (1993).

The advent of selective serotonin reuptake inhibitors (SSRI) represented a further evolution in antidepressant agents (Figure 4). Fluoxetine, the first agent approved by the U.S. Food and Drug Administration (FDA) for major depressive disorder (MDD), was followed by sertraline and paroxetine. Fluvoxamine (Luvox) has most recently come into clinical use, but it has been approved only for treatment of obsessive compulsive disorder (OCD).

Although chemically dissimilar, these agents seem to exert their effects by blocking the reuptake of 5-HT, which leads to an increase in serotonin in the synaptic cleft [21]. The fact that these agents exhibit minimal binding to any specific neuroreceptor system contributes to their favorable side-effect profile [22]. They also differ in a number of ways pharmacologically, specifically in their binding affinity to the serotonin carrier, in half-life, in degree of protein binding, and in their effect on the cytochrome P450 system. In preferential serotonin binding affinity, weakest to strongest affinity is found in fluoxetine, sertraline, fluvoxamine, and paroxetine, in that order (Table 2) [23, 24]. No relationship between binding affinity and pharmacological effect has been verified.

Half-life ($t_{1/2}$) varies greatly among these newer agents, as do active metabolites. Fluoxetine has a $t_{1/2}$ of 1.9 days and an active metabolite, norfluoxetine, with a $t_{1/2}$ of seven days; it does not reach a steady state for 30 days [25, 26]. In contrast sertraline, fluvoxamine, and paroxetine are not believed to have active metabolites [27]. Sertraline has a $t_{1/2}$ of about 26 hours [28] and reaches a relatively steady state in one to two weeks. Paroxetine has a $t_{1/2}$ of 24 hours and reaches a steady state also in one to two weeks [29]. Fluvoxamine has the shortest $t_{1/2}$, 14.6 hours, reaching a steady state in

Table 3.
Relative Potency (K_i, μm) of three different serotonin selective reuptake inhibitors and their metabolites for inhibiting the functional integrity of the hepatic isoenzyme IID*†

Drug	Crewe et al.	Von Moltke et al.	Sellers	Otton et al.
Paroxetine	0.15	–	0.065	–
M2	0.50	–	–	–
Fluoxetine	0.60	3.0	0.15	0.17
Norfluoxetine	0.43	3.5	–	0.19
Sertraline	0.70	22.7	1.2	1.5
Desmethylsertraline	–	16.9	–	–

* Based on *in vitro* studies using human hepatic microsomes.
† K_i: inhibition constant, the smaller the value, the greater the potency on a molar basis.
Reprinted with permission from S. Preskon: J. Clin. Psychiatry *54*(9) (suppl.), 14–34 (1993).

about seven days [30]. Because of fluvoxamine's shorter half-life, it is the only SSRI given in a multi-dose schedule of twice a day.

Most of the SSRI's are highly protein-bound; fluoxetine, sertraline, and paroxetine are more than 95% protein-bound [25], thereby displacing such other highly protein-bound drugs as warfarin. Fluvoxamine is 77% protein-bound, thereby making this somewhat less of a concern, but a concern nevertheless [22].

Paroxetine, sertraline, fluoxetine, and their metabolites inhibit the cytochrome P450 IID6 isoenzyme to varying degrees [31] (Table 3). This may lead to higher levels of medications such as TCA, codeine, and phenytoin [32]. Since fluvoxamine has been associated with inhibition of the P450 IIIA4 isoenzyme, concomitant use of the new antihistamines terfenadine and astemizole and the anxiolytic drug alprazolam requires great care [33]. Terfenadine and astemizole are also metabolized by the P450 IIIA4 isoenzyme and have a narrow therapeutic index; relatively low supratherapeutic levels have been associated with supraventricular tachyarrhythmias. The combination of any SSRI and MAOI is contraindicated. Seven deaths have been reported in cases in which the temporal proximity of MAOI and fluoxetine administration was close [34]. An SSRI should not, therefore, be administered within two weeks of the patient's receiving an MAOI. Depending on the half-life of the SSRI, a washout of as long as five weeks is recommended before an MAOI is administered.

The superiority of the SSRI side-effect profile and the lower risk of death from overdose distinguishes the SSRI from the MAOI and TCA [35]. Typical side effects include transient nausea, headache, and an occasional

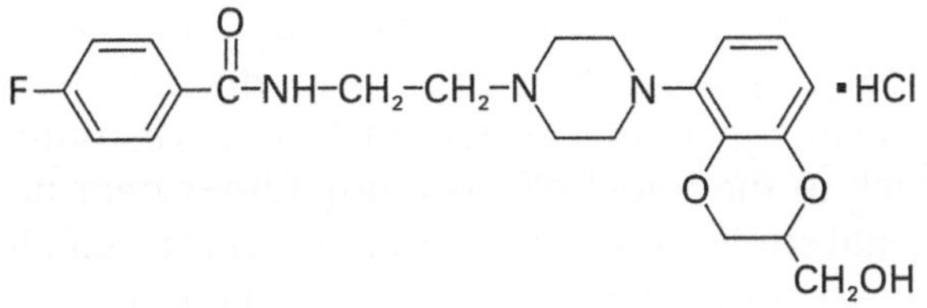

Flesinoxan hydrochloride

Fig. 5.

increase in nervousness. TCA side effects, typically associated with the drugs' anticholinergic and histamine-blocking effects, are much reduced with the SSRI [36].

The efficacy of SSRI in the management of patients with mild to moderate depression has been well established in outpatient trials [37]. What continues to be called into question is their efficacy in treatment for severe depression. Severely depressed patients typically score well above 25 on the 17-item HAM-D rating scale and often require hospitalization. Few studies address this question [38]. Three studies, in which SSRI were found equivalent to TCA in treating severely depressed patients, had significant experimental design flaws that limit their usefulness. Specific criticisms were the grouping together of inpatients and outpatients, and the patients' high dropout rates [39–41].

2   Flesinoxan

Flesinoxan hydrochloride (Figure 5) is a Solvay Pharmaceutical compound currently in phase II development trials for use as an antidepressant and/or anxiolytic agent. The compound is a heteroaryl-piperazine.

Pharmacologically, flesinoxan is similar to buspirone [42]. It binds potently to the 5-HT-$_{1a}$ receptor (Ki = 1.7 nM), and is a highly selective serotonin receptor subtype. Its next highest affinity is to the 5-HT-$_{1D}$ receptor (Ki = 160 nM). It also binds significantly to the D2 receptor (Ki = 140 nM) and the alpha 1-adrenergic receptor (Ki = 380 nM) [42].

In models of depression flesinoxan prolongs the active resistance to aversive stimuli for as long or longer than do traditional antidepressants [43]. It seems to decrease the function of noradrenergic activity but has no effect on the β-adrenergic receptor. It has no psychostimulatory or neuroleptic properties [43]. 5-HT-$_{1a}$ agonists have been recognized to have antidepressant properties in human beings as demonstrated in a number of clinical trials dating back to the mid-1980s [44–46]. Other pharmacological effects noted in animal studies indicate a lowering of arterial blood pressure, inhibition of aggression, and an analgesic effect [43].

2.1   Pharmacokinetics and pharmacodynamics of flesinoxan

To date more than 1000 subjects have been exposed to flesinoxan. Orally administered, it is rapidly absorbed from the gastrointestinal tract and reaches peak plasma concentrations one to two hours after administration. The drug's mean plasma half-life is 5.5 to 7.9 hours; it seems to be 90% protein-bound, and is metabolized by at least three pathways in the liver [47, 48]. In six phase I studies of single doses and three phase I studies of multiple doses, the primary pharmacodynamic findings were modest lowering of blood pressure in some studies; no consistent changes in physical examinations, weight, temperature, electrocardiograms; transient increase in prolactin levels; and electroencephalographic changes similar to those seen with buspirone [47, 49–56].

The efficiency of flesinoxan in the treatment of major depressive disorder has been evaluated in one European and one Canadian study, although only data from the European study are currently available [57]. The study included 369 patients who were randomly assigned to flesinoxan (0.4, 1.2, or 4.0 mg), imipramine (150 mg) or placebo for six weeks; 259 patients of 369 patients completed the study. Significant differences were noted in ITT inpatient analyses of the MADRs, CGI, and HAM-D rating scales between patients on the 1.2-mg flesinoxan dose and those on placebo. More patients in the 4.0-mg flesinoxan group reported treatment-emergent adverse effects than did patients in the placebo group. Most common adverse effects were dizziness, headache, dry mouth, and nausea. No significant changes were noted in laboratory, body weight, electrocardiogram, or vital signs.

To date the number of subjects exposed to flesinoxan has been too low to arrive at a judgment concerning possible adverse effects. One overdose occurred at 20 mg without significant sequelae. About 0.9% of 1,375 patients developed "hallucinations" – either hypnogogic illusions or visual disturbances. All patients recovered spontaneously.

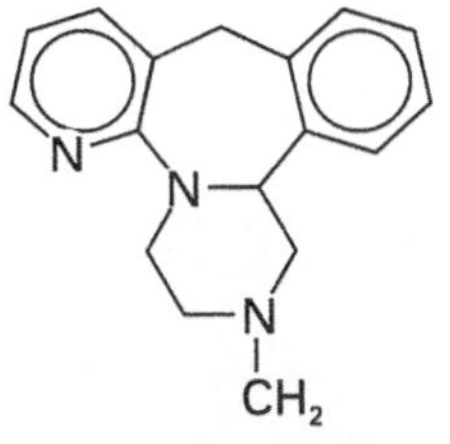

Mirtazapine
(Remeron)

Fig. 6.

3   Remeron [mirtazapine]

Remeron [mirtazapine] is an antidepressant medication currently available in Austria and The Netherlands. Its structural formula is shown in Figure 6. Readily absorbed, with linear absorption kinetics, it reaches peak plasma concentrations within approximately two hours and has an elimination half-life ranging from 20 to 40 hours. Extensively metabolized by oxidative and demethylation routes, it is a centrally active presynaptic alpha-2 antagonist that enhances serotonin neurotransmission indirectly. Because it antagonizes the 5-HT-$_2$ and 5-HT-$_3$ receptors specifically, it stimulates the 5-HT-$_1$ receptor. It is an antihistamine with sedative effects. Ninety percent of the administered dose of Remeron [mirtazapine] is excreted – 75% in the urine and 15% in the feces; 85% is protein-bound in nonspecific and reversible binding. The drug's pharmacokinetics are generally linear in dosages ranging from 15 mg to 80 mg. The presence of food in the stomach has little effect on the absorption of Remeron. In women, who have higher AUCs than men, the drug has a longer elimination half-life. In clinical trials of 2,796 patients treated with Remeron, two patients (one of whom had Sjögren's syndrome and one patient who was treated with imipramine) developed reversible agranulocytosis. Caution should be observed, therefore, concerning the development of sore throat, fever, stomatitis, or other signs of infection accompanied by a low white blood count. Of the known metabolites – demethyl ORG 3770, 8-hydroxy ORG 3770, 8-hydroxy demethyl ORG 3770, N[2]-oxide of ORG 3770, glucuronide of 8-hydroxy ORG 3770, and N[2]-sulphonate of

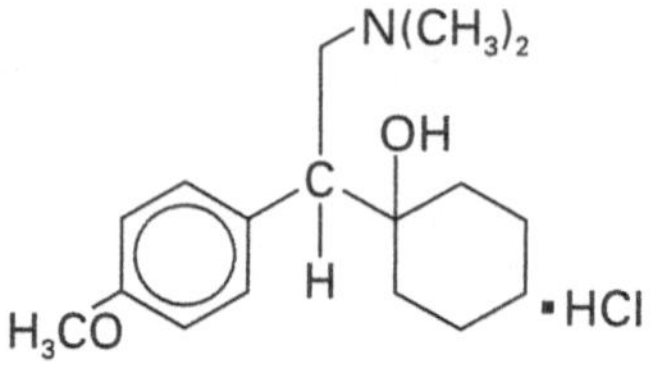

Venlafaxine
(Effexor)

Fig. 7.

demethyl ORG 3770 – only the demethyl metabolite is known to enter the brains of rats, the species in which the most extensive tests have been performed. This metabolite showed antianxiety activity in the conflict-punishment test in rats, but was less active than the parent compound in the rat electroencephalographic profile of antidepressant activity. It was also less active in *in vivo* tests of alpha-2 blockade and 5-HT-$_2$ antagonistic activity. In a series of preclinical studies, which included varying numbers of patients treated with a placebo, amitriptyline, trazodone, clomipramine, diazepam, doxepin, and maprotyline, 2,796 patients received Remeron. Comparable efficacy was seen in all active treatments in most studies. Remeron is yet another example of a trend to develop drugs with simultaneous noradrenergic and serotonergic effects. Unique among the newly developed drugs is its blockade of the 5-HT-$_2$ and 5-HT-$_3$ receptors, which renders the serotonergic effect specific to the 5-HT-$_1$ receptor.

4   Venlafaxine

Recently introduced in the United States under the brand name Effexor, venlafaxine is an antidepressant of the phenylethylamine group (Figure 7). Unlike the traditional SSRI, it inhibits the reuptake of both serotonin and norepinephrine. At doses above 375 mg per day, venlafaxine also seems to inhibit dopamine uptake. With virtually no affinity for the muscarinic,

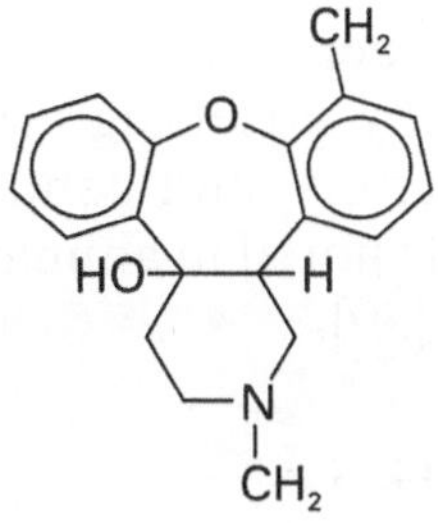

CH$_2$

O

HO— —H

N

CH$_2$

ORG 4428

Fig. 8.

histaminergic, or alpha-1 adrenergic receptors, the drug has few sedative or cardiovascular adverse effects. Its principal metabolite in humans, O-desmethylvenlafaxine (ODV), seems to inhibit potently both serotonin and norepinephrine reuptake. Food has no significant effect on the absorption and metabolism of venlafaxine. Absorption is fast, mean half-life being about five hours for venlafaxine and 11 hours for ODV. Protein-binding is low, about 27%, and steady-state plasma concentrations are reached within 72 hours. In experimental trials in which venlafaxine was compared to trazodone, imipramine, and placebo, the active agents showed comparable efficacy, each being superior to placebo. Generally, placebo differences were evident during the second and third weeks of treatment on most major rating indices, such as the Hamilton-D, MADRS, and CGI scales.

5   ORG 4428

ORG 4428 (cis-1, 2, 3, 4, 4a, 13b-hexahydro-2, 10-dimethyldiben-[2,3:6,7] oxepino [4,5-c] pyridin-4a-ol) is a tetracyclic compound currently undergoing early phase III testing for use as an antidepressant agent (Figure 8). In addition to preclinical antidepressant-like properties, it also exhibits rapid eye movement (REM)-suppressant activity.

Pharmacologically, ORG 4428 selectively inhibits neuronal reuptake of norepinephrine, without affecting dopamine or serotonin reuptake. It is not an antagonist of the adrenergic, histaminergic, or dopaminergic receptors [58], but it has modest affinity for the 5-HT-_{2c} receptor [58]. In preclinical studies with animal models of depression, ORG 4428 was noted to exhibit antidepressant properties by offsetting acquired immobility behavior, reserpine-induced hypothermia, and conditioned avoidance behavior. Other pharmacologic effects noted in animals include possible induction of orthostatic hypotension [59].

5.1   Pharmacokinetics of ORG 4428

In a single rising-dose safety study, ORG 4428 displayed linear kinetics over a broad range, with a dose-independent t_{max} of one to four hours and a $t_{1/2}$ of 11 to 15 hours following doses of 10 to 500 mg [60]. Steady-state pharmacokinetic parameters obtained in healthy normal subjects, who participated in a multiple rising-dose safety and tolerance study [61], showed that at doses of 50 to 800 mg, t_{max} was 1.17 hours, and $t_{1/2}$ varied from 12 to 14 hours. No important adverse effects were observed in healthy volunteers who received up to 800 mg/day.

Outcome data from early phase II trials of ORG 4428 are limited. In the phase IIA studies of patients hospitalized for depression, two-thirds of patients had a moderate to good response, based on HAM-D score reduction [62]. Non-emergency adverse effects, in order of frequency, were headache, insomnia, dry mouth, nausea, dizziness, constipation, nervousness, dyspepsia, and somnolence. So far, five patients have experienced serious adverse effects believed to be possibly related to ORG 4428. These include hypomania, gastrointestinal bleeding, overdose, vertigo, and suicidal ideation. Currently, several phase III studies are in progress that include long-term relapse prevention as well as an examination of how the drug affects elderly patients.

6   Nefazodone

Nefazodone hydrochloride (Serzone®), a phenylpiperazine derivative, has recently received a USFDA indication for the treatment of depression (Figure 9). Nefazodone has a unique chemical structure, separate from SSRI's, TCA's, MAOI's, venlafaxine and bupropion.

Pharmacologically, nefazodone affects both the serotonin and norepinephrine systems [63, 64]. Specifically, nefazodone blocks 5-HT-_2 receptors postsynaptically and inhibits 5-HT reuptake presynaptically. Within the norepinephrine synapse, norepinephrine reuptake is blocked presynaptically.

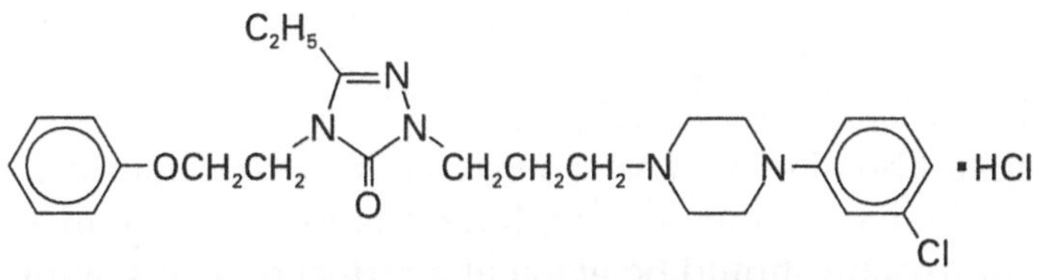

Nefazodone hydrochloride
(Serzone)

Fig. 8.

6.1 Pharmacokinetics of nefazodone

Nefazodone is almost completely absorbed following oral administration. Food does not alter clinically significantly the bioavailability of the compound. Nefazodone is highly but loosely protein bound. Interactions with other highly protein bound medications may occur and should be approached with caution. Nefazodone has three active metabolites: OH-nefazodone, triazole dione, and M-chlorophenylpiperazine (M-CPP). The OH-nefazodone metabolite is considered to have significant clinical activity which is similar to that of the parent compound. Nefazodone has a $t_{1/2}$ of 2–6 hours and is given as a twice-a-day medication.

6.2 Efficacy of nefazodone

Several double-blind, placebo-controlled trials have established nefazodone as an effective treatment for depression in outpatients. The compound was well-tolerated, superior to placebo and equivalent to imipramine [66]. In several published studies involving 283 outpatients and 180 outpatients respectively [67, 68], nefazodone was shown to be as effective as imipramine but with a significantly lower side effect profile. The average effective dose of nefazodone was between 400–500 mg/D. Nefazodone appears to have a favorable effect on sleep with apparent decrease in wake time and fragmental sleep [69].

6.3 Safety of nefazodone [66]

Nefazodone had been extensively evaluated in over 1400 patients. No significant EKG changes, renal or hepatic impairments were noted. In seven reports of overdose (1000 mg–11,200 mg), no deaths occurred. The most common adverse events were dry mouth, somnolence, nausea and dizziness. No significant effects upon nocturnal penile tumescence time compared to placebo has been noted [70].

Nefazodone inhibits P450 IIIA4 isoenzyme *in vitro*. Therefore the compound is not given in conjunction with terfenadine and astemizole. Triazolam and alprazolam should be given at a reduced dose. Caution should also be used when MAOI's are considered for patients exposed to nefazodone. One should discontinue nefazodone one week prior to starting MAOI's and wait two weeks prior to initiating nefazodone in a patient who has come off MAOI's.

7   Discussion

During the past 35 years, theoretical explanations for depression have been based on a variety of interpretations of how the neurotransmitters, serotonin and norepinephrine, regulate mood. Of the available hypotheses, deficiency in norepinephrine-regulated neurotransmission was believed to play a critical role. Prien [71] and colleagues, in an attempt to explain the benefits of L-tryptophan in treating patients for manic episodes, concluded that when serotonin levels were diminished norepinephrine was the controlling neurotransmitter. When norepinephrine was similarly reduced, the result was depression. If it was not reduced, the patient would have a manic episode. Perplexing to investigators has been the speed with which most available drugs change neurotransmitter levels. With most agents, these effects occurred almost immediately, while clinical changes required two to four weeks to be evident. An explanation was necessary. The characterization by Vetulani [72] and others of the down regulation of beta receptors offered a plausible explanation. Since that time, theoreticians have tended to look more closely at defects in homeostatic regulation and the role of pharmaceutical products in restoring adaptive balance. In all these theories norepinephrine and serotonin are recognized as playing important roles. The lack of specificity of available agents has fuelled the discovery process, beginning with the monamine oxidase inhibitors and the tricyclic antidepressants, which nonspecifically affect a wide variety of receptors, including the histamine, muscarinic, and dopamine receptors that produce sedation, anticholinergic effects, and dyskinesias. Among the SSRI group of drugs, which seem to drive the serotonin system selectively and as effectively as their predecessors but with fewer adverse events, of interest was the singular benefit in treatment of obsessive-compulsive disorders. Unlike the nonserotonin-selective agents, these drugs, except for clomipramine, seem singularly effective in treating these troublesome disorders. We see now an ever greater precision in development of new agents. Remeron [mirtazapine], for example, is capable of blocking certain serotonin-sensitive receptors that are not directly related to the depression syndrome. By blocking the 5-HT_2 and 5-HT_3 receptors, as well as not stimulating the muscarinic receptors, an even more precise neurotransmitter effect can be achieved. By renewing the simultaneous augmentation of both systems, venlafaxine rekindles the search for dual-channel agents that are comparatively free of troublesome adverse effects. We expect to see more of this kind of sophisticated neuroregulation growing out of basic research in characterizing the broadening family of neuroamine receptors.

References

1   Practice guidelines for major depression disorders in adults. Am. J. Psychiatry (suppl) *150*, 1-26 (1993).

2   Guze S., Robins E.: Suicide and primary affective disorders. Br. J. Psychiatry *117*, 437–438 (1970).

3   Block R., Dooneieff A., Buchberg A., Spellman S.: The clinical effects of isoniazid and iproniazid in the treatment of pulmonary tuberculosis. Ann. Intern. Med. *40*, 881–900 (1954).

4   Kline N.S.: Clinical experience with iproniazid (Marsilid). J. Clin. Exp. Psychopathol. *19* (suppl.), 72–78 (1958).

5   Potter W., Rudorfer M., Manji H.: The pharmacological treatment of depression. N. Engl. J. Med. *325*, 633–642 (1991).

6   Baldessarini R.: Chemotherapy in Psychiatry. Harvard University Press, Cambridge 1985.

7   Kuhn R.: The treatment of depressive states with G22355 (imipramine hydrochloride). Am. J. Psychiatry *115*, 459–464 (1958).

8   Potter W.Z.: Psychotherapeutic drugs and biogenic amines: Current concepts and therapeutic implications. Drugs *28*, 127–43 (1984).

9   Richelson E.: The new antidepressants: Structures, pharmacokinetics, pharmacodynamics, and proposed mechanisms of action. Psychopharmacol. Bull. *20*, 213–23 (1984).

10   Richelson E., Nelson A.: Antagonism by antidepressants of neurotransmitter receptors of normal human brain *in vitro*. J. Pharmacol. Exp. Ther. *230*, 94–102 (1984).

11   Joyce P.R., Paykel E.S.: Predictors of drug response in depression. Arch. Gen. Psychiatry *46*, 89–99 (1989).

12   Bech P.: A review of the antidepressant properties of serotonin re-uptake inhibitors. Adv. Biol. Psychiatry *17*, 58–69 (1988).

13   Rudorfer M.V., Potter W.Z.: Antidepressants: A comparative review of the clinical pharmacology and therapeutic use of the "newer" versus the "older" drugs. Drugs *37*, 713–38 (1989).

14   Richelson E.: The pharmacology of antidepressants at the synapse: Focus on newer compounds. J. Clin. Psychiatry *55*, 9 (suppl. A) 34–39 (1994).

15   Clements-Jewery S., Robson P.A., Chidley L.J.: Biochemical investigations into the mode of action of trazodone. Neuropharmacology *19*, 1165–1173 (1980).

16   Caccia S., Ballalio M., Samanin R. et al.: (–)M-chlorophenyl-piperazine, a central 5-hydroxytryptamine antagonist, is a metabolite of trazodone. J. Phar. Pharmacol. *33*, 477–78 (1981).

17   Laizure S.C., Devane C.L., Stewart J.T. et al.: Pharmacokinetics of bupropion and its major basic metabolites in normal subject after a single dose. Clin. Pharmacol. Ther. *38*, 586–589 (1985).

18   Perumal A., Smith T., Suckow R. et al.: Effect of plasm from patients containing bupropion and its metabolites on the up-take of norepinephrine. Neuropharmacology *25*, 199–202 (1986).

19   Rudorfer M.V., Golden R.N., Potter W.Z.: Second Generation Antidepressants. Psychiatric Clin. of North Am. *7*, 519–534 (1984).

20   Davidson M.: Seizures and bupropion: A review. J. Clin. Psychiatry *50*, 256–261 (1989).

21   Grimsley S.R., Jann M.W: Paroxetine, sertraline, and fluvoxamine: New selective serotonin re-uptake inhibitors. Clin. Pharmacol. *2*, 930–957 (1992).

22   Van Harten J.M.: Clinical pharmacokinetics of selective serotonin re-uptake inhibitors. Clin. Pharmacokinet. *24*/3, 203–220 (1993).

23   Johnson A.M.: The comparative pharmacological properties of selective serotonin re-uptake inhibitors in animals. In: Selective Serotonin Re-Uptake Inhibitors. Feighner and Boyers (eds.), pp. 37–70. John Wiley & Sons, Chichester 1991.

24   Thomas D.R., Nelson D.R., Johnson A.M.: Biochemical effects of the antidepressant paroxetine, a specific 5-hydroxy-tryptamine uptake inhibitor. Psychopharmacology *93*, 193–200 (1987).

25   Bergstrom R.F., Lemberger L., Farid N.A., Wolen R.L.: Clinical pharmacology and pharmacokinetics of fluoxetine: A review. Br. J. Psychiatry *153* (suppl. 3), 47–50 (1988a).

26   Benfield P., Heel R.C., Lewis S.P.: Fluoxetine: A review of its pharmacodynamic and pharmacokinetics properties and therapeutic efficacy in depressive illness. Drugs *32*, 481–508 (1986).

27   Hevm J., Koe B.K.: Pharmacology of sertraline: A review. Clin. Psychiatry *495*, 40–45 (1988).

28   Pages L.J., Garg D.C., Martinez J.J. et al.: Safety and pharmokinetics of sertraline in healthy young males. J. Clin. Pharmacological. *28*, 920 (abstract) (1988).

29   Kay C.M., Haddock R.E., Langley P.F. et al.: A review of the metabolism and pharmacokinetics of paroxetine in man. Acta Psychiatr. Scand. *80* (suppl 350), 60–73 (1989).

30   Devane C.L.: Pharmacokinetics of the selective serotonin re-uptake inhibitors. J. Clin. Psychiatry *53*/2 (suppl), 13–20 (1992).

31   Preskon S.H.: Pharmacokinetics of antidepressants: Why & How They are Relevant to Treatment. J. Clin. Psychiatry *54*(9) (suppl), 14–34 (1993).

32   Greenblatt D.J.: Basic pharmacokinetic principles and their application to psychotropic drugs. J. Clin. Psychiatry *54*(9) (suppl), 8–13 (1993).

33   Fleishaker J.C., Hulst L.K.: Effect of fluvoxamine on the pharmacokinetics and pharmacodynamics of alprazolam in healthy volunteers. Pharmacol. Res. *9* (suppl), S292 (1992).

34   Beasley C., Masica D.N., Heilegenstein J.A., Wheadon D.E., Zerve R.L.: Possible

MAOI-SSRI interaction: Fluoxetine clinical data and preclinical findings. J. Clin. Psychiatry *13*, 312–20 (1993).

35   Leonard B.E.: Comparative pharmacology of new antidepressants. J. Clin. Psychiatry *54*, 8 (suppl), 3–15 (1993).

36   Tollefsan G.D.: Antidepressant treatments and side effect consideration. J. Clin. Psychiatry *52*, 5 (suppl), 4–13 (1991).

37   Bech P:. Acute therapy of depression. J. Clin. Psychiatry *54*, 8 (suppl) (1993).

38   Nievenberg A.A.: The treatment of severe depression: Is there an efficacy gap between SSRI and TCA antidepressant generations? J. Clin. Psychiatry *55*, 9 (suppl. A) (1994).

39   Beasley C.M., Holman S.L., Potvin J.H.: Fluoxetine compared with imipramine in the treatment of inpatient depression: A multicenter trial. Ann. Clin. Psychiatry *5*, 199–208 (1993).

40   Bowden C.L., Schatzberg A.F., Rosenbaum A. et al.: Fluoxetine and desipramine in major depressive disorder. J. Clin. Psychopharmacol. *13*, 305–310 (1993).

41   Pande A., Sayler M.: Severity of depression and response to fluoxetine. Int. Clin. Psychopharmacol. *8*, 243–245 (1993).

42   Report H.128.112. Pharmacological properties of flesinoxan. The Netherlands: DuPhar, 1990, pp. 1–31.

43   Report H.128.113. Pharmacological properties of flesinoxan. Effects on the central nervous system. The Netherlands: DuPhar, 1990, pp. 1–42.

44   Amsterdam J.D., Berwish N., Potter L., Rickels K.: Open trial of gepirone in the treatment of major depressive disorder. Curr. Ther. Res. *41*, 185–193 (1987).

45   Cott J.M., Kurtz N.M., Robinson D.S., Copp J.E.: A 5-HT_{1a} ligand with both antidepressant and anxiolytic activity. Psychopharmacol. Bull. *24*, 164–167 (1988).

46   Schweizer E.E., Amsterdam J., Rickels K., Kaplan M., Droba M.: Open trial of buspirone in the treatment of major depressive disorder. Psychopharmacol. Bull. *22*, 183–185 (1986).

47   Report H.128.6001. Pharmacokinetics of flesinoxan hydrochloride after single oral dosing in healthy volunteers. The Netherlands: DuPhar, No. H.128.623.

48   Report H.128.6002. Pharmacokinetics of flesinoxan hydrochloride in healthy volunteers after single intravenous infusion: A pilot study. DuPhar Report No. H.128.630.

49   Report H.128.5012. The effects of oral flesinoxan, placebo and buspirone in healthy male volunteers: A pharmaco EEG, safety and tolerance cross-over study (protocol H.128.5012).

50   Report H.128.5001. Disposition of the radioactivity of (14c)DU 29373 after oral administration to healthy male volunteers. DuPhar Report No. H.128.611.

51   Report H.128.5002. The effects of DU 29373 in healthy male volunteers. A randomized, double-blind, placebo-controlled, rising-single-oral-dose study (protocol No. H.128.5002/M).

52   Report H.128.5003/M. The effects of DU 29373 in healthy male volunteers. A randomized, double-blind, oral placebo-controlled, cross-over study (protocol No. H.128.5003/M).

53   Report H.128.5009/A. Effects of oral flesinoxan in healthy volunteers. A randomized, double-blind, placebo-controlled pilot single-rising-dose study and multiple dose study. Part A: The single-rising-dose study.

54   Report H.128.5009B. Effects of oral flesinoxan in healthy volunteers. A randomized, double-blind, placebo-controlled pilot single-rising-dose study and multiple dose study. Part B: The multiple dose study.

55   Report H.128.6007. The influence of different dose levels and multiple dosing of flesinoxan on its pharmacokinetics in healthy male subjects. An oral multiple-dose/dose-proportionality study).

56   Report H.128.5004. Effects of oral flesinoxan in healthy male volunteers. A randomized, double-blind, placebo-controlled, multiple-dose study.

57   Report H.128.5020. Oral flesinoxan and imipramine treatment in patients with major depressive disorder. A double-blind, placebo-controlled, multi-center study. The Netherlands: Solvay DuPhar, 1993, pp. 1–98.

58   Ruigt G.: Effects of ORG 4428 on the central and autonomic nervous systems – *in vivo* studies (SDG RR 3597).

59   Zandberg P., Santegoets W.: Cardiovascular effects in anesthetized cats (SDGRR 2729).

60   Altman J.F.B., Mant T.G.K., Morrison P.J.: A phase I, double-blind, placebo-controlled, single-rising-oral-dose study with ORG 4428 in healthy male volunteers to assess its tolerance and safety as well as its pharmacokinetics profile (protocol 25801) Part I: Safety and tolerance at dose levels of 10, 25, 35, 50, 200, 350, 500, 750, and 1000 mg. SDG Release Report No. 3065.
     Part II: Pharmacokinetics profile of ORG 4428 after doses of 10–500 mg. SDG Release Report No. 3007.

61   Mant T.G.K., Morrison P.J., Altman J.F.B.: A phase I, double-blind, placebo-controlled, multiple-dose study with ORG 4428 in healthy male volunteers to assess its tolerance and safety as well as its effects on EEG-monitored sleep characteristics (protocol 28502).

62   Sennef C., Kramer J.: Pilot efficacy studies in depressed hospitalized patients. SDG Release Report No. 3675.

63   Eison A.S., Eison M.S., Torrente J.R., Wright R.N., Yocca F.D.: Nefazodone: preclinical pharmacology of a new antidepressant. Psychopharmaco.l Bull. *26*, 311–315 (1990).

64   Fontaine R.: Novel serotonergic mechanisms and clinical experience with nefazodone. Clin. Neuropharmacol. *16* (suppl 3), S45–S50 (1993).

65   Shukla U.A., Shea J.P., Gammans R.E.: Single and multiple dose pharmacokinetics of nefazodone and two metabolites in healthy volunteers. Clin. Pharmacol. Ther. *41*, 205 (1987).

66   Data on file: Bristol-Myers Squibb Company; Princeton, NM, 1992.

67   *Fontaine R., Ontiveros A., Elie R., Kensler T.T., Roberts D.L. et al.: A double-blind comparison of nefazodone, imipramine, and placebo in major depression. J. Clin. Psychiatry *55*, 234–241 (1994).

68   *Rickels K., Schweizer E., Clary C. et al.: Nefazodone and imipramine in major depression: a placebo-controlled trial. Br. J. Psychiatry *1644*, 802–805 (1994).

69   Armitage R., Rush A.J., Trivedi M., Cain J., Roffwarg H.P.: The effects of nefazodone on sleep architecture in depression. Neuropsychopharmacol. *10*, 123–127 (1994).

70   Ware J.C., Rose F.V., McBrayer R.H.: The acute effects of nefazodone, trazodone, and buspirone on sleep and sleep-related penile tumescence in normal subjects. Sleep *17*(6), 544–550 (1994).

71   Prange A.J., Wilson I.C., Lynn C.W. et al.: L-tryptophan in mania. Arch. Gen. Psych. *30*, 56–62 (1974).

72   Vetulani J., Stawarz R.J., Dingell J.V. et al.: A possible common mechanism of action of antidepressant treatments: reduction in the sensitivity of the noradrenergic cyclic AMP generating system in the rat limbic forebrain. Naunyn-Schmiedeberg's Arch. Pharmacol. *293*, 109–114 (1976).

Progress in Drug Research, Vol. 46 (E. Jucker, Ed.)
© 1996 Birkhäuser Verlag, Basel (Switzerland)

Immunopharmacological and biochemical bases of Chinese herbal medicine

By Eric J. Lien[1], Arima Das[1] and Linda L. Lien[2]

[1] Department of Pharmaceutical Sciences, School of Pharmacy, University of Southern California, Los Angeles, CA 90033, and
[2] R.Ph. 10728 Kelmore St., Culver City, CA 90230

1   Introduction

In the practice of traditional Chinese medicine (TCM), many drugs are described as having properties like Fu-Zhen Ku Ban (扶正固本); tonic action) or Chien-Liang Chie-Du (清涼解毒); cooling and toxin-clearing). These types of herbal preparations have been used in the treatment of various types of cancer, infections and other diseases. In recent years, through the process of analysis of active ingredients and testing with sensitive *in vitro* and *in vivo* models, the positive effects of these herbs on the immune system and the growth of cancer cells have been elucidated. Some have been proven effective in clinical trials in humans.

In this report, selected examples of the positive findings on the immunopharmacological and biochemical bases of the natural products derived from Chinese medicinal herbs will be presented. It is hoped that through systematic analysis of the old literature and new chemical and biological information, useful new leads can be discovered for the development of novel therapeutic agents.

1.1   Immunostimulating polysaccharides (ISPs) from fungi

In the practice of traditional oriental and folk medicine, different kinds of fungi belonging to *basidiomycetes* have been used as remedies for cancer. Following this lead, Chihara of the National Cancer Center Research Institute of Japan and his coworkers in 1969 first reported marked antitumor activity of a polysaccharide from the edible mushroom (Shiitake, Hsiang-Ku) *Lentinus edodes* and named it lentinan [1–4]. In the same year Ikehawa et al. reported that the antitumor activities of aqueous extracts of seven different edible mushrooms against sarcoma-180 ascites tumor in mice [5, 6]. The structure of lentinan has been established to be a glucan made of repeating units of five β (1,3)-glucopyranoside linear linkage with two β (1,6)-glucopyranoside branchings, with molecular weight of up to 10^6 [3, 6]. Lentinan exists as a right-handed triple helical structure in the solid state [6, 7], with a possibility of hydrogen bonds between adjacent glucose units [6] (see Figure 1).

Since then many different immunopolysaccharides with immunostimulating properties have been found in many species of fungi used as Chinese Medicine: *Poria cocos* (Hoelen), *Polyporus umbellatus* (Chu-ling), *Ganoderma lucidium* (Ling zhi, red), *G. japonicum* (Ling zhi, purple), *Cordyceps ophigoglossoides* (Tung-chung hsia tsao), *Cordyceps sinensis* (Tung-chung hsin tsao), *Cordyceps cicadae* (Chan-hua), *Polyporus versicolar* (Coriolus, Kawaratake), *Omphalia lepidescense* (Lei-wan),

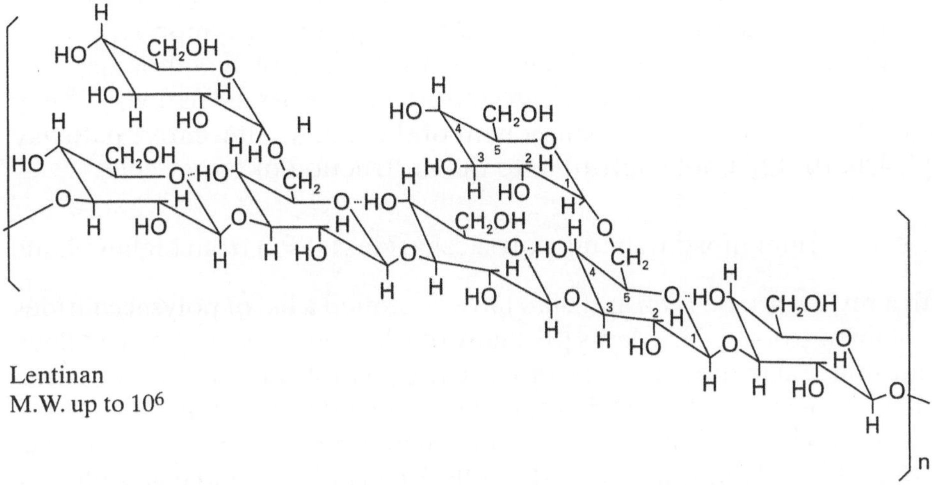

Lentinan
M.W. up to 10^6

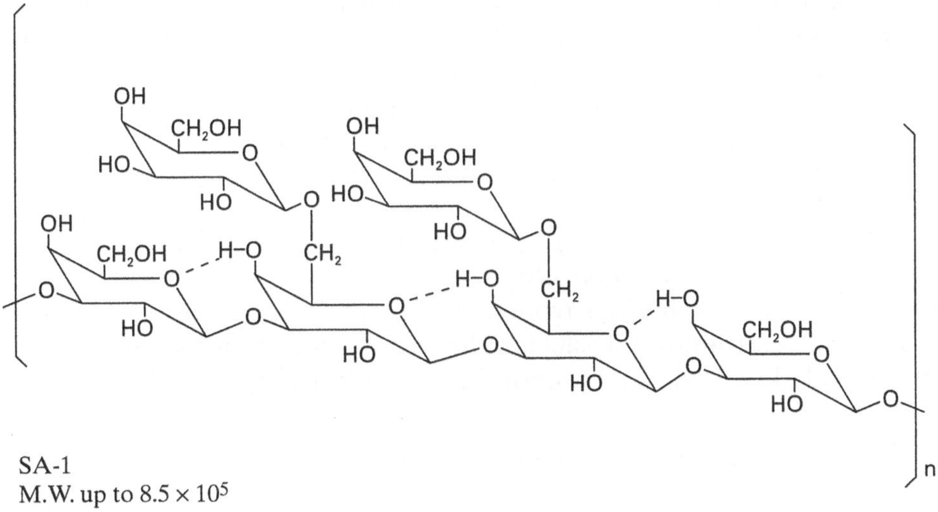

SA-1
M.W. up to 8.5×10^5

Fig. 1
The primary structure of Lentinan from *L. edodes* and SA-1 from Sam-qu-ginseng (*Panax notoginseng*) (adapted from [6] and [12]).

Dictyphora indusiata (Zhu sun, Kinugasatake), *Schizophyllum commune* (Tricholomataceae), *Sclerotium glucanicum*, etc. [6, 9]. Fungal polysaccharides like lentinan can stimulate macrophages, T-lymphocytes and B-lymphocytes leading to increased production of lymphokines and immunoglobins (IgG, IgM, etc., via the adaptive, classical pathway). They can also stimulate the C3 component of the innate, alternative pathway [3, 4, 6, 10–12], both contribute to the destruction of tumor cells.

1.2   Immunostimulating polysaccharides (ISPs) from higher plants

In a review article Lien and Gao have compiled a list of polysaccharides obtained from higher plants [8], many of which have been shown to have antitumor activities in animal models. The possible mechanisms of action of polysaccharides from higher plants include: lymphoproliferation, increased colony-stimulating factors, increased interferon production, stimulation of natural killer (NK) cells, T-cells, B-cells and macrophages, and stimulation of the complement system. The plants studied include: *Abelmoschus glutinotextilis*, *Abelmoschus manihot*, *Acanthopanax senticosus*, *Aconitum camichaellii*, *Althaea officinalis*, *Althaea rosea*, *Angelica acutiloba*, *Arctium lappa*, *Artemisia princeps*, *Aucanacua carmizulis*, *Bryonia alba*, *Bryonia diocia*, *Codonopsis pilosula*, *Coffee* sp., *Coix lachryma- jobi var. ma yuen*, *Colchicum autumnale*, *Cucumis melo cantalupensis*, *Eryngium creticum var. oblongum*, *Ginkgo biloba*, *Hydrangea paniculata*, *Lithospermum euchromum*, *Nicotiana sp.*, *Oryza sativa* (rice bran), *Panax ginseng*, *Panax notoginseng* (see Figure 1), *Pinus* sp. (pine cone), *Plantago major*, *Rumex acetosa*, *Saccharum officinarum* (sugar cane), *Solidago* sp., *Spiraea ulmaria*, *Trifolium pratense*, *Yucca schidegera*, *Zizyphus jujuba*, etc.

In general, polysaccharides from higher plants are complex heteroglycans. Many antitumor polysaccharides are soluble D-glucans which are not quickly hydrolyzed by humoral D-glucanases [9].

2.1   Cancer preventing agents

Various ways of carcinogenesis and different stages of chemoprevention of cancer are summarized in Figure 2. As the individual ages, accumulated events of changes in DNA and compromised immunity caused by environmental factors and intake of harmful chemicals, the chance of developing cancer increases. It is important to balance this with various chemopreventive measures in order to prevent the onset of cancer. These measures include consumption of fresh vegetables and fruits

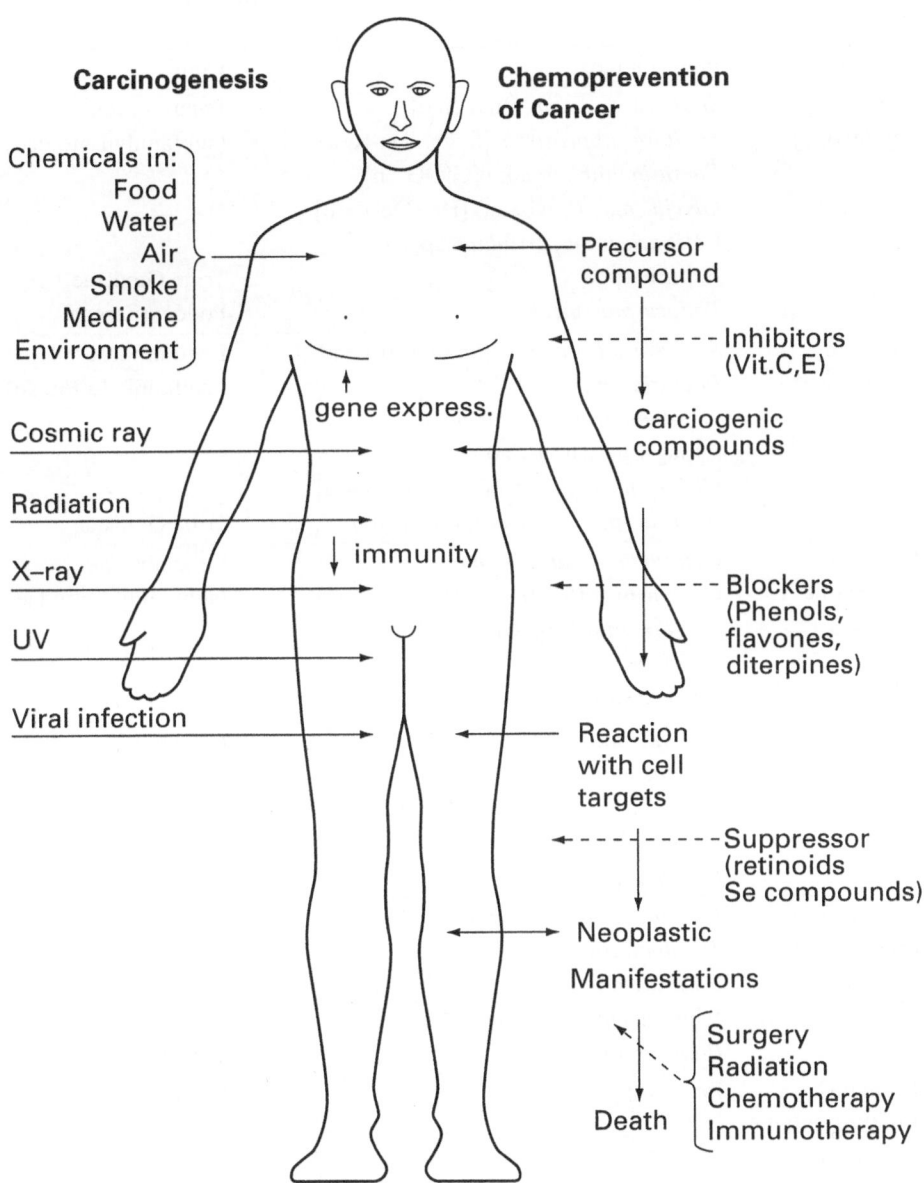

Fig. 2
Carcinogenesis and different stages of chemoprevention (adapted from [13]).

Table 1.
Chinese medicinal plants known to contain isoflavonoids (adapted and expanded from [17]).

Compound	Plant sources	Family
Genistein (isoflavone)	*Sophora japonica* [Huai-Jiao] *Sophora subprostrata* [Shan-Tou-Ken] *Pueraria thunbergiana* [G'e-G'en] *Glycine max* (Soybean) [Hei-Da-Dou] *Cicer arietinum, Trifolium* spp., *Baptisia* spp. *Podocarpus spicatus*	Leguminosae (subfamily Lotoidae) Tribe Genistae Podocarpaceae
Daidzein (isoflavone)	*Sophora subprostrata* [Shan-Tou-Ken] *Pueraria* spp. *Trifolium pratense* (red clover) [Hong-Che-Zhou-Cao] *Glycine max* (Soybean) [Hei-Da-Dou] *Baptisia* spp., *Machaerium villosum*	Leguminosae (subfamily Lotoidae) Tribe Genistae
Genistin (isoflavone glucoside)	*Genista tinctoria, Ulex nanus* *Glycine max* (Soybean) [Hei-Da-Dou] *Pueraria thunbergiana* [G'e-G'en] *Trifolium* spp., *Thermopsis* spp. *Baptisia* spp.	Leguminosae (subfamily Lotoidae) Tribe Genistae
Daidzin (isoflavone glucoside)	*Pueraria* spp., *Thermopsis* spp. *Glycine max* (Soybean) [Hei-Da-Dou] *Trifolium pratense* (red clover) *[Hong-Che-Zhou-Cao]* *Baptisia* spp.	Leguminosae (subfamily Lotoidae) Tribe Genistae
Biochanin A (methoxylated (isoflavone)	*Pueraria thunbergiana* [G'e-G'en] *Trifolium* spp., *Dalbergia* spp., *Cicer arietinum* *Sophora japonica* [Huai-Jiao] *Baptisia* spp.	Leguminosae (subfamily Lotoidae) Tribe Genistae
Prunetin (methoxylated isoflavone)	*Prunus* spp.	Rosaceae
Formononetin (methoxylated isoflavone)	*Glycyrrhiza glabra* (Licorice) [Kan-Tsaõ] *Dalbergia paniculata, Trifolium* spp. *Wisteria floribunda* [Fugikobu] *Sophora angustifolia* [Ku-Shen] *Diplotropis pupurea, Machaerium villosum*	Leguminosae (subfamily Lotoidae) Tribe Genistae

rich in Vitamins C and E and β-Carotene (Vitamin A, retinoids), fibers, complex carbohydrates and flavonoids [14]. Many of these active ingredients are antioxidant/free radical scavengers. According to Boutwell [15] the carcinogenic process involves two phases, initiation and promotion.

Cancer preventing agents include anti-initiation compounds and anti-promotion agents. Anti-initiation compounds like ellagic acid, flavonoids, indoles, vitamins (Vitamin A and its analogues, Vitamins C and E), sulfur compounds, selenium compounds, unsaturated fatty acids, extracts of *Spirulina-Dunaliella* algae and of *Piper betle* have been shown to have many varying degrees of biological activities in different systems [14]. Anti-promotion compounds include coumarins, flavonoids, selenium compounds, retinoids, sarcophytol A and B, curcumin and unsaturated fatty acids [14]. For a detailed discussion of the structure-activity relationship of these cancer preventive natural products, ref. [14] should be consulted. Various flavonoids with polyhydroxy/hydroquinone functions have been shown to inhibit the mutagenic effect of benzo[2]pyrene7,8-diol-9,10-epoxide [14, 16].

2.2   Phytoestrogen isoflavonoids

Many Chinese medicinal herbs are known to contain isoflavonoids; they are listed in Table 1 [17]. We have reported that the estrogenic activities of many isoflavonoids can be attributed to their structural similarities with estradiol and diethylstilbestrol [DES] [16]. Additional isoflavonoids with similar structures and phytoestrogenic activities have been included in Figure 3. Among the physicochemical properties (log P, dipole moment, O–O distance, and molecular weight) were compared. The O–O distance appears to be within 11 ± 1 Å (see Table 2) for all the estrogenic compounds examined [17]. Figure 4 shows the near perfect overlapping of estradiol/diethylstilbestrol, daidzein/estradiol, genistein/estradiol and coumestrol/estradiol based on molecular modeling [17].

2.3   Antiestrogenic flavonoids

Several bioflavonoids found in many Chinese herbs as well as other plants have structures different from those of isoflavonoids or estradiol. These flavonoids include quercetin (found in 86 herbs), luteolin (found in 45 species), hesperidin (found in 13 herbs), hesperitin and pelargonidin [18] (Figure 5). Scambia et al. [19] have reported that the synthetic

Table 2.
Physicochemical properties of estrogens and phytoestrogen isoflavonoids. Note the similar O–O distances found [17].

Compound	calc. LOG P	Dipole moment μ	O–O distance	Molecular weight
17-β Estradiol (steroid)	3.784	2.710 Debyes	10.83 Å	272.39
Diethylstilbestrol (stilbene)	4.956	0.095 Debyes	12.07 Å	268.36
Coumestrol (coumestan)	3.125	6.140 Debyes	11.28 Å	268.23
Genistein (isoflavone)	0.979	4.240 Debyes	12.00 Å	270.24
Daidzein (isoflavone)	1.646	4.450 Debyes	12.00 Å	254.24
Formononetin (methoxylated isoflavone)	2.232	4.440 Debyes	12.02 Å	268.27
Biochanin A (methoxylated isoflavone)	1.565	4.840 Debyes	12.02 Å	284.27
Equol (a metabolite in mammalian urine)	2.859	1.960 Debyes	12.04 Å	242.28

antiestrogen tamoxifen (TAM) and the flavonoids quercetin and rutin competed for [^{3}H]-E$_2$ binding to type-II EBS. The relative binding affinity of quercetin, rutin, DES and TAM for type-II EBS (K_D = 18–24 nM) correlated well with their potency as lymphoblastoid cell growth inhibitors [20]. Because of the wide distribution of these bioactive flavonoids, careful epidemiological study with respect to their consumption and cancer incidence is warranted [21, 22]. Markaverich et al. reported that some of these bioflavonoids specifically inhibited the binding of [^{3}H] estradiol to type II sites but did not interact with the rat uterine estrogen receptor [23]. Quercetin (5–10 μg/ml) inhibited the growth of MCF-7 cells in a dose-dependent manner. Injection of quercetin or luteolin in immature rats blocked estradiol stimulation of nuclear type II sites which may be involved in cell growth regulation [23].

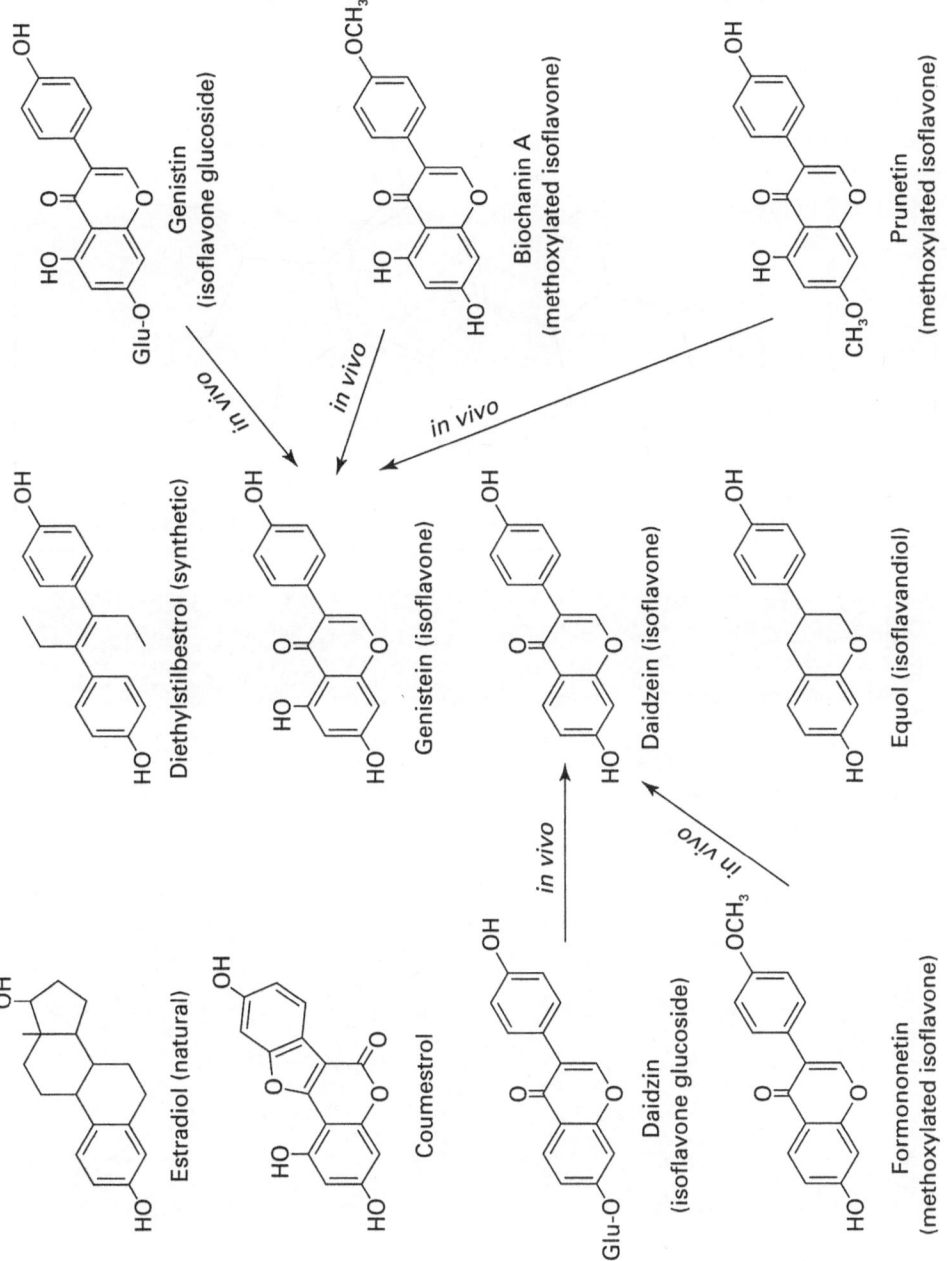

Fig. 3
Structural similarity of estrogens and phytoestrogen isoflavonoids.

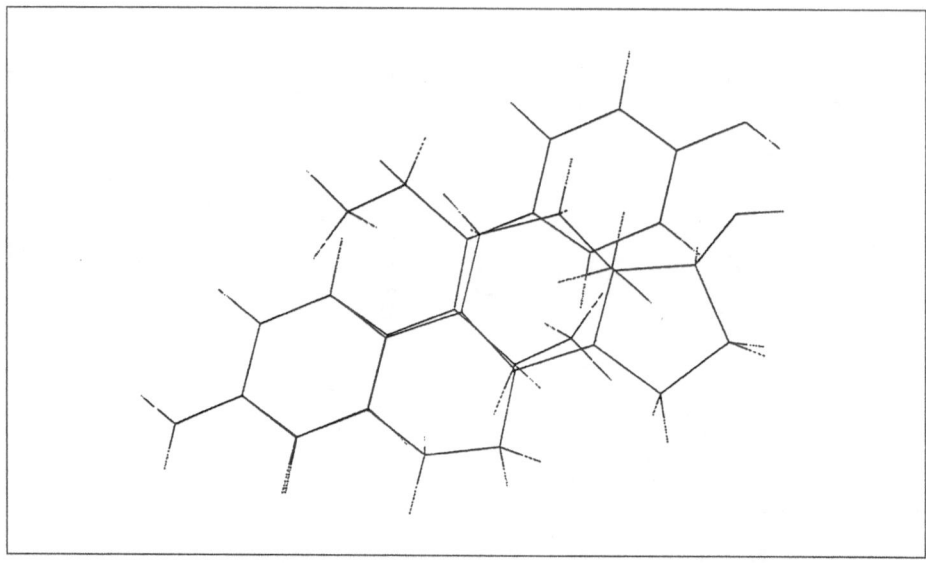

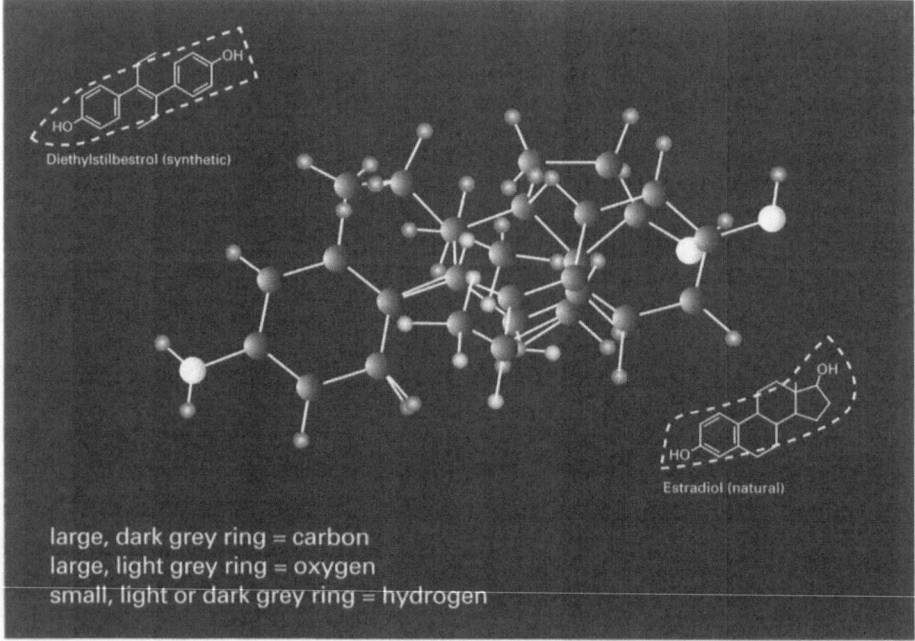

Fig. 4
Molecular modeling of estrogenic compounds, showing their overlapping backbones and very close O–O distance.

(A) estradiol/diethylstilbestrol

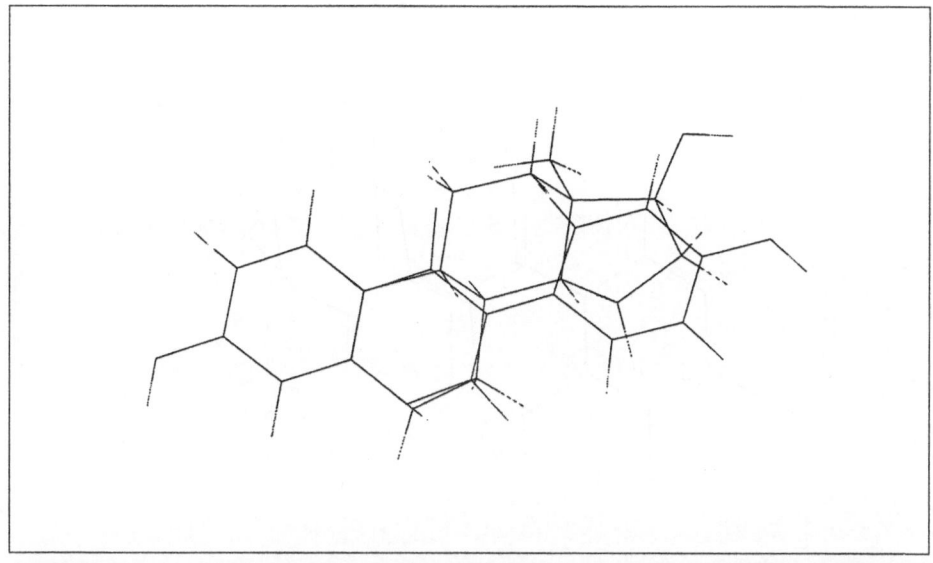

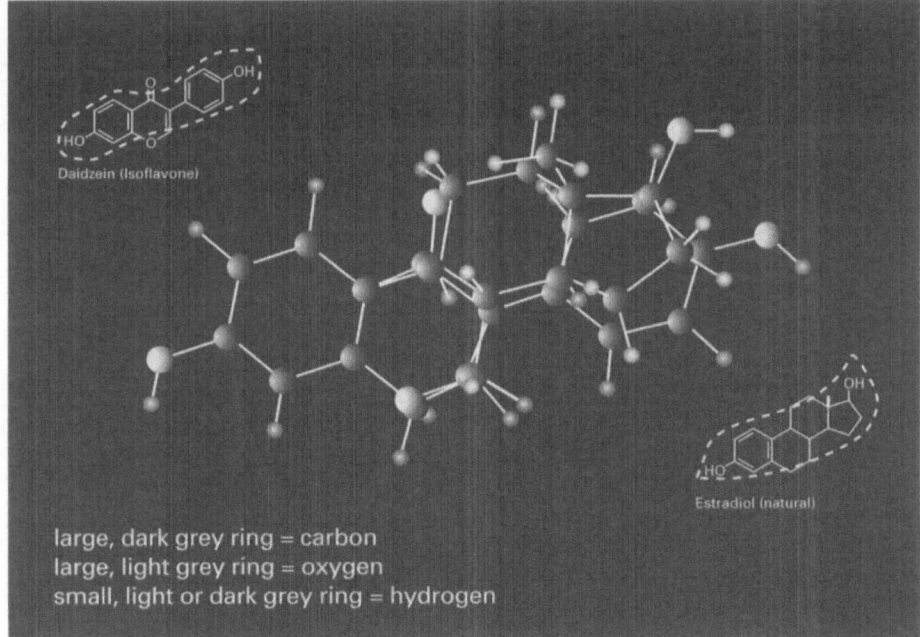

Daidzein (Isoflavone)

Estradiol (natural)

large, dark grey ring = carbon
large, light grey ring = oxygen
small, light or dark grey ring = hydrogen

(B) daidzein/estradiol

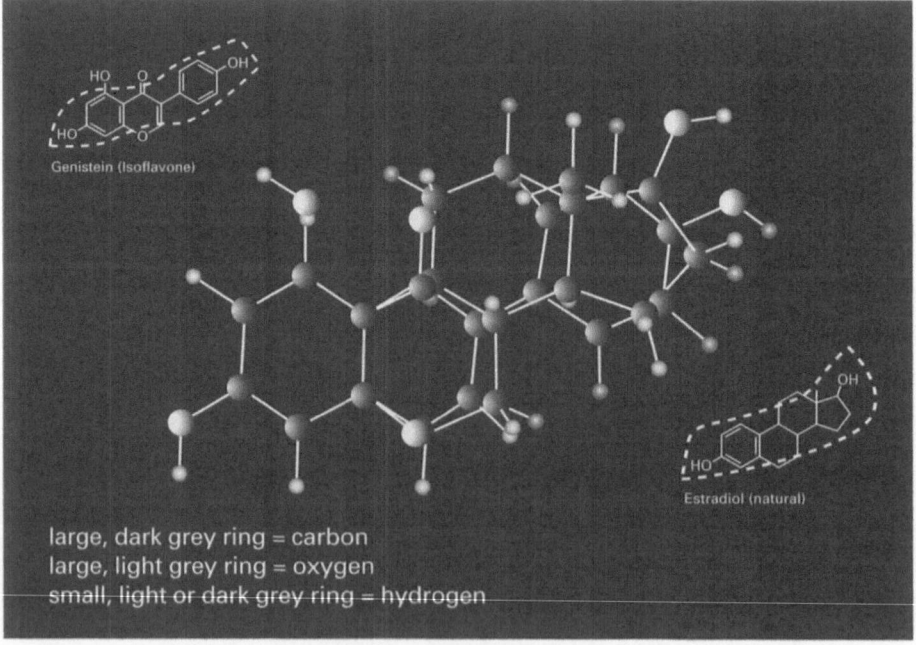

large, dark grey ring = carbon
large, light grey ring = oxygen
small, light or dark grey ring = hydrogen

(C) genistein/estradiol

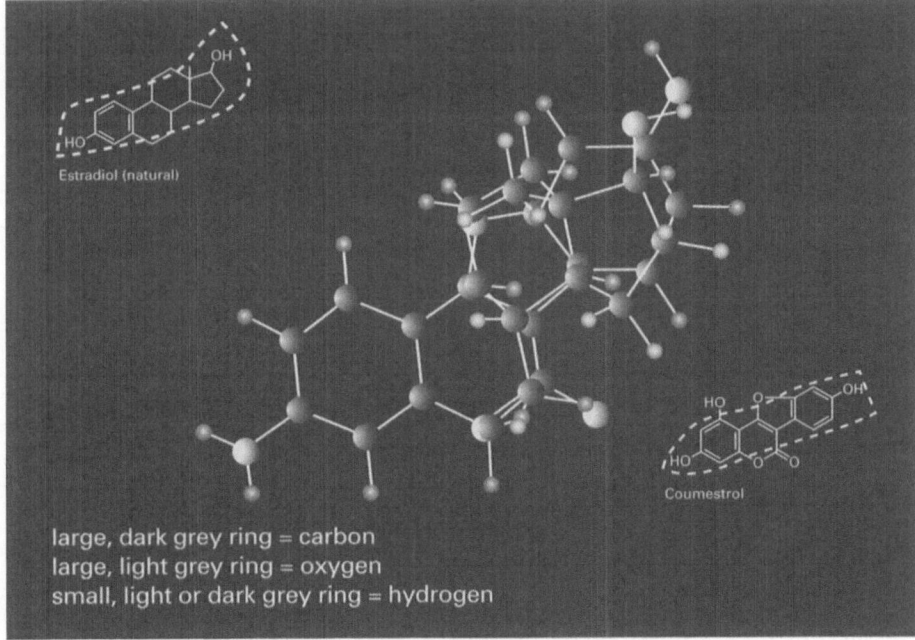

large, dark grey ring = carbon
large, light grey ring = oxygen
small, light or dark grey ring = hydrogen

Estradiol (natural)

Coumestrol

(D) coumestrol/estradiol

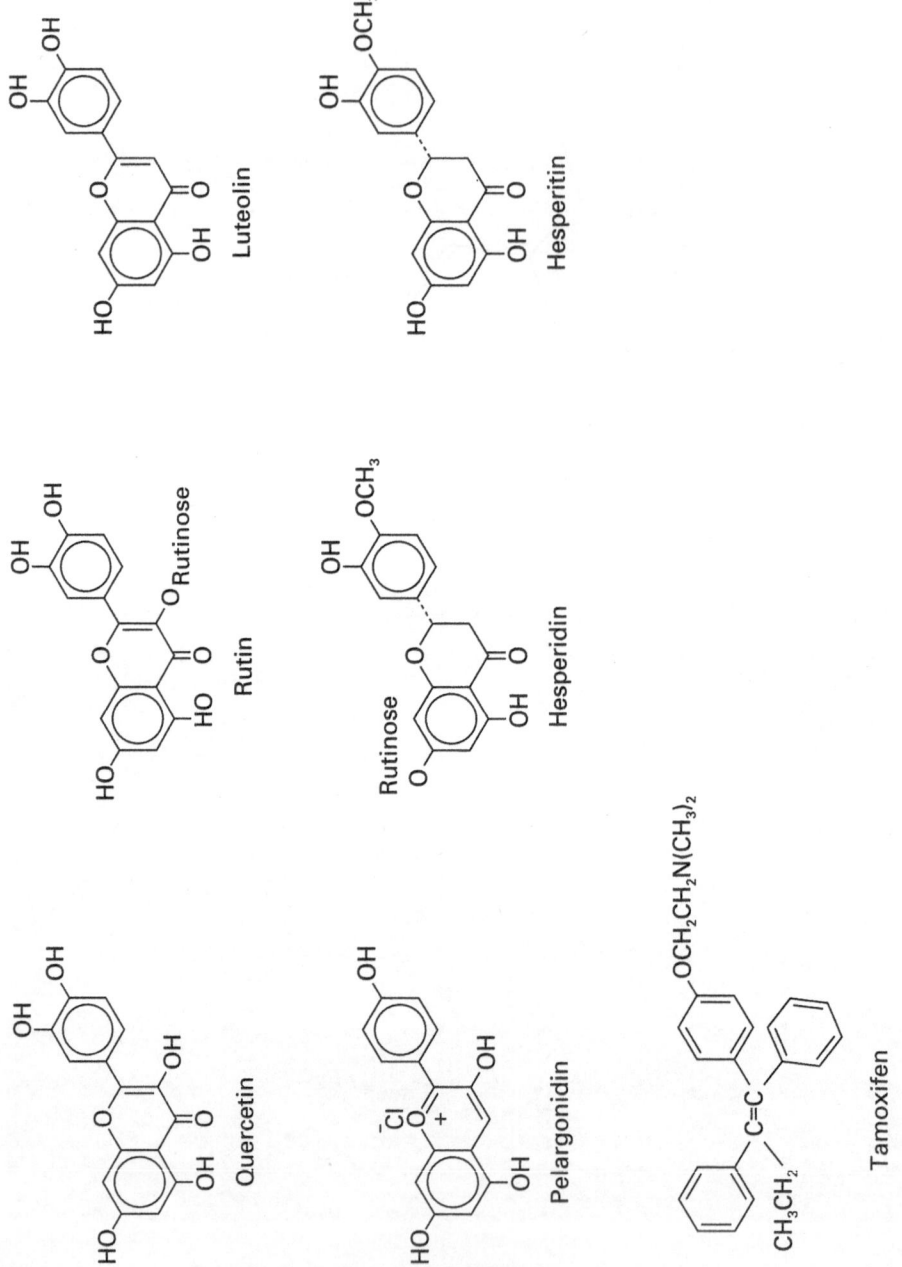

Fig. 5

Structures of antiestrogenic flavonoids found in many plants and tamoxifen. Note the absence of two OH groups equivalent to those in estradiol.

3　Cancer chemotherapeutic agents

In China, many plants with "Cooling and Toxin-Clearing" or "Toxin-Clearing and Heat Dissipating" properties are used in the treatment of various forms of cancer (see Table 3). Some of the active ingredients are known [24–28], while others remain to be identified. Many of the active ingredients have been modified and are undergoing extensive investigation [24–29].

Besides these seventeen herbs there are additional thirteen herbs used for blood regulation in cancer patients [27]. These include: *Curcuma zedoaria* (é zhú), *Sarcandra glabra* (jiú jié chá), *Cudrania tricuspidata* (zhé shū), *Polygonium cuspidatum* (hŭ zhàng), *Tylophora floribunda* (wá ér téng), *Actinidia chinensis* (mî hóu taó), *Sparganium stoloniferum* (sān léng), *Rubia cordifolia* (qian tsao gén), *Cirsium japonicum* (dà jì), *Cephalanoplos segetum* (xiăo jì), *Agrimonia pilosa* (xiān hé), *Akebia trifoliata* (bā yue zhá), and *Rheum officinale* (dā huáng).
Additional nine herbs are used for their tonic (immunostimulating) properties [24, 26]: *Ganoderma lucidium* (líng zhí), *Asparagus officinalis* (lu shun), *Phaseolus vulgaris* (tsai dōu), *Lentinus edodes* (hsing ku), *Panax ginseng* (jen shen), *Gossypium herbaceum* (*G. arboreum* and *G. hirsutum*) (mian hua), *Acanthopanax senticosus* (wŭ jia pí), *Helianthus annuns* (xiang rìkuí), and *Asparagus cochinchinensis* (tian men dong).

4　Longevity-promoting Chinese herbal preparations

Many of the above-mentioned cancer preventive agents (antioxidants, free-radical scavengers), tonic drugs (Fu-Cheng Ku-Ban, immunostimulating) are frequently used in combination to promote longevity in traditional Chinese medicine [26–29]. For a detailed description of the components of ten commonly used longevity-promoting preparations, and some experimentally proven biological activities, the readers should consult a review by Lien et al. [29] and the references cited therein. In general these preparations have been used in humans for many generations. There are little or no major side effects if these preparations are used properly. Since their actions are mild, prolonged use may be necessary to achieve the desired effects.

Table 3.
Toxin-clearing and heat-dissipating plants used to treat various forms of cancer in China
[23–27].

Plant(s)	Active ingredients (preparation)	Treatment of
Cephalotaxi hainanensis	Harringtonine Homoharringtonine	Non-lymphocytic leukemia, chronic granulocytic leukemia, malignant lymphoma, polycythemia vera
Indigo naturalis *Isatis tinctoria* *Baphicacanthus cusia* *Indigofera tinctoria* (or *Polygonium tinctorium*)	Indirubin	Chronic granulocytic leukemia, primary eosinophilia, eosinophilic lympho-granuloma, and nasopharyngeal carcinoma
Camptothecae acuminatae	Camptothecine Hydroxycamptothecine	Stomach cancer, urinary bladder cancer, head and neck cancer, lymphoma, leukemia, sarcoma
Andrographis paniculata	(1% Chloroform or alcohol extract)	Malignant hydatidiform mole and trophoblastoma
Trichosanthes kirilowii	Trichosanthin	Malignant hydatidiform mole and chorionic epithelioma
Brucea javanica	Brueosides A and B Brusatel Brucein D (Capsules, 50% emulsion or 30% injection)	Carcinoma of esophagus, stomach, rectum, lung, cervix and skin papilloma of larynx, vocal cord, external auditory meatus and gum
Catharanthus roseus	Vinblastine Vincristine	Hodgkin's disease, chorionic epithelioma, acute lymphocytic leukemia, acute monocytic leukemia, lymphocarcinoma, reticulum cell sarcoma
Scutellaria barbata	(Decoction)	Tumor of digestive tract, carcinoma of liver, lung, cervix and breast, malignant hydatidiform mole, and chorionic epithelioma
Maytenus hookeri	(Methanol extract) Maytansine, Maytanvalin	Carcinoma of esophagus, stomach, liver, uterus, lung and nasopharynx

Table 3. (Cont.)

Plant(s)	Active ingredients (preparation)	Treatment of
Hydyotis diffusa	(Decoction)	Tumors of digestive tract lymphosarcoma, carcinoma of liver and larynx
Taraxacum mongolicum	(Decoction) (Tablet) (Syrup)	Tumors of the digestive system (esophagus, stomach, intestine, liver and pancreas), carcinoma of mammary gland, lung, cervix, uteri and gum, and chronic granulocytic leukemia
Sophora flavescens	(Decoction) (Tablet of total alkaloids) (Tablet of crude drug) Matrine Oxymatrine l-Maackianin	Carcinoma of intestine and cervix, malignant hydatidiform mole, and chorionic epithelioma diform mole, and chorionic epithelioma
Duchesnea indica	(Decoction)	Carcinoma of urinary bladder, lung, larynx, esophagus and thymus
Prunella vulgaris	(Decoction) Polysaccharides	Carcinoma of thyroid, breast, liver, larynx and rectum, thyroid adenoma and thyroid cyst
Solanum lyratum	(Decoction)	Carcinoma of lung, vocal cord, cervix, liver, stomach and thyroid
Hibiscus mutabilis	(Decoction) (Powder) (Ointment)	Carcinoma of esophagus, cardia, stomach, lung, mammary gland and skin
Adina rubella	(Decoction) (Tablet containing extract) (Suppositories) (Syrup)	Carcinoma of esophagus, stomach, intestine, cervix, uteri, trophoblastoma and malignant hydatidiform mole

References

1   G. Chihara, Y.Y. Maeda, J. Harnuro, et al.: Nature *222*, 687 (1969).
2   G. Chihara, J. Hamuro, Y.Y. Maeda, et al.: Nature *225*, 943 (1970).
3   G. Chihara: In: Manipulation of host defense mechanisms, Excerta Medica. Eds. T. Aoki, I. Urushizaki, and E. Tsubura (1981).
4   G. Chihara, J. Hamuro and Y.Y. Maeda: Can. Detect. Prev. Suppl. *1*, 423 (1987).
5   T. Ikekawa, N. Uehara, Y. Maeda, et al.: Can. Res. *29*, 734 (1969).
6   E.J. Lien: Prog. Drug Res. *34*, 395 (1990).
7   T.L. Bluhm and A. Sarko: Can J. Chem. *55*, 293 (1977).
8   E.J. Lien and H. Gao: Int. J. Orient. Med. *15*, 123 (1990).
9   R.L. Whistler, A.A. Bushway and P.P. Singh: Adv. Carbohy. Chem. and Biochem. *32*, 235 (1976).
10 H. Miyakoshi and T. Aoki: Int. J. Immunopharmac. *6*, 365 (1984).
11 H. Miyakoshi, T. Aoki and M. Mizukoshi: Int. J. Immunopharmac. *6*, 373 (1984).
12 I.M. Roitt, J. Brostoff and D.K. Male: "Immunology". The C.V. Mosby Co., St. Louis, 1985, p. 710.
13 E.J. Lien: Orient. Healing Arts Int. Bull. *13*, 59 (1988).
14 H. Gao and E.J. Lien: Int. J. Orient. Med. *16*, 55 (1991).
15 R.K. Boutwell: CRC Critical Rev. Toxicol. *2*, 419 (1974).
16 A. Das, J.H. Wang and E.J. Lien: Prog. Drug Res. *42*, 133 (1994).
17 A. Das and E. Lien: Pharm. Res. *11*, S118 (1994).
18 Chiang Su New Medical College: Chon Yao Da Tze Dian, Shanghai Science Technology Publisher, 1979.
19 G. Scambia, F.O. Ranelleti, P.B. Panici, et al.: Int. J. Cancer. *46*, 1112 (1990).
20 H. Adlercrentz: Scand. J. Clin. Lab Invest. *50*, Suppl. 201, 3 (1990).
21 H. Adlercrentz, Y. Mousani, J. Clark, et al.: J. Steroid Biochem. Molec. Biol. *4*, 331 (1992).
22 H.P. Lee, L. Gourley, S. Duffy, et al.: Lancet *337*, 1197 (1991).
23 B.M. Markaverich, R.R. Roberts, M.A. Alejandro, et al.: J. Steroid. Biochem. *30*, 71 (1988).
24 K.H. Lee: Kaohsiung J. Med. Sci. *3*, 234 (1987).
25 K.H. Lee and T. Yamagishi: Abs. Chinese Med. *1*, 606 (1987).
26 E.J. Lien and W.Y. Li: Structure-Activity Relationship Analysis of Anticancer Chinese Drugs and Related Plants, Oriental Healing Arts Institute, Long Beach, 1985. pp. l–150.
27 M.Ou, H.H. Xu, Y.N. Li, H.S. Luo: An Illustrated Guide to Antineoplastic Chinese Herbal Medicine, The Commercial Press, Hong Kong, 1990, pp.1–210.
28 E.J. Lien and H. Gao (Unpublished data).
29 E.J. Lien and H. Gao, C.S. Hsu and F.Z. Wang: Int. J. Orient. Med. *17*, (1992).

Index Vol. 46

The references of the Subject Index are given in the language of the respective contribution.
Die Stichworte des Sachregisters sind in der jeweiligen Sprache der einzelnen Beiträge aufgeführt.
Les termes repris dans la Table des Matières sont donnés selon la langue dans laquelle l'ouvrage est écrit.

Index of titles
Verzeichnis der Titel
Index des titres
Vol. 1–46 (1959–1996)

Author and paper index
Autoren- und Artikelindex
Index des auteurs et des articles
Vol. 1–46 (1959–1996)

Recent developments in disease-modifying antirheumatic-drugs *24*, 101 (1980)	I. M. Hunneyball
The pharmacology of homologous series *7*, 305 (1964)	H. R. Ing
Progress in the experimental chemotherapy of helminth infections. Part. 1. Trematode and cestode diseases *17*, 241 (1973)	P. J. Islip
Pharmacology of the brain: The hippocampus, learning and seizures *16*, 211 (1972)	I. Izquierdo A. G. Nasello
Cholinergic mechanism – monoamines relation in certain brain structures *16*, 334 (1972)	J. A. Izquierdo
The development of antifertility substances *7*, 133 (1964)	H. Jackson
Development of novel anti-inflammatory agents: A pharmacological perspective on leukotrienes and their receptors *46*, 115 (1996)	William T. Jackson Jerome H. Fleisch
Agents acting on central dopamine receptors *21*, 409 (1977)	P. C. Jain N. Kumar
Recent advances in the treatment of parasitic infections in man *18*, 191 (1974) The levamisole story *20*, 347 (1976)	P. A. J. Janssen
Recent developments in cancer chemotherapy *25*, 275 (1981)	K. Jewers
Search for pharmaceutically interesting quinazoline derivatives: Efforts and results (1969–1980) *26*, 259 (1982)	S. Johne
A review of advances in prescribing for teratogenic hazards *29*, 121 (1985)	E. Marshall Johnson
A comparative of bitoscanate, bephenium hydroxynaphthoate and tetrachlor-ethylene in hookworm infection *19*, 70 (1975)	S. Johnson

Epidemiology of diphtheria *19*, 336 (1975)	L. G. Marquis
Biological activity of the terpenoids and their derivatives *6*, 279 (1963)	M. Martin-Smith T. Khatoon
Biological activity of the terpenoids and their derivatives – recent advances *13*, 11 (1969)	M. Martin-Smith W. E. Sneader
Antihypertensive agents 1962–1968 *13*, 101 (1969) Fundamental structures in drug research – Part I *20*, 385 (1976)	A. Marxer O. Schier
Fundamental structures in drug research – Part II *22*, 27 (1978) Antihypertensive agents 1969–1980 *25*, 9 (1981)	A. Marxer O. Schier
Relationships between the chemical structure and pharmacological activity in a series of synthetic quinuclidine derivatives *13*, 293 (1969)	M. D. Mashkovsky L. N. Yakhontov
Further developments in research on the chemistry and pharmacology of synthetic quinuclidine derivatives *27*, 9 (1983)	M. D. Mashkovsky L. N. Yakhontov M. E. Kaminka E. E. Mikhlina S. Ordzhonikidze
Role of neutrotransmitters in the central regulation of the cardiovascular system *35*, 25 (1990) Neurotransmitters involved in the central regulation of the cardiovascular system *46*, 43 (1996)	Robert B. McCall
On the understanding of drug potency 13, 123 (1971) The chemotherapy of intestinal nematodes *16*, 157 (1972)	J. W. McFarland
Non-steroidal menses-regulating agents: The present status *44*, 159 (1995)	P.K. Mehrotra Sanjay Batra A.P. Bhaduri

High resolution nuclear magnetic resonance spectroscopy of biological samples as an aid to drug development *31*, 427 (1987)	J. K. Nicholson Ian D. Wilson
Antibody response to two cholera vaccines in volunteers *19*, 554 (1975)	Y. S. Nimbkar R. S. Karbhari S. Cherian N. G. Chanderkar R. P. Bhamaria P. S. Ranadive B. B. Gaitonde
Surface interaction between bacteria and phagocytic cells *32*, 137 (1988)	L. Öhman G. Maluszynska K. E. Magnusson O. Stendahl
Die Chemotherapie der Wurmkrankheiten *1*, 159 (1959)	H.-A. Oelkers
Structural modifications patterns from agonists to antagonists and their application to drug design – A new serotonin(5HT$_3$)antagonist series *41*, 313 (1993)	Hiroshi Ohtaka Toshio Fujita
Serenics *42*, 167 (1994)	Berend Olivier Jan Mos Maikel Raghoeba Paul de Koning Marianne Mak
GABA-Drug interactions *31*, 223 (1987)	Richard W. Olsen
Drug research and human sleep *22*, 355 (1978)	I. Oswald
Effects of drugs on calmodulin-mediated enzymatic actions *33*, 353 (1989)	Judit Ovádi
An extensive community outbreak of acute diarrhoeal diseases in children *19*, 570 (1975)	S. C. Pal C. Koteswar Rao
Drug and its action according to Ayurveda *26*, 55 (1982)	Madhabendra Nath Pal
Oligosaccharide chains of glycoproteins *32*, 163 (1990)	Y. T. Pan Alan D. Elbein
Pharmacology of synthetic organic selenium compounds *36*, 9 (1991)	Michael J. Parnham Erich Graf

Moral challenges in the organisation and management of drug research *42*, 9 (1994)	Michael J. Parnham
3,4-Dihydroxyphenylalanine and related compounds *9*, 223 (1966)	A. R. Patel A. Burger
Mescaline and related compounds *11*, 11 (1968)	A. R. Patel
Experience with bitoscanate in adults *19*, 90 (1975)	A. H. Patricia U. Prabakar Rao R. Subramaniam N. Madanagopalan
The impact of state and society on medical research *35*, 9 (1990)	C. R. Pfaltz
Transfer factor in malignancy *42*, 401 (1994)	Giancarlo Pizza Caterina De Vinci H. Hugh Fudenberg
Monoaminoxydase-Hemmer *2*, 417 (1960)	A. Pletscher K. F. Gey P. Zeller
Antifungal therapy: Are we winning? *37*, 183 (1991)	A. Polak P. G. Hartman
What makes a good pertussis vaccine? *19*, 341 (1975) Vaccine composition in relation to antigenic variation of the microbe: Is pertussis unique? *19*, 347 (1975) Some unsolved problems with vaccines *23*, 9 (1979) Eradication by vaccination: The memorial to smallpox could be surrounded by others *41*, 151 (1993)	N. W. Preston
Antibiotics in the chemotherapy of malaria *26*, 167 (1982)	S. K. Puri G. P. Dutta
Potassium channel openers: Airway pharmacology and clinical possibilities in asthma *37*, 161 (1991)	David Raeburn Jan-Anders Karlsson
Isozyme-selective cyclic nucleotide phosphodiesterase inhibitors: Biochemistry, pharmacology and therapeutic potential in asthma *40*, 9 (1993)	David Raeburn John E. Souness Adrian Tomkinson Jan-Anders Karlsson

Clinical study of diphtheria, tetanus and pertussis *19*, 356 (1975)	V. B. Raju V. R. Parvathi
Epidemiology of cholera in Hyderabad *19*, 578 (1975)	K. Rajyalakshmi P. V. Ramana Rao
Adenosine receptors: Clinical implications and biochemical mechanisms *32*, 195 (1988)	Vickram Ramkumar George Pierson Gary L. Stiles
New synthetic ligands for L-type voltage-gated calcium channels *40*, 191 (1993)	David Rampe David J. Triggle
Problems of malaria eradication in India *18*, 245 (1974)	V. N. Rao
Pharmacology of migraine *34*, 209 (1990)	Neil H. Raskin
The photochemistry of drugs and related substances *11*, 48 (1968)	S. T. Reid
Orale Antikoagulantien *11*, 226 (1968)	E. Renk W. G. Stoll
Mechanism-based inhibitors of monoamine oxidase *30*, 205 (1986)	Lauren E. Richards Alfred Burger
The hopanoids, bacterial triterpenoids, and the biosynthesis of isoprenic units in prokaryote *37*, 271 (1991)	Michael Rohner Philippe Bisseret Bertrand Sutter
Tetrahydroisoquinolines and β-carbolines: Putative natural substances in plants and animals *29*, 415 (1985)	H. Rommelspacher R. Susilo
Functional significance of the various components of the influenza virus 18, 253 (1974)	R. Rott
Drug receptors and control of the cardiovascular system: Recent advances *36*, 117 (1991)	Robert R. Ruffolo Jr J. Paul Hieble David P. Brooks Giora Z. Feuerstein Andrew J. Nichols
Behavioral correlates of presynaptic events in the cholinergic neurotransmitter system *32*, 43 (1988)	Roger W. Russell

Epidemiology of pertussis *19*, 257 (1975)	J. A. Sa
Surgical amoebiasis *18*, 77 (1974)	A. E. de Sa
Role of beta-adrenergic blocking drug propranolol in severe tetanus *19*, 361 (1975)	G. S. Sainani K, L. Jain V. R. D. Deshpande A. B. Balsara S. A. Iyer
Studies on *Vibrio parahaemolyticus* in Bombay *19*, 586 (1975)	F. L. Saldanha A. K. Patil M. V. Sant
Leukotriene antagonists and inhibitors of leukotriene biosynthesis as potential therapeutic agents *37*, 9 (1991)	John A. Salmon Lawrence G. Garland
Pharmacology and toxicology of axoplasmic transport *28*, 53 (1984)	Fred Samson Ralph L. Smith J. Alejandro Donoso
Clinical experience with bitoscanate *19*, 96 (1975)	M. R. Samuel
Tetanus: Situational clinical trials and therapeutics *19*, 367 (1975)	R. K. M. Sanders M. L. Peacock B. Martyn B. D. Shende
Epidemiological studies on cholera in non-endemic regions with special reference to the problem of carrier state during epidemic and non-epidemic period *19*, 594 (1975)	M. V. Sant W. N. Gatlewar S. K. Bhindey
Epidemiological and biochemical studies in filariasis in four villages near Bombay *18*, 269 (1974)	M. V. Sant W. N. Gatlewar T. U. K. Menon
Hookworm anaemia and intestinal mal- absorption associated with hookworm infestation *19*, 108 (1975)	A. K. Saraya B. N. Tandon
The effects of structural alteration on the anti-inflammatory properties of hydrocortisone *5*, 11 (1963)	L. H. Sarett A. A. Patchett S. Steelman
The impact of natural product research on drug discovery *23*, 51 (1979)	L. H. Sarett

Chemotherapy of cestode infections *24*, 217 (1980)	Satyavan Sharma S. K. Dubey R. N. Iyer
Chemotherapy of hookworm infections *26*, 9 (1982)	Satyavan Sharma Elizabeth S. Charles
Ayurvedic medicine – past and present *15*, 11 (1971)	Shiv Sharma
Mechanisms of anthelmintic action *19*, 147 (1975)	U. K. Sheth
Aspirin as an antithrombotic agent *33*, 43 (1989)	Melvin J. Silver Giovanni Di Minno
Immunopharmacological approach to the study of chronic brain disorders *30*, 345 (1986) Implications of immunomodulant therapy in Alzheimer's disease *32*, 21 (1988)	Vijendra K. Singh H. Hugh Fudenberg
Neuroimmune axis as a basis of therapy in Alzheimer's disease *34*, 383 (1990) Immunoregulatory role of neuro- peptides *38*, 149 (1992) Neuropeptides as native immune modul- ators *45*, 9 (1995)	Vijendra K. Singh
Natural products as anticancer agents *42*, 53 (1994)	Shradha Sinha Sudha Jain
Biologically active quinazolones *43*, 143 (1994)	Shradha Sinha Mukta Srivastava
Some often neglected factors in the control and prevention of communicable diseases *18*, 277 (1974)	C. E. G. Smith
Tetanus and its prevention *19*, 391 (1975)	J. W. G. Smith
Growth of *Clostridium tetani in vivo* *19*, 384 (1975)	J. W. G. Smith A. G. MacIver
The biliary excretion and enterohepatic circulation of drugs and other organic compounds *9*, 299 (1966)	R. L. Smith

Biologische Oxydation und Reduktion am Stickstoff aromatischer Amino- und Nitroderivate und ihre Folgen für den Organismus *8*, 195 (1965) Stoffwechsel von Arzneimitteln als Ursache von Wirkungen, Nebenwirkungen und Toxizität *15*, 147 (1971)	H. Uehleke
Mode of death in tetanus *19*, 439 (1975)	H. Vaishnava C. Bhawal Y. P. Munjal
Comparative evaluation of amoebicidal drugs *18*, 353 (1974) Comparative efficacy of newer anthelmintics *19*, 166 (1975)	B. J. Vakil N. J. Dalal
Cephalic tetanus 19, 443 (1975)	B. J. Vakil B. S. Singhal S. S. Pandya P. F. Irami
The effect and usefulness of early intravenous beta blockade in acute myocardial infarction *30*, 71 (1986)	Anders Vedin Claes Wilhelmsson
Methods of monitoring adverse reactions to drugs *21*, 231 (1977)	J. Venulet
Aspects of social pharmacology *22*, 9 (1978)	J. Venulet
The current status of cholera toxoid research in the United States *19*, 602 (1975)	W. F. Verwey J. C. Guckian J. Craig N. Pierce J. Peterson H. Williams Jr
Systemic cancer therapy: Four decades of progress and some personal perspectives *34*, 76 (1990)	Charles L. Vogel
Cell-kinetic and pharmacokinetic aspects in the use and further development of cancerostatic drugs *20*, 521 (1976)	M. von Ardenne

Krebswirksame Antibiotika aus Actinomyceten *3*, 451 (1961)	Kh. Zepf
Developments in histamine H_1-receptor agonists *44*, 49 (1995)	V. Zingel C. Leschke W. Schunack
Fifteen years of structural modifications in the field of antifungal monocyclic 1-substituted 1 H-azoles *27*, 253 (1983)	L. Zirngibl
Lysostaphin: Model for a specific enzymatic approach to infectious disease *16*, 309 (1972)	W. A. Zygmunt P. A. Tavormina